*To staff nurses everywhere who really make the
critical difference for immunocompromised patients.*

Nursing Care

Of The

Immunocompromised

Patient

M. Linda Workman, PhD, RN, ONC

Frances Payne Bolton School of Nursing
Case Western Reserve University
Cleveland, OH

Jan Ellerhorst-Ryan, MSN, RN CS

Clinical Specialist
Critical Care America
Cincinnati, OH

Victoria Hargrave-Koertge, MSN, RN, OCN

Hospice of Cincinnati
Cincinnati, OH

W.B. SAUNDERS COMPANY
Harcourt Brace Jovanovich, Inc.
Philadelphia • London • Toronto • Montreal • Sydney • Tokyo

W.B. SAUNDERS COMPANY

Harcourt Brace Jovanovich, Inc.

The Curtis Center
Independence Square West
Philadelphia, Pennsylvania 19106

Library of Congress Cataloging-in-Publication Data

Workman, M. Linda.
    Nursing care of the immunocompromised patient / M. Linda Workman,
Jan Ellerhorst-Ryan, Vicki Hargrave-Koertge.
        p.   cm.
    ISBN 0-7216-3213-0
    1. Immunodeficiency—Nursing. 2. Immunocompromised Host.
I. Ellerhorst-Ryan, Jan. II. Hargrave-Koertge, Vicki. III. Title.
    [DNLM: 1. Immunity—nurses' instruction. 2. Immunologic
Deficiency Syndromes—nursing. 3. Immunosuppression—nursing. WY
150 W926n]
RC606.W93   1993
616.97'0024613—dc20
DNLM/DLC   92–49980

NURSING CARE OF THE IMMUNOCOMPROMISED PATIENT   ISBN 0–7216–3213–0

Printed in Mexico

Last digit is the print number: 9   8   7   6   5   4   3   2   1

ABOUT THE AUTHORS

M. Linda Workman, RN, PhD, OCN, received her BSN and MSN from the College of Nursing and Health at the University of Cincinnati. She then earned a PhD in Developmental Biology from the College of Arts and Science at the University of Cincinnati. Dr. Workman is an Associate Professor and Chairperson for the Department of Acute and Critical Care Nursing at the Frances Payne Bolton School of Nursing, Case Western Reserve University in Cleveland, Ohio. In addition, she is an American Cancer Society Professor of Oncology Nursing for the Ohio Division.

Jan M. Ellerhorst-Ryan, RN, MSN, CS, is a graduate of the University of Cincinnati College of Nursing and Health and the Indiana University School of Nursing. She is certified as a Medical-Surgical Clinical Nurse Specialist by the American Nurses Association and is currently employed as a nurse clinician by Critical Care America, Cincinnati, Ohio.

Victoria "Vicki" Hargrave-Koertge, RN, MSN, OCN, received her BSN from Northern Illinois University and her MSN from the College of Nursing and Health at the University of Cincinnati. She is certified in oncology nursing by the Oncology Nursing Certification Corporation. Her nine years of clinical experience in oncology nursing include: staff nurse and assistant manager positions on medical oncology and bone marrow transplant units, on-call and home care RN for hospice, and an oncology clinical nurse specialist for a private oncology practice. She is currently an optional home care RN for Hospice of Cincinnati, Inc.

A special thanks to:

Mary Ann Battles, BSN, who provided special input to Chapter 10. Ms. Battles has a BSN from the University of Pittsburgh School of Nursing and is a pre-medical student at the University of Cincinnati. Currently she is the Antepartum Coordinator at the University Women's Health Service, University of Cincinnati.

ACKNOWLEDGMENT

The authors wish to acknowledge the unfailing support of the men in their lives toward the finalization of this work. Husbands Tom, Steve, and John, together with sons David, Greg, Jake, and Ben have made the hard times easier and the good times even better. Thanks guys!

PREFACE

This book is meant to be a resource for practicing nurses who find more and more of their patients to have health problems associated with altered immune function, specifically immunosuppression. In a large sense this book was written for those nurses who are caught in the middle of change in health care. Many of us received our basic nursing educations at a time when the biologic sciences were not emphasized in nursing and the immune system, if it was presented at all, was briefly introduced as mysterious but not of any specific importance to nursing. In fact, it often was relegated into the "nice to know" or even the "nuts to know" category.

Now nurses are expected to care for individuals whose immune systems have been compromised to some degree. Advancing technology has successfully controlled severe immune system problems that in the past did not permit long-term survival. Other technologies not directly related to immune response are now commonly available, and many of these suppress immune function at least temporarily. As a result, more patients are at risk for infection and other complications of immunosuppression than ever during the second half of the twentieth century. Nurses are expected to know the specific risks for each patient and provide the safest environment possible. However, because of a lack of previous education in this area, a nurse's knowledge may be deficient at a time when the need for this information has dramatically increased.

This book is designed to increase the nurse's knowledge of immune function and immunosuppression. The first four chapters present an overview of specific immune function and how each component interacts with the others to prevent or limit infection. This section assumes no prior knowledge about the immune system and clearly presents basic immune function, using common terms and everyday examples. The rest of the chapters provide information about specific types of immunosuppression, including syndromes of congenital immunosuppression, acquired immunosuppression, immunosuppression as a primary treatment, and immunosuppression resulting as a side effect of other treatments or illnesses.

Because different aspects of immune function are affected by these different etiologies, the degree of immunosuppression and risk for complications varies with the specific cause of the immunosuppression. For example, the immunosuppression caused by chemotherapeutic agents causes different immune impairment than does the immunosuppression caused by drugs prescribed for long-term use following solid organ transplants. The chapters on individual causes of specific types of immunosuppression provide an overview of the etiology, pathophysiology, manifestations, and usual treatment for the condition and the immunosuppression. The information is further enhanced by a case presentation. Terms are defined as they are presented in the text and are grouped together in a glossary. A comprehensive nursing care plan for patients with specific types of immunosuppression is presented in the last chapter.

Information is presented at the depth needed by a nurse who has little previous familiarity with the condition rather than for the clinical nurse specialist in that field. For example, the information about solid organ transplantation is presented for the nurse working on a general medical-surgical unit who is faced with an admission of a patient 2 years status post kidney transplant who now has cholecystitis. This level of presentation would not be appropriate for a solid organ transplant coordinator.

We hope this book is helpful to you in providing the best possible care to your patients.

M. LINDA WORKMAN

JAN ELLERHORST-RYAN

VICTORIA HARGRAVE-KOERTGE

CONTENTS

UNIT I

BASIC CONCEPTS OF IMMUNOLOGY

I

INTRODUCTION

Today's nurses and other health care professionals are becoming increasingly aware of the vast and rather complex role played by immune function in maintaining good health and homeostasis. Many disease states, injuries, and physiologic changes alter immune function to some degree. In addition, many types of traditional medical therapy also alter immune function. These alterations in immune function may be temporary or permanent, but they always have an impact on the overall health and well-being of the individual. We also now know that specific alterations in immune function permit and, at times, even cause other diseases or health problems to develop.

Virtually all patients in acute-care settings experience some degree of alteration in immune function. The majority of these alterations are suppressive in nature. Significant suppression of immune function increases the patient's risk for serious potential complications, such as infection and debilitation. Nurses need a strong working knowledge of specific areas of immune function in order to provide a safe environment, adequate patient support, and appropriate early interventions to minimize the risk of complications.

PURPOSE

The purpose of this book is to serve as a reference and guide for the nurse in acquiring, assimilating, and applying critical concepts in regard to suppressed immune function. The contents of the book are designed to provide the nurse with sufficient background knowledge of the biology of immune function as well as the clinical consequences of general and specific immunosuppression. Such knowledge can assist the nurse in providing appropriate care to patients who are experiencing problems that result in suppression of one or more components of the immune system.

3

The book is divided into two parts. Unit I, the first four chapters, presents the anatomy, physiology, and biology involved in normal immune function. Unit II is divided into specific conditions that result in suppression of immune responses. These chapters include discussion of the underlying pathophysiology, clinical manifestations and assessment findings, interpretation of laboratory data, and risks and potential complications. Chapter 15 contains a comprehensive nursing care plan for people with immunosuppression. This information can help nurses recognize common suppressive changes in immune function.

OVERVIEW

General immunity is divided into the two broad categories of *innate immunity* and *acquired immunity*. Innate immunity is a genetically determined characteristic of an individual, group, or species. An individual either does or does not have innate immunity. This type of immunity cannot be developed after birth and is not an adaptive response to injury or invasion by foreign proteins.

Acquired immunity is the immunity that every individual's body normally makes (or can receive) as an adaptive response to invasion by foreign proteins. The major function of the immune system is to participate in activities that result in the development of immune protection. Acquired immunity occurs either naturally or artificially and is either active or passive.

Proper acquired immune function provides humans with protection against the side effects that can accompany invasion or injury. People interact with many other living organisms in the environment. These organisms vary in size from quite large (other humans and animals) to microscopic and submicroscopic (bacteria, viruses, molds, spores, pollens, protozoa, and cells from other people or animals). Generally, we can exist in harmony with many of these other living organisms as long as they do not actually enter our internal environment. The body has many defenses to prevent such organisms from gaining access to the internal environment; however, these defenses are not completely foolproof, and invasion of the internal environment does occur relatively frequently. The fact that invasion occurs much more frequently than does the expression of an actual disease or illness is a result of proper immune function.

The ultimate purpose of the cells that compose the immune system is to neutralize, destroy, or eliminate the microorganisms that penetrate or invade the internal environment before the invaders have a chance to multiply and overwhelm bodily defenses. In order to accomplish this, the cells that make up the immune system must be able to distinguish "undesirable invaders" from normal healthy cells. This ability to distinguish "self" from "nonself" (necessary so that normal healthy body cells are not neutralized, destroyed, or eliminated along with the invaders) is called *self-tolerance*. Nonself cells include infected or debilitated body cells, self cells that have undergone malignant transformation into cancer cells, and all foreign cells (Gallucci, 1987; Groenwald, 1980; Workman, 1989). Recognition and self-tolerance are possible because of the unique ability of immune system cells to examine and interpret the surface proteins present on any cell or organism they contact directly.

All organisms are made up of cells. Each cell is surrounded by a plasma membrane (Fig. 1–1). Protruding through the membranes of all cells are a variety of proteins. For example, your liver cells all have many different proteins present on the surface (protruding through the membrane). Each protein differs from all other protein types in its amino acid sequence. Some of these proteins are found on the liver cells of all animals (including humans) that have livers because these proteins are liver-specific and are considered a "marker" for liver tissue. Other proteins are found only on the liver cells of human beings because these protein types are human-specific markers. Still other proteins are found only on the liver cells of people with a specific blood type. In addition, your liver cells have proteins on them that are unique to you and would only be absolutely identical to the same proteins of an identical twin. In a sense, these "you" proteins, present on the surface of all your body cells, serve as a cellular fingerprint or a "universal product code" for you. These universal product codes are as unique as the individual and would only be exactly the same on the surfaces of cells from identical twins and other mon-

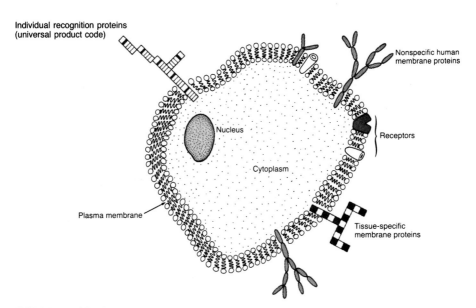

FIGURE I–I. Membrane proteins of a typical normal cell. (From *Medical-Surgical Nursing: A Nursing Process Approach* [p. 528, Fig. 23–1] by D. Ignatavicius and M. Bayne, 1991, Philadelphia: W.B. Saunders.)

ozygotic multiple births (Guyton, 1991). The proteins that make up your universal product code can be recognized as foreign by the immune system of another person; these proteins are called *antigens*.

Part of this unique universal product code is composed of the *human leukocyte antigens* (HLAs). The term "leukocyte antigen" is not actually correct, as these antigens also are present on the surfaces of all cells containing a nucleus, not just on leukocytes. These antigens form the specific "tissue type" of the individual. Other names for these antigens include *human transplantation antigens, human histocompatibility antigens,* and *Class I antigens.*

Chromosome 6 has a region that contains the genes that code for an individual's human leukocyte antigens. This gene region is called the *major histocompatibility complex* (MHC). The complex contains three different classes of genes responsible for at least three different types of activities related to immune function. Class I genes code for the human leukocyte antigens. Class II genes, which also code for part of the leukocyte antigens, primarily code for proteins that control or regulate immune function (Ir [immune regulation] proteins). Class III genes code for proteins that regulate complement synthesis and activity.

Class I antigens are coded for by the human leukocyte antigen genes HLA-A, HLA-B, and HLA-C. At each of the three gene locations on chromosome 6 for HLA, more than one alternative form can exist for each of the genes (these alternative gene forms are called "alleles"). For example, HLA-A has 27 known different possible alleles and HLA-B has 47 known different possible alleles (Roitt, 1991). Therefore, because all normal humans have a pair of number 6 chromosomes and each chromosome of the pair contains three HLA Class I genes, any one person can only have up to six different HLA Class I proteins on the surfaces of all their nucleated cells. However, more than 80 different forms of these three genes have been identified among the human population (Roitt, 1991). For any one person, three of the HLA genes were inherited from the father (and the father had up to six gene forms to choose from) and three were inherited from the mother (who also had up to six HLA gene forms to choose from). Therefore, the HLA Class I proteins present on a child's cells may not be exactly the same as either the father's, the mother's, or the sibling's.

These six Class I proteins form the most obvious or major part of a person's universal product code. In addition, it is thought that a number of minor antigens also compose part of each person's universal product code. Immunologists speculate that the number of minor antigens may far exceed the number of major antigens and that these are also genetically determined. It is the major HLA antigens that must be closely matched between donor and recipient for the best outcome of solid organ transplantation. At present, matching the minor antigens is not possible, although mismatched minor antigens are likely to be responsible for some degree of rejection among recipients of solid organ transplants.

The universal product code is a key feature for recognition and self-tolerance. The cells of your immune system constantly come into contact with other body cells and with any invader that enters your internal environment At each encounter, your immune system cell attempts to match up its surface protein universal product code with the universal product code of the encountered cell to determine whether the encountered cell really belongs in the internal environment (Fig. 1–2). If the encountered cell's universal product code is a perfect match for all human leukocyte antigens to the universal product code on the immune system cell, the encountered cell is considered "self" and is not further molested by the immune-system cell. If the encountered cell's universal product code is not a perfect match with that of the immune system cell, the encountered cell is considered "nonself" or "foreign," and the immune system cell will take steps to neutralize, destroy, or eliminate the foreign invader.

ORGANIZATION OF THE IMMUNE SYSTEM

The immune system does not reside in any one organ or area of the body. Instead, the cells of the immune system originate in the bone marrow. Some of these cells mature in the bone marrow whereas others mature in other specific body sites. After maturation, most of the immune system cells are released into the blood, where they circulate to all areas of the body and exert their specific effects.

The bone marrow is the ultimate source of all cells found in the blood. It produces a very immature, undifferentiated cell called a *stem cell* (Kemp, 1986). This immature stem cell also is referred to by such adjectives as *pluripotent,*

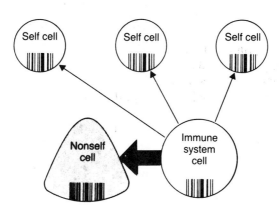

FIGURE I–2. Recognition of self versus nonself by immune-system cell. (From *Medical-Surgical Nursing: A Nursing Process Approach* [p. 528, Fig. 23–2] by D. Ignatavicius and M. Bayne, 1991, Philadelphia: W.B. Saunders.)

multipotent, totipotent, and even *omnipotent.* These adjectives actually describe the potential future of the stem cell. At the time the stem cell is created in the bone marrow, it is undifferentiated; it has not yet committed itself to differentiating into a specific cell type. Thus, at this stage, the stem cell is flexible and has the potential to become any of a variety of different mature cells. Figure 1–3 presents a scheme showing the major possible maturational outcomes for the stem cell. The specific cell type into which the stem cell ultimately matures depends on which specific maturational pathway it selects.

The selection of or commitment to a maturational pathway appears to be an irreversible event. For instance, if a stem cell commits to the platelet pathway and becomes a megakaryocyte it does not appear to be able to revert back to the pluripotent state and later become a T lymphocyte. It is possible for the cell to stop the process and never completely mature, but once commitment to a specific maturational pathway occurs the cell remains with that choice. The maturational pathway that a stem cell becomes committed to depends, to some extent, on body needs at the time and also on the presence of specific proteins (termed *factors* or *poietins*) that stimulate specific commitment and induce maturation. For example, erythropoietin is synthesized in the kidney. When immature stem cells are exposed to erythropoietin the immature stem cells commit to the erythrocyte maturational pathway and eventually become mature red blood cells.

White blood cells, leukocytes, are the cells that actually protect the body from the side effects of invasion by foreign microorganisms. These cells are the actual immune system cells. The leukocytes are able to provide protection through a variety of defensive actions (Abernathy, 1987; Grady, 1988; Roitt, 1991; Smith, 1986). These actions include the following:

1. Recognition of self versus nonself.
2. Phagocytic destruction of foreign invaders, cellular debris, and unhealthy self cells.
3. Lytic destruction of foreign invaders and unhealthy self cells.
4. Production of antibodies directed against foreign invaders.
5. Stimulation of complement activity.
6. Production of chemicals that stimulate increased formation of leukocytes by the bone marrow.
7. Production of chemicals that increase specific leukocyte growth and activity.

Not all leukocytes are capable of performing every defensive function listed. Leukocytes are divided into different categories based on appearance, structure, and specific activity. Table 1–1 summarizes the categories of leukocytes. First, leukocytes are categorized based on the appearance of the cytoplasm.

Granulocytic Leukocytes

Some leukocytes have many small granules and vesicles within the cytoplasm, giving them a rough or granular appearance under the microscope.

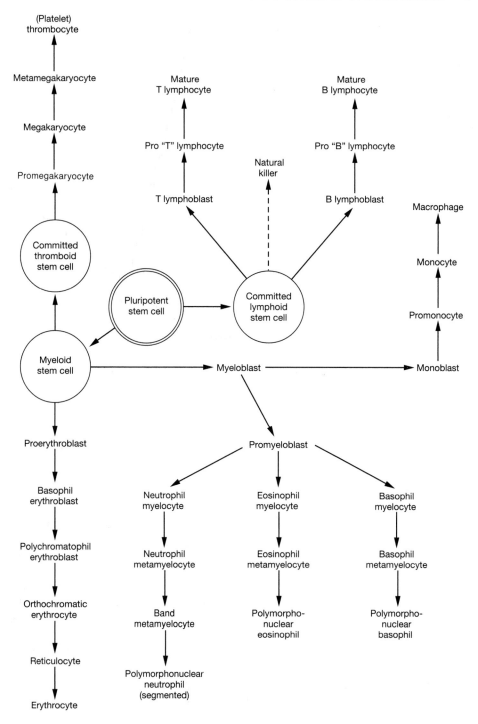

FIGURE I-3. Stem-cell differentiation and maturation pathways.

TABLE I-I. Specific Leukocyte Immune Functions.

Immune Division	Leukocyte	Cell Action
Inflammation	Neutrophil	Nonspecific ingestion and phagocytosis of microorganisms
	Macrophage	Nonspecific recognition of foreign proteins and microorganisms; ingestion and phagocytosis
	Monocyte	Destruction of bacteria and cellular debris; matures into macrophage
	Eosinophil	Weak phagocytic action; releases histamines during allergic reactions
	Basophil	Releases histamines and heparin in areas of tissue damage
Antibody-mediated	B lymphocyte	Becomes sensitized to foreign cells and proteins
	B-lymphocyte plasma cell	Secretes immunoglobulins in response to the presence of a specific antigen
	B-lymphocyte memory cell	Remains sensitized to a specific antigen and can secrete increased amounts of immunoglobulins specific to the antigen
Cell-mediated	T-lymphocyte helper cell	Enhances immune activity through the secretion of various factors, cytokines, and lymphokines
	T-lymphocyte cytotoxic T cell	Selectively attacks and destroys nonself cells, including virally infected cells, grafts, and transplanted organs
	Natural killer cell	Nonspecifically attacks nonself cells, especially body cells that have undergone mutation and become malignant; will also attack grafts and transplanted organs

These cells are called *granulocytes* and the granules are called *lysosomes.* Lysosomes are intracellular bags of enzymes that can digest or degrade proteins and cellular debris. These enzymes are contained within the lysosomes so that the enzymes do not digest essential parts of the immune system cell. Granulocytes are categorized by the pH of the cytoplasm. Cytoplasmic pH is determined by the color the cytoplasm stains when immersed in a solution called Wright's stain. This stain has an acid-seeking component that is red and a base-seeking component that is blue.

Cells with an acidic cytoplasm preferentially take up the acid-seeking component (the red dye, *eosin*) and appear red under the microscope. These cells are called *eosinophils* or *acidophils* (old terminology). Eosinophils normally make up a very small percentage of the total white-cell count (about 1 to 2 per cent) except during allergic reactions. These cells are relatively weak phagocytes and function most prominently in reactions that destroy or remove parasitic larvae from humans. In addition, eosinophils participate in specific inflammatory reactions that assist in generating allergic manifestations in sensitive individuals.

Cells with a basic cytoplasm preferentially absorb the base-seeking component (the blue dye, *hematoxylin*) and appear blue under the microscope. These cells are called *basophils* and make up less than 0.5 per cent of the total white-cell count. Basophils release histamine, heparin, and a variety of vasoactive amines in areas of tissue damage. They appear important in the generation of acute inflammatory reactions.

Cells with a neutral cytoplasm take up the acid- and base-seeking components equally and appear light purple under the microscope. These cells are the *neutrophils*. Other names for neutrophils are derived from the unusual shape of the nucleus and include *polymorphonuclear cells* ("polys"), *banded neutrophils* ("bands" or "stabs"), and *segmented neutrophils* ("segs"). These cells are normally the most numerous of leukocytes, making up 55 to 70 per cent of the total circulating white blood cells. Neutrophils are very efficient at the process of phagocytosis. Neutrophils are much smaller than most of the other leukocytes, but because they are so numerous they are critically important in the destruction and removal of many foreign invaders.

Nongranulocytic Leukocytes

The group of leukocytes that have smooth-appearing cytoplasm under low-powered microscopic examination have been categorized previously as *agranulocytes,* although this term is inaccurate and rarely used today. Most textbooks include the *lymphocytes, monocytes,* and *macrophages* as agranulocytes even though the monocytes and macrophages do contain relatively large amounts of fine lysosomal granules in the cytoplasm.

Lymphocytes are divided into B and T lymphocytes. These cells are critically important in providing specific sustained protection against a vast array of microorganisms capable of invading our bodies. Normally, lymphocytes make up 25 to 30 per cent of the total white-cell count. B lymphocytes secrete antibodies and participate in humoral immunity (antibody-mediated). T lymphocytes participate in a wide variety of activities to provide cell-mediated immunity. Detailed descriptions of the actions of lymphocytes are presented in Chapters 3 and 4.

Monocytes are immature cells released into circulation from the bone marrow before functional maturation is complete. Normally, monocytes comprise only 2 to 4 per cent of the total white-cell count. These cells are committed to ultimate maturation and differentiation into macrophages. Until they mature, monocytes are not functionally efficient components of the immune system. Monocytes are capable of limited bacterial phagocytosis and can stimulate the activation of complement. The name *monocyte* is derived from the appearance of these cells as relatively large entities each with a single, large nucleus.

Macrophages are the final maturation stage of monocytes. They are large, efficient at recognition of self versus nonself, and exceptionally competent at the process of phagocytosis. Usually, maturation of monocytes into macro-

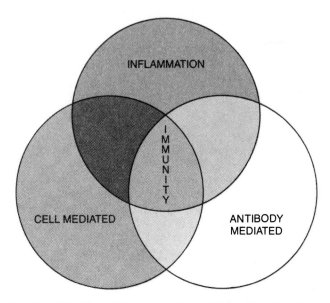

FIGURE 1-4. Functional divisions of immunity. (From *Medical-Surgical Nursing: A Nursing Process Approach* [p. 532, Fig. 23–4] by D. Ignatavicius and M. Bayne, 1991, Philadelphia: W.B. Saunders.)

phages occurs after the monocytes migrate into the tissues. Therefore, the circulating population of white blood cells normally has very few macrophages, and this value does not reflect the enormous number of active macrophages stored in many body tissues.

SUMMARY

Immunity is the protection provided to us by the ability of the cells of the immune system to recognize the body's own healthy cells (self) from all other cells (nonself) and to mount a defense against those nonself cells, resulting in their removal or destruction. Nonself cells include infected or debilitated normal cells, self cells that have undergone malignant transformation, and foreign cells such as bacteria, viruses, fungi, protozoa, pollens, helminths, and spores, as well as cells from other people or animals. The overall protection of immunity occurs through the interactions of the various leukocytes and specific chemical products made by some leukocytes. A number of different types of leukocytes are involved in immune function. Although they all share some characteristics, they each have additional specialized functions to perform that contribute to the protection the immune system provides against the side effects of foreign invaders. The bone marrow is the site of origin for all immature leukocytes; final differentiation and maturation of specific leukocytes occurs at other body sites.

The processes of immunity and the involved cells can be categorized into the following three divisions: inflammation (the inflammatory response), antibody-mediated immunity, and cell-mediated immunity (Fig. 1–4). These three divisions represent diverse defensive actions. Some of these defensive actions are nonspecific and provide immediate but short-term protection. Other defensive actions are very specific and provide long-lasting immunity. Full immunity or immunocompetence requires the adequate function and interaction of all three divisions, even though some functions of each division appear to overlap with functions of the other divisions.

SELECTED BIBLIOGRAPHY

Abernathy, E. (1987). How the immune system works. *American Journal of Nursing, 87*(4), 456.

Barrett, J. (1988). *Textbook of immunology* (5th ed.). St. Louis: C.V. Mosby.

Fischbach, F. (1988). *A manual of laboratory diagnostic tests* (3rd ed.). Philadelphia: J.B. Lippincott.

Gallucci, B. (1987). The immune system and cancer. *Oncology Nursing Forum, 14*(suppl.), 3.

Grady, C. (1988). Host defense mechanisms: An overview. *Seminars in Oncology Nursing, 4*(2), 86.

Groenwald, S. (1980). Physiology of the immune system. *Heart and Lung, 9*(4), 645.

Guyton, A. (1991). *Textbook of medical physiology* (8th ed.). Philadelphia: W.B. Saunders.

Huffer, T., Kanapa, D., & Stevenson, G. (1986). *Introduction to human immunology.* Boston: Jones and Bartlett.

Kemp, D. (1986). Development of the immune system. *Critical Care Quarterly, 9*(1), 1.

Roitt, I. (1991). *Essential immunology* (7th ed.). Boston: Blackwell Scientific.

Price, S., & Wilson, L. (1986). *Pathophysiology* (3rd ed.). St. Louis: McGraw-Hill.

Smith, S. (1986). Physiology of the immune system. *Critical Care Quarterly, 9*(1), 7.

Stites, D., Stobo, J., & Wells, J. (Eds.) (1987). *Basic and clinical immunology* (6th ed.). Norwalk, CT: Appleton & Lange.

Tizard, I. (1984). *Immunology: An introduction.* Philadelphia: Saunders College Publishing.

Workman, M. (1989). Immunologic late effects of cancer therapy. *Seminars in Oncology Nursing, 5*(1), 36.

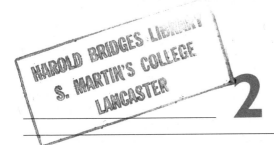
2

THE INFLAMMATORY RESPONSES

The division of immunity that comprises inflammation or the inflammatory responses is not always considered a true part of the immune system. Differences in mechanisms of action and duration of action between inflammation and antibody-mediated and cell-mediated immunity are responsible for the inconsistent classification of inflammatory responses within immunity. Inflammation differs somewhat from antibody-mediated and cell-mediated immunity in two primary ways. First, inflammation is a nonspecific response to invasion or injury. Second, the inflammatory responses are not capable of "remembering" the universal product code of an invader or injuring organism. As a result, the inflammatory responses provide immediate but short-term protection against the effects of injury or foreign invaders rather than sustained, long-term immunity on repeated exposures to the same foreign invader(s).

Inflammatory responses also result in tissue actions that generate observable and frequently uncomfortable symptoms. In spite of the discomfort, these inflammatory reactions are beneficial to the individual and also are crucial processes involved in the neutralization, destruction, and elimination of microorganisms. Moreover, interaction of inflammatory responses with both antibody-mediated actions and cell-mediated actions appears necessary to initiate the more specific immune processes provided by these other two divisions of immunity. Without proper function of the inflammatory processes, individuals are at grave risk of succumbing to the effects of tissue injury and invasion by overwhelming numbers of microorganisms.

The concept that the process of inflammation occurs in response to tissue injury as well as in response to invasion by microorganisms or other foreign proteins confuses many health care professionals. Inflammation can occur without the accompanying presence of foreign proteins or microorganisms, although, under normal conditions, infection is always accompanied by inflammation. A few examples of inflammatory responses not associated with infection include sprain injuries to joints, myocardial infarction, sterile surgical incisions, thrombophlebitis, and blister formation as a result of exposure to temperature extremes or mechanical trauma. Examples of inflammatory responses associated with noninfectious invasion by foreign proteins include allergic rhinitis, some types of contact dermatitis, and other immediate allergic reactions. Examples of inflammatory responses associated with invasion by pathogenic (disease-causing) microorganisms include otitis media, appendicitis, bronchitis, bacterial peritonitis, viral hepatitis, bacterial myocarditis, and many other infections. These clinical examples of inflammation also may involve concurrent stimulation of either of the other two components of immunity.

Inflammation is considered a nonspecific body defense against the side effects of injury or invasion. This defense is nonspecific because the same tissue-level responses occur as a result of any type of injury or invasion, regardless of the location or the specific initiating agent. Therefore, the inflammatory processes stimulated by a scald burn to the hand are virtually the same as the inflammatory processes stimulated by either the reflux of hydrochloric acid stomach contents into the esophagus or bacteria present in the middle ear. The extent of the physical reactions to inflammation is dependent on the intensity, severity, duration, and extent of exposure to the initiating injury or invasion as well as on individual host characteristics (such as age and general immunocompetence).

CELLULAR COMPONENTS

The leukocytes responsible for the generation of inflammatory responses are the myeloid-origin cells—neutrophils, macrophages, basophils, and eosinophils. The neutrophils and macrophages primarily participate in phagocytosis actually destroying and eliminating foreign invaders. The action of eosinophils and basophils generally is directed on specific cells within the vascular system to initiate tissue-level inflammatory responses. Figure 2–1 describes the differentiation and maturation pathways of these cells.

Neutrophils

Mature neutrophils (polymorphonuclear cells) normally compose between 55 and 70 per cent of the total white-cell count. Neutrophils originate from the pluripotent stem cells and complete the maturation process in the bone marrow (Fig. 2–2). Under normal conditions, maturation from the undifferentiated-stem-cell stage to functional segmented neutrophils requires 12 to 14 days. This maturation time can be shortened considerably by certain conditions that stimulate the body to synthesize and release specific chemical factors such as GM-CSF (granulocyte–macrophage colony-stimulating factor) and G-CSF (granu-

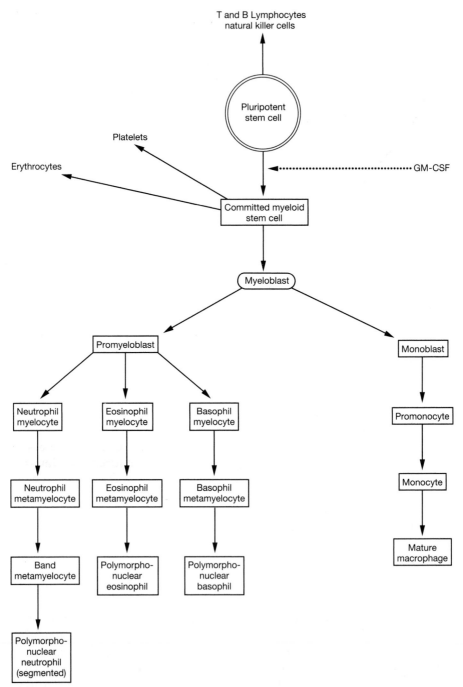

FIGURE 2–1. Granulocyte–macrophage maturational pathway. GM-CSF = granulocyte–macrophage colony-stimulating factor.

locyte colony-stimulating factor) (Haeuber & DiJulio, 1989; Sieff, 1987). In the immunocompetent, healthy individual more than 100 billion mature neutrophils are released from the bone marrow into systemic circulation daily. This massive generation of neutrophils is necessary since the lifespan of a circulating neutrophil is extremely short, averaging only about 12 to 18 hours. Once in the blood, neutrophil movement is ameboid. They are capable of penetrating the endothelial lining of small blood vessels, especially capillaries, and then also can exert their effects in interstitial fluid.

Although the neutrophils, as a group, compose the largest number of circulating leukocytes, the physical size of an individual neutrophil is very small. This army of powerful little cells provides the first line of defense through the process of phagocytosis against foreign invaders, particularly bacteria, in blood and extracellular fluids. The specific structures of neutrophils, which allow successful completion of the phagocytic process, are the granules. The cytoplasm of mature neutrophils is filled with large numbers of two distinctly different types of enzyme-filled granules. Primary granules (azurophilic) contain myeloperoxidase, lysozyme, acid hydrolases, and β-glucuronidase. Secondary granules, devoid of myeloperoxidase, contain alkaline phosphatase and general aminopeptidases. Each of these specific enzymes and enzyme groups helps to degrade different components of foreign invaders that are ingested by neutrophils.

Neutrophils have a finite energy supply, usually in the form of adenosine triphosphate (ATP), and no internal mechanism for replenishing chemical energy substances or the enzymes used in degradation. For this reason, each neutrophil is capable of only one episode of phagocytic destruction before its supplies are exhaused and its death ensues.

A concept important in understanding the protection provided by inflammation is the fact that the mature, segmented neutrophil is the only neutrophil stage capable of immediate, effective phagocytosis. Because this cell is responsible for providing continuous, on-the-spot, nonspecific protection against invasion by microorganisms, the percentage and actual number of circulating white blood cells that are mature neutrophils is a reliable measure of a patient's susceptibility to infection. The higher the numbers of mature neutrophils, the greater resistance the patient has against infection. This measurement is the absolute neutrophil count (sometimes called the absolute granulocyte count [AGC] or the total granulocyte count [TGC]). This count is calculated by first adding the percentage of fully mature segmented neutrophils together with the percentage of the slightly less mature "band" neutrophils (see Fig. 2–2) listed on the differential count. The sum of these two percentages is multiplied by the total white-cell count. For example:

if a patient has a total white-cell count of 8000 cells/cu mm of blood with a differential that includes 60 per cent segmented neutrophils and 2 per cent band neutrophils, the absolute neutrophil count is 62 per cent of 8000 (0.62 × 8000) or 4960/cu mm.

The percentage of circulating band neutrophils is included in this count because even though these immature neutrophils are not yet capable of phago-

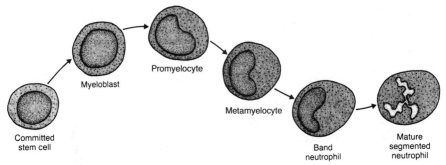

FIGURE 2-2. Neutrophil maturation. (From: *Medical-Surgical Nursing: A Nursing Process Approach* [p. 533] by D. Ignatavicius and M. Bayne, 1991, Philadelphia: W.B. Saunders.)

cytic action as "bands," they will mature rapidly (within a few hours) while circulating in the blood and become segmented neutrophils. The absolute neutrophil count is an important number because it represents the number of cells actually able to mount a defense against invading microorganisms. It is this count that determines whether an immunocompromised patient should be placed in reverse isolation.

Normally, the differential white-cell count indicates that most of the neutrophils released into the blood from the bone marrow are segmented neutrophils, with only a very small percentage being band neutrophils (Tizard, 1984). The less mature forms of neutrophils (metamyelocytes, myelocytes) should not be present in the blood. Some infectious conditions cause the major population of neutrophils present in the blood to change from being mostly segmented neutrophils to being mostly a less mature form of neutrophils. This situation is termed a *left shift* or a *shift to the left* of neutrophils because the greatest number of circulating neutrophils is no longer the segmented neutrophil depicted at the far right of the neutrophil maturational pathway (see Fig. 2-2). Instead, the major circulating population is one of the cell types depicted further left on the maturational pathway. This situation is an ominous clinical sign, as it indicates that the patient's bone marrow production of mature neutrophils cannot keep pace with the continuing presence of infectious microorganisms; thus, the bone marrow is releasing immature neutrophils into the blood. Unfortunately, many of these immature neutrophils are of no benefit to the patient, as they are not functional phagocytic cells and do not further mature in the blood.

Macrophages

These interesting multifunctional cells originate in the bone marrow from the committed myeloid stem cell. Under the influence of specific factors, such as GM-CSF, this cell begins to differentiate into a monocyte and is released into the blood at this stage. Most monocytes migrate into various tissues where they complete the maturation process into macrophages. Macrophages in various tissues have slightly different appearances (morphologies) and different names. Table 2–1 summarizes the names of the different tissue macrophages. Figure 2–3 shows the distribution and concentration of the tissue macrophages throughout the body. Although most tissues contain some macrophages, the liver and spleen contain the greatest concentration of these cells.

At one time, the tissue macrophage system was referred to as the reticuloendothelial system (RES) and thought to be a new body system. Later, this name was deemed inappropriate, and the system was renamed the mononuclear phagocytic system.

The lifespan of the macrophage is primarily dependent on the nature of the substances ingested by phagocytosis. Generally, tissue macrophages have relatively long lifespans, lasting from months to years. Macrophages are the largest of all the leukocytes, contain large amounts of cytoplasm, and have a single nonlobulated nucleus. Macrophage granules contain a wide variety of proteolytic and hydrolytic enzymes, including catalase instead of myeloperoxidase.

Macrophage activity is complex, and these cells have more than one role in providing protection against the effects of invasion and tissue injury. Macrophages are critically important in the inflammatory responses and also are capable of participating in the stimulation of more long-lasting immune responses associated with antibody-mediated immunity and cellular-mediated immunity. Specific macrophage functions include phagocytosis, repair of injured tissues, antigen processing, and secretion of chemical substances that participate in the regulation of overall immune function.

The major macrophage function associated with inflammation is phagocytosis. Macrophages are efficient at recognition of self versus nonself. Many tissue macrophages have large cytoplasmic extensions to assist in physically trapping foreign proteins. Unlike neutrophils, macrophages have the intracellular machinery necessary to regenerate chemical energy supplies in the form of ATP and can also continuously generate all of the enzymes needed to degrade foreign protein. Therefore, each macrophage is quite capable of participating in many different phagocytic events during the course of its life.

TABLE 2–1. Names of Tissue Macrophages.

Tissue	Macrophage
Lung	Alveolar macrophage
Connective tissue	Histiocyte
Brain	Microglia
Liver	Kupffer cell
Peritoneum	Peritoneal macrophages
Bone	Osteoclasts
Joints	Synovial type A cells
Kidney	Mesangial cells

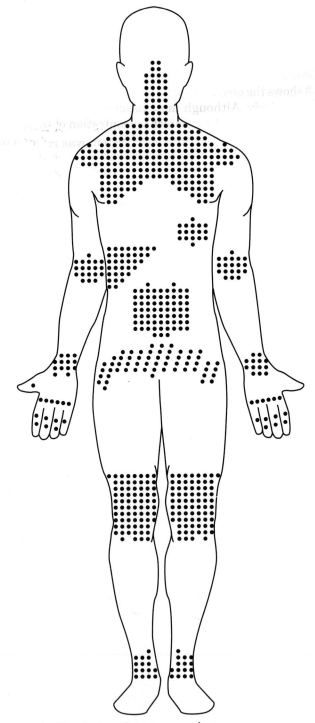

FIGURE 2-3. Concentration/distribution of tissue macrophages.

Basophils

Basophils are the smallest of all the leukocytes and the most rare. They are derived from myeloid stem cells and released from the bone marrow after a short maturation period. Even though they are rare, basophils largely are responsible for the obvious signs and symptoms associated with inflammation. Basophils do not have the capacity for ameboid movement and cannot engage in phagocytic actions. Structurally and functionally basophils resemble mast cells, although basophils have a completely different known origin from mast cells. Mast cells are special connective tissue cells that contain histamine and heparin. Although these cells do not arise from the bone marrow and do not circulate in the blood, they do mediate inflammatory responses in connective tissue. Both cell types contain enormous numbers of cytoplasmic granules and have binding sites for IgE attached to their membrane surfaces. It is thought that the attached IgE molecules have a role in assisting the basophils to recognize nonself cells.

Basophilic granules contain heparin and a variety of vasoactive amines, including histamine, serotonin, kinins, and leukotrienes. The actions of most of these vasoactive amines, when they are released into the blood, affect the integrity and function of many types of smooth muscle and vascular endothelium. Heparin inhibits coagulation of blood and other protein-containing extracellular fluids. Histamine constricts the smooth muscles of the respiratory system and venules. Constriction of respiratory smooth muscle narrows the lumens of airways and restricts pulmonary ventilation. Constriction of venule smooth muscle inhibits blood flow through small veins and diminishes venous return. This effect causes blood to dam up in capillaries and small arterioles, increasing the hydrostatic pressure within these vessels. Kinins cause slow vasodilation of arterioles. Together, kinins and serotonin dramatically enhance capillary permeability, permitting the plasma portion of the blood to leak into the interstitial space, leading to edema in the involved tissue areas.

Eosinophils

Eosinophils are myeloid-origin cells that require 6 days in the bone marrow to differentiate and mature. After maturation they are released into circulation. Free eosinophils in the blood have a half-life of from 30 to 60 minutes, while those that migrate into tissues can live 2 weeks or longer. Eosinophils are not efficient at the process of phagocytosis, although they do perform a modification of this function against parasitic larvae infestations and also appear to have an important role in preventing pulmonary infections.

The primary function of eosinophils is to modulate and regulate tissue-level inflammatory reactions. The cytoplasm of eosinophils contains a variety of granules. Some of these granules contain histamine and kinins just like those of the basophils. In addition, eosinophil granules contain special enzymes to degrade the vasoactive amines and other agents released by basophils and mast cells. These enzymes limit the activity of the vasoactive amines and thus control the extent of inflammatory reactions generated in response to invasion or tissue injury.

PHAGOCYTOSIS

Phagocytosis is the key mechanism for the successful outcome of inflammation in the destruction of nonself cells. It is the process by which leukocytes engulf cellular debris and foreign proteins and destroy them through a series of intracellular degradative events. When inflammation is initiated purely by tissue injury, leukocyte phagocytic action removes cellular debris. When inflammation is initiated purely through invasion by foreign organisms or proteins, leukocyte phagocytic action destroys and removes the invaders. Although all mature leukocytes (except for basophils) are capable of performing phagocytic actions to some extent, the neutrophils and macrophages are most efficient at this process. Phagocytosis occurs in a predictable manner and involves the following seven steps: (1) exposure/invasion, (2) attraction, (3) adherence, (4) recognition, (5) cellular ingestion, (6) phagosome formation, and (7) degradation. Figure 2–4 presents these seven steps schematically. Although these seven steps are described individually, considerable interaction occurs in the early stages.

Exposure/Invasion

Leukocytes capable of engaging in phagocytosis and of stimulating inflammation are present in extracellular fluids. Therefore, phagocytosis generally occurs in the body's internal environment. In order to initiate phagocytosis, leukocytes capable of engaging in phagocytic events must first be exposed to substances released by internal tissue damage or to foreign proteins.

Events that cause tissue damage can be externally or internally generated. Tissue damage occurs as a result of direct mechanical and chemical disruption of cellular integrity. Such events include wounds created by pressure, temperature extremes, and movement of chemicals normally confined to a specific body area into a different body area.

Some tissue-damaging events allow simultaneous penetration of foreign proteins into the body's internal environment. Such events include cuts, puncture wounds, abrasions, and any tissue injury that results in loss of integrity of the skin or mucous membranes.

Foreign proteins can also enter the body's internal environment through routes that do not involve tissue damage. Some "internal" body areas come into direct contact with the external environment. These areas include the entire oral–gastrointestinal tract, the nasorespiratory tract, and the genitourinary tract. When these areas are exposed to foreign proteins in excessive

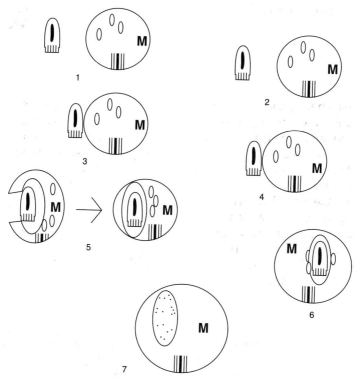

FIGURE 2-4. Steps of phagocytosis. 1 = exposure/invasion; 2 = attraction; 3 = adherence; 4 = recognition; 5 = cellular ingestion; 6 = phagosome formation; 7 = degradation; M = macrophage.

amounts, the normal surface defenses may be overwhelmed and thus the foreign proteins gain entry into the body's internal environment.

Attraction

Phagocytosis is effective only when the phagocytic cell comes into direct contact with the target or victim cell. Because tissue injury or invasion by foreign proteins can occur at sites somewhat remote from the presence of either neutrophils or macrophages, mechanisms to unite phagocytic cells with their intended targets are necessary.

Special chemical substances have the capacity to act as chemical magnets that attract a variety of leukocytes, including neutrophils and macrophages. These substances are called *chemotaxins* or *leukotaxins*. Damaged tissues excrete chemotaxins. In addition, elements present in plasma and other extracellular fluids as a result of blood vessel injury also attract neutrophils and macrophages. These elements include fibrin, collagen, and plasminogen activator. Bacterial endotoxins often are powerful chemotaxins. In addition, substances that combine with surface components of invading foreign proteins also serve as chemotaxins. This mechanism is described more completely in the section on opsonins and opsonization.

Adherence

Because phagocytosis requires direct contact of the phagocyte with its intended target, the phagocytic cell first must bind to the surface of the target. In living systems many substances suspended in the blood cannot come into direct contact with each other because the surfaces of these substances all carry an overall negative charge. Because like charges repel each other, two particles or cells that both have negative surface charges would have great difficulty overcoming the repelling forces of the negative charges and coming into contact with each other. Because opposite charges attract or pull toward each other, direct contact is enhanced when the surface charge of one cell is changed to neutral or to an overall positive charge. Adherence of phagocytic cells to targets is enhanced by a process called *opsonization,* which changes the surface charge of target cells to neutral or positive.

Opsonins

The word *opsonin* is derived from Greek and literally means to cover food with a sauce in preparation for eating. In biology, opsonins coat a target cell, changing its surface charge, in preparation for eating by phagocytic cells. A variety of substances can act as opsonins and change the surface charge of cellular debris and foreign proteins so that they are more easily trapped and adhered to by phagocytic cells. Some of these substances include residual particles from dead neutrophils, antibodies, and fixated complement components.

Neutrophils, by virtue of their numbers, more easily bind to many foreign proteins than do macrophages. However, neutrophils are small and usually are destroyed in the phagocytic process. Upon destruction, neutrophil particles can remain attached to the surface of a target foreign protein, change the protein's charge, and enhance subsequent macrophage adherence to that target foreign protein.

Antibodies do not carry an overall positive or negative charge and thus are electrically "neutral." When antibodies surround and bind to a target foreign protein they change the foreign protein's surface charge and directly enhance adherence of phagocytic cells to it. In addition, binding of some antibodies indirectly assists with this adhering process through stimulation of the complement cascade.

Complement Fixation

Complement fixation is a well-characterized mechanism of opsonization and enhancement of phagocytic adherence to target cellular debris or foreign proteins. Within the blood are approximately 20 different inactive protein components of the complement system (Roitt, 1991). The major complement proteins are labeled C1 through C9. Some of the nine major complement proteins have subsets (for example, C1 protein can be separated into C1q, C1r, and C1s) so that the number of currently identified complement components is 20. These components are primarily synthesized by the liver although some are also synthesized by macrophages. Under the correct stimulation, these complement proteins are activated rapidly and then act together to cause dramatic biologic actions as a result of fixation to specific tissues. Because the biologic actions of complement fixation usually are needed quickly but can have devastating effects if exerted at the wrong time or in the wrong place, the complement system functions as a "cascade" reaction, with multiple sites of activation and control through various feedback integration points.

Cascade reactions are actually chain reactions in which events must occur in a specific sequence In the case of the complement cascade for complement activation and fixation, a specific component of complement must be activated first. Activation of this component leads to activation of the next component, which leads to the activation of the next component, and so on.

In the classical complement pathway or cascade sequence (Fig. 2–5), the complement component that must be activated first is C1q. Because it is not desirable to stimulate the complement cascade unnecessarily, only a few specific circumstances lead to the activation of C1q. The primary event stimulating the activation of C1q is the binding of some types of antibody to antigen. This binding provides a critical site for the binding of C1q to the antigen-antibody complex. The binding of C1q to the special site created on the antigen–antibody complex activates C1q, which in turn activates the next complement protein in the cascade. When all components of complement are bound or fixated on the surface of the target foreign protein, causing activation of the complement components, the surface charge of the target is changed and phagocytic cells adhere more easily (Barrett, 1988).

In addition to the classical complement pathway, complement fixation and activation can also occur through an alternate complement pathway. Stimulation for activation of this cascade is somewhat different and is initiated with complement protein C3 rather than C1q. A triggering event for this pathway is the presence of certain carbohydrate groups on the surface of many microorganisms. These carbohydrate groups allow conversion of C3 into C3a and C3b. C3b binds to the surface of the micoorganism, and this binding stimulates the activation of the next complement protein in the series. It is thought that this alternate pathway exists as a shortcut to allow more rapid complement fixation in limited areas in response to invasion by microorganisms without having specific antibodies present. The overall result of complement fixation by this alternate activation pathway is the same as by the classical activation pathway. Activation of the alternate complement pathway also may assist phagocytic cells in the process of distinguishing self cells from nonself cells.

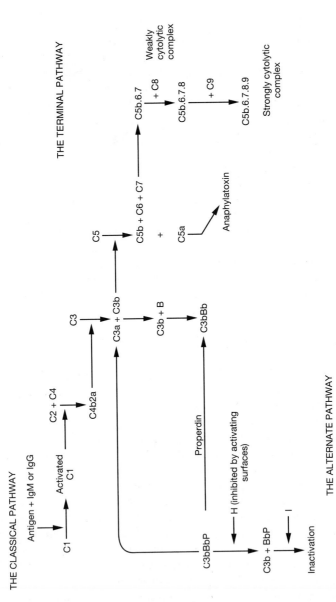

FIGURE 2-5. Pathway of complement activation. (Adapted from *Veterinary Immunology*, 3rd ed. [p. 118, Fig. 10-3] by I. Tizard, 1987, Philadelphia: W.B. Saunders.)

Recognition

When the phagocytic cell is adhering to the surface of the target cell, recognition of self as opposed to nonself occurs. The mechanism for recognition at this point is identical to the mechanism described earlier in this chapter for self-tolerance and involves examination of universal product codes (defined in Chapter 1). Recognition of nonself is slightly enhanced by the presence of opsonins on the surface of the target cell. Under normal circumstances, phagocytic cells proceed with the process of phagocytosis only if the target cell is recognized either as "foreign" or as self-cell debris.

Cellular Ingestion

Because phagocytic destruction is an intracellular process, the target cell or foreign protein must be brought inside the phagocytic cell. The primary mechanism for cellular ingestion of target cells or debris by phagocytic cells is absorptive endocytosis. This mechanism permits ingestion without disruption of the integrity of the phagocytic cell's membrane.

After adherence to and recognition of the target cell, the phagocytic cell changes shape and allows its membrane to invaginate the target. Some areas of the phagocytic membrane appear better able to carry out this maneuver than other areas. These areas are called *coated pits* and may also be more efficient at adherence to the target. Once the target is surrounded, the touching edges of the phagocytic cell's membrane fuse together, effectively sealing the target within a vesicle inside the phagocytic cell, forming a vacuole. Other less-refined mechanisms for cellular ingestion of target cells also may function within phagocytic cells.

Phagosome Formation

If some of the phagocyte's cytoplasmic granules are inside the vacuole, the structure is called a *phagosome*. When these cytoplasmic granules degranulate and release enzymes and other lytic substances within the fluid of the phagosome, some destruction of the ingested target begins. Assistance from lysosomes enhances this intracellular destruction. Lysosomal membranes have the same composition as phagosomal membranes. Therefore, lysosomes can fuse with phagosomes to form a special destructive organelle termed by some cell biologists as a *phagolysosome*. Fusion of lysosomes with a phagosome allows lysosomal degradative products to be incorporated within the phagosome. These products enhance the destruction of the target.

Degradation

The granular and lysosomal enzymes within the phagolysosome exert their specific effects on various components of the ingested target. Specific enzymes split carbohydrate and lipid moieties from the target, allowing better degradation of the target by proteolytic enzymes. Nonspecific proteolytic enzymes first degrade the large target molecule into many much smaller molecules that are more sensitive to specific and nonspecific degradation by other enzymes. Destruction of the target also occurs through the formation of oxygen metabolites (some of which are oxygen free radicals) capable of exerting oxidation damage to target cells. This entire process is known as the "respiratory burst" and begins at the time a target cell first adheres to the phagocyte's membrane. This adherence stimulates several membrane-level biochemical reactions to occur that increase the phagocytic cell's consumption of oxygen. This intracellular oxygen is acted on by myeloperoxidase and superoxide dismutase to form damaging oxidation products. These products weaken many of the forces holding the target molecule together and increase its susceptibility to further degradation.

INFLAMMATORY RESPONSES

Inflammatory responses for protecting the body from side effects of tissue injury or invasion by foreign proteins occur in a predictable sequence. The sequence is the same regardless of the initiating stimulus. The responses of inflammation can be divided into three distinctly different functional stages, although the timing of the stages may overlap.

Stage I

Stage I is called the *vascular stage* because most of the early effects of this response involve physiologic changes at the vascular level. When inflammation occurs as a result of tissue injury, this stage has two phases.

The first phase is an immediate but short-term vasoconstriction of arterioles and venules as a direct result of physical trauma to vascular smooth muscle. This phase lasts only seconds to minutes and may be of such short duration that the individual undergoing the response is unaware of the vasoconstriction.

The second phase is characterized by hyperemia and swelling at the site of injury or invasion. Injured tissues and the leukocytes in this area secrete vasoactive amines (histamine, serotonin, and kinins) that cause constriction of the venules and dilation of the arterioles in the immediate area. The effects of these changes in blood vessel dilation cause the symptoms of redness and increased warmth of the tissues in the area. The purpose of this response is to enhance healing by increasing nutrients at the tissue level through increased blood flow to the area.

Some of the same vasoactive amines also increase capillary permeability, allowing blood plasma to leak into the interstitial space. This response causes the symptoms of swelling (edema formation), as fluid collects, and pain, as both the pressure of increased fluid in the area and chemicals in the fluid stimulate local sensory nerve endings. Edema formation at the site of injury or invasion is overall a helpful event. This swelling can protect the area from further injury by creating a fluid cushion. The extra fluid also can dilute any toxins or microorganisms that enter the area. The plasma that leaks into the interstitial space contains fibrin and other protein factors that can clot the interstitial fluid in the area of injury or invasion, literally walling off the site and confining the effects largely to the immediate area. The duration of these responses is dependent on the severity of the initiating event.

The major leukocyte involved in this stage of inflammation is the tissue macrophage. The response of the tissue macrophages is immediate since they are already in place at the site of injury or invasion. However, this response is limited since their numbers are so few. In addition to phagocytosis, the tissue macrophages secrete several granulocyte substances to enhance inflammation. One substance is colony-stimulating factor (G-CSF), which stimulates the bone marrow to decrease leukocyte generation time from 14 days to just a matter of hours. In addition, tissue macrophages secrete substances that will stimulate the release of neutrophils from the bone marrow and attract them to the site of injury or invasion, leading to the next stage of inflammation.

Stage II

This stage of inflammation also is called the *cellular exudate stage*. It is characterized by neutrophilia, the secretion of many factors into the interstitial fluid and the formation of exudate.

The leukocyte most prominent in this stage is the neutrophil. Under the influence of chemotactic agents and substances that increase the number and rate of maturation of neutrophils, the actual neutrophil count can increase up to fivefold within 12 hours of the onset of inflammation. The purposes of the neutrophils at the site of inflammation are to (1) attack and destroy foreign materials and (2) remove dead and dying tissue. Both of these functions are accomplished through phagocytosis.

During acute inflammatory responses of short duration, the otherwise healthy individual can synthesize enough mature neutrophils to keep pace with the effects of injury and invasion and eventually overcome the ability of invaders to multiply. At the same time, these leukocytes secrete colony-stimulating factors that cause reproduction of tissue macrophages and increase bone marrow production of monocytes (Werb, 1987). Although this reaction is slower to start, its effects are relatively long-lasting.

When infectious processes stimulating inflammation are of longer duration (chronic), the bone marrow's capacity to synthesize and release mature neutrophils into the blood is not able to keep pace with the ability of microorganisms to multiply. In this situation, the bone marrow begins to release immature neutrophils, many of which are unable to phagocytize and cannot complete maturation out of the bone marrow. Such depletion of functional phagocytic neutrophils limits the effectiveness of inflammation and dramatically increases the susceptibility of the individual to new and recurring microbial infections.

Stage III

This stage of inflammation also is called the *stage of tissue repair and replacement.* Although this stage is completed last, it actually is initiated at the time of injury and is critical to the ultimate function of the inflamed area.

Some of the leukocytes involved in inflammation are capable of stimulating repair of lost or damaged tissues by inducing the remaining normal, healthy tissue to divide. In tissues that are not mitotically active (nondividing tissues), leukocytes stimulate revascularization and the laying down of different types of collagen to form scar tissue. Because scar tissue does not behave in the same manner as normal differentiated tissue, some functional loss occurs in areas where damaged tissues are replaced with scar tissue. The extent of the functional loss is determined by the percentage of tissue replaced by scar tissue.

SUMMARY

Inflammation provides immediate protection against the effects of tissue injury and invading foreign proteins. However, because the inflammatory responses are nonspecific and the response is the same even on reexposure to the same initiating factors, inflammation does not provide sustained immunity. Although generally beneficial, some inflammatory responses are accompanied by unpleasant and even tissue-damaging actions. The capacity for inflammation is a critical component to the overall health and well-being of an individual.

SELECTED BIBLIOGRAPHY

Abernathy, E. (1987). How the immune system works. *American Journal of Nursing, 87*(4), 456.

Barrett, J. (1988). *Textbook of immunology* (5th ed.). St. Louis: C.V. Mosby.

Carrieri, V., Lindsey, A., & West, C. (1986). *Pathophysiological phenomena in nursing: Human responses to illness.* Philadelphia: W.B. Saunders.

Colten, H. (1985). Complement biosynthesis. *Clinics in Immunology and Allergy, 5*(2), 287.

Cooper, N. (1987). The complement system. In D. Stites, J. Stobo, & J. Wells (Eds.), *Basic and clinical immunology* (6th ed.) (p. 114). Norwalk, CT: Appleton & Lange.

Dawson, M. (1988). Immunology: non-specific immunity. *Nursing Times 84*(17), 75.

Gallucci, B. (1987). The immune system and cancer. *Oncology Nursing Forum, 14*(6), Suppl., 3.

Goldstein, E. (1983). Hydrolytic enzymes of alveolar macrophages. *Review of Infectious Diseases, 5,* 1078.

Grady, C. (1988). Host defense mechanisms: An overview. *Seminars in Oncology Nursing, 4*(2), 86.

Groenwald, S. (1980). Physiology of the immune system. *Heart and Lung, 9*(4), 645.

Gurevich, I., & Tafuro, P. (1986). The compromised host. *Cancer Nursing, 9*(5), 263.

Gurevich, I. (1985). The competent internal immune system. *Nursing Clinics of North America, 20,* 151.

Guyton, A. (1991). *Textbook of medical physiology* (8th ed.). Philadelphia: W.B. Saunders.

Haeuber, D., & DiJulio, J. (1989). Hemopoietic colony stimulating factors: An overview. *Oncology Nursing Forum, 16*(2), 247.

Huffer, T., Kanapa, D., & Stevenson, G. (1986). *Introduction to human immunology.* Boston: Jones and Bartlett.

Jett, M., & Lancaster, L. (1983). The inflammatory immune response: The body's defense against invasion. *Critical Care Nurse,* 64.

Kemp, D. (1986). Development of the immune system. *Critical Care Quarterly, 9*(1), 1.

Roitt, I. (1991). *Essential immunology* (7th ed.). Boston: Blackwell Scientific.

Sieff, C. (1987). Hemopoietic growth factors. *Journal of Clinical Investigation, 79*(6), 1549.

Smith, S. (1986). Physiology of the immune system. *Critical Care Quarterly, 9*(1), 7.

Stites, D., Stobo, J., & Wells, J. (Eds.) (1987). *Basic and clinical immunology* (6th ed.). Norwalk, CT: Appleton & Lange.

Tami, J., Parr, M., & Thompson, J. (1986). The immune system. *American Journal of Hospital Pharmacy, 43,* 2483.

Tizard, I. (1984). *Immunology: An introduction.* Philadelphia: Saunders College Publishing.

Werb, Z. (1987). Phagocytic cells: Chemotaxis & effector functions of macrophages and granulocytes. In D. Stites, J. Stobo, & J. Wells (Eds.), *Basic and clinical immunology* (6th ed.) (p. 96). Norwalk, CT: Appleton & Lange.

Workman, M. (1989). Immunologic late effects of cancer therapy. *Seminars in Oncology Nursing, 5*(1), 36.

3

ANTIBODY-MEDIATED IMMUNITY

Antibody-mediated immunity (AMI) is a very specific type of acquired immunity. AMI was formerly known as humoral-mediated immunity because the actual substances that conferred the immunity, the antibodies, were released and freely circulating in the blood and other extracellular fluids (body humors). Antibody-mediated immunity primarily involves antigen–antibody actions to neutralize, eliminate, or destroy substances containing foreign proteins. These actions are accomplished directly by populations of B lymphocytes, although assistance with these actions is also needed from several other lymphocytes and macrophages.

CELLULAR COMPONENTS

The leukocytes that have the most direct role in antibody-mediated immunity are the B lymphocytes. Because B lymphocytes have limited specific functions and are not efficient at recognition of self versus nonself, major interactions with cells responsible for inflammation (macrophages along with helper T cells) are required to initiate and complete antigen–antibody actions. In addition, special T lymphocytes (helper T-cells) secrete products that regulate the activity of B lymphocytes and assist with recognition of nonself. Therefore, in order for antibody-mediated immunity to be optimal, the entire immune system must be functioning adequately.

B lymphocytes originate from the pluripotent stem cells in the bone marrow (see Chapter 1). The pluripotent stem cells destined to become B lymphocytes commit early to the lymphocyte maturational pathway (Fig. 3–1), pos-

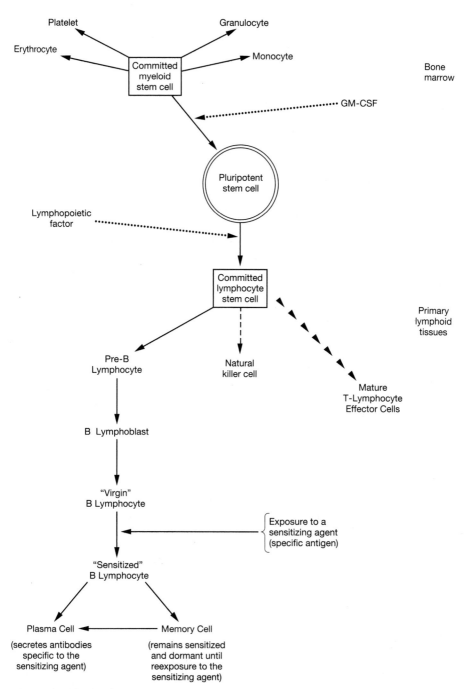

FIGURE 3–1. Maturation pathway of B lymphocytes. GM-CSF = granulocyte–macrophage colony-stimulating factor.

sibly under the influence of a specific lymphopoietic factor. At this point, committed lymphocyte stem cells are no longer pluripotent, but now are limited to lymphocyte differentiation. The committed lymphocyte stem cells are released from the bone marrow into the blood, where they migrate into various lymphoid tissues.

In birds, this maturation and differentiation of committed lymphocyte stem cells into B lymphocytes occurs in a special area of lymphoid tissue called the bursa of Fabricius (hence the designation "B"). Humans do not have any one tissue or organ analogous to the bursa of Fabricius. Instead, the committed lymphocyte stem cells that mature and differentiate into human B lymphocytes first must migrate into germinating centers of lymph nodes, tonsils, Peyer's patches of the intestinal tract, the white pulp of the spleen, and possibly other lymphoid areas. Once maturation has occurred, the B lymphocytes are released into general circulation.

The primary function of B lymphocytes is to become sensitized to a specific foreign protein (antigen) and synthesize an antibody directed specifically against that protein. The antibody, rather than the actual B lymphocyte, then participates in one of a variety of actions to neutralize, eliminate, or destroy that antigen.

ANTIGEN–ANTIBODY INTERACTIONS

Generating sufficient quantities of a specific antibody to provide an individual with long-lasting immunity against the specific microorganisms or toxins responsible for causing a disease requires time and a series of special interactions. These interactions revolve around the actions of B lymphocytes but also include specific and nonspecific activities of other leukocytes. Developing the capacity to secrete a unique and specific antibody directed against a unique and specific antigen whenever the individual is exposed to that antigen involves the following seven steps: (1) exposure/invasion, (2) antigen recognition, (3) lymphocyte sensitization, (4) antibody production and release, (5) antibody–antigen binding, (6) antibody-binding reactions, and (7) sustained immunity/memory. Each step of the antigen–antibody interaction and antibody-mediated immunity is explained below in detail. Figure 3–2 is a schematic drawing depicting the sequence of events necessary for successful antibody-mediated immunity.

Exposure/Invasion

Antigen–antibody interactions occur in the body's internal environment. In order to make an antibody that can exert its effects on a specific antigen, the body must first be exposed to that antigen to the degree that the antigen penetrates the body's external defensive barriers (primarily the skin and mu-

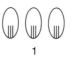

1

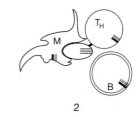

2

FIGURE 3-2. Sequence of events required to initiate antibody-mediated immunity.

(1) Invasion of the body by new antigens in sufficient numbers to stimulate an immune response. (2) Interaction of macrophage (M) and T helper (T_{H}) cell in the processing and presenting of the antigen to the unsensitized "virgin" B lymphocyte (B). (3) Sensitization of the virgin B lymphocyte to the new antigen. (4) Antibody production by the B lymphocyte. These antibodies are directed specifically against the initiating antigen. The antibodies are released from the B lymphocyte and float freely in the blood and some other fluids. (5) Antibodies bind to the antigen, forming an immune complex. (6) Antibody binding causes cellular events and attracts other leukocytes to the complex. The interaction of other leukocytes along with the cellular events results in the neutralization, destruction, or elimination of the antigen. (7) On reexposure to the same antigen, the sensitized lymphocytes and their progeny produce large quantities of the antibody specific to the antigen. In addition, new "virgin" B lymphocytes become sensitized to the antigen and also begin antibody production.

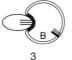

3

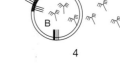

4

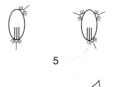

5

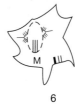

6

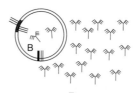

7

cous membranes). Not all exposures result in the stimulation of antibody production, even when exposure includes penetration and invasion into the body's internal environment. The invasion by the antigen must occur in such a way that some of the antigen is able either to evade detection by the normal nonspecific defenses or to overwhelm the abilities of the inflammatory responses to neutralize, eliminate, or destroy the invading antigen.

An example of a successful first step would be the case of an individual who has never contracted or been exposed to the childhood viral disease chickenpox babysitting for children who erupt with chickenpox lesions within the next 10 hours. In the preeruption stage, these children are shedding many millions of live chickenpox viruses through the droplets of their upper aerodigestive tracts. Because small children often are unconcerned about the finer points of infection control, these children drink out of the babysitter's soft drink can, kiss the sitter directly (and wetly) on the lips, and both sneeze and cough directly into the sitter's face. After spending 5 hours with the children at close range, the babysitter has been overwhelmingly invaded by the chickenpox virus (varicella–zoster) and will become sick with this disease within 14 to 21 days. While this individual is incubating the virus and chickenpox is actually developing, the exposed lymphocytes are participating in the next steps in the series to prevent the sitter from contracting the chickenpox more than once.

Antigen Recognition

In order to begin to make antibodies against an antigen, the "virgin" or previously unsensitized B lymphocyte must first recognize the antigen as nonself. B lymphocytes are the least efficient of all the leukocytes at differentiating self cells from nonself cells and, in fact, actually may not be able to carry out this important function alone. For this reason, antigen recognition by B lymphocytes requires the interactions of macrophages and helper T cells.

This cooperative effort for B-lymphocyte antigen recognition appears to be primarily initiated by the macrophages. The macrophages, after the membrane of the antigen has been altered somewhat by opsonization (discussed in Chapter 2), recognizes the invading foreign protein (antigen) as nonself and physically attaches itself to the antigen, "processing" it in some way. This particular macrophage attachment to the antigen does not result in complete phagocytosis or immediate destruction of the antigen. Instead, the "processing" appears to enhance exposure of the antigen's universal product code. While this antigen processing is a macrophage function, some other cells can also process the antigen. After processing, the macrophage presents the attached processed antigen to a helper T cell. After recognizing the processed antigen, the helper T cell brings it into contact with the virgin B lymphocyte in such a way that the B lymphocyte is able to recognize the antigen as nonself. An additional important role of the helper T cell in antibody production is to secrete special proteins that induce the B lymphocyte to initiate and continue the processes that eventually result in antibody production.

Lymphocyte Sensitization

Once the B lymphocyte recognizes the antigen as nonself, the B lymphocyte carries out special steps to become sensitized to this antigen. An individual virgin B lymphocyte can undergo sensitization only once. Therefore, in theory, each B lymphocyte can be sensitized to only one antigen.

The exact mechanisms of the extracellular and intracellular events that result in B-lymphocyte sensitization are not precisely known. The result of sensitization is that this B lymphocyte is able to respond to any substance that carries the identical antigenic determinants or universal product codes as the original antigen. Once sensitized to a specific antigen, the B lymphocyte remains sensitized to that specific antigen. More importantly, all future progeny of that sensitized B lymphocyte also are sensitized to that specific antigen.

Immediately after sensitization, the sensitized B lymphocyte divides and forms two different types of lymphocytes, each remaining sensitized to the specific antigen (Fig. 3–3). One new cell becomes a *plasma cell* and starts the immediate production of antibody directed specifically against the antigen that originally sensitized the B lymphocyte. The other new cell becomes a *memory cell*. The plasma cell functions immediately and has a rather short lifespan. The memory cell remains sensitized but functionally dormant until the next exposure to the same antigen. This memory forms the basis for administration of immunization "booster shots." The production of antibody is at least 50 times greater and much faster after the booster than after the first immunization.

Antibody Production and Release

Antibody production is the responsibility of the plasma cell. When fully stimulated, each plasma cell can produce as many as 300 molecules of antibody per second. Each plasma cell is capable of producing antibody specific only to the antigen that originally sensitized the parent B lymphocyte. For example, in the case of the babysitter exposed to and invaded by chickenpox viruses, the plasma cells derived from the B lymphocytes sensitized at that time to the chickenpox virus can only produce antichickenpox antibodies. The exact class of antibody the plasma cell can produce (IgG, IgM, etc) may vary with time and circumstances, but the specificity of that antibody remains forever directed against chickenpox virus. Individual plasma cells have lifespans of approximately 1 week.

Most of the antibody molecules produced by the plasma cells are secreted into the blood and other extracellular fluids as free antibody by the process of exocytosis. The lifespan of free antibody varies with the type of antibody generated. IgG has the longest lifespan (half-life of approximately 30 days) and IgD has the shortest (half-life, 2 to 3 days). Because the antibody circulates in body fluids (or body "humors") separate from the B lymphocytes, the immunity provided was once called humoral-mediated immunity. Circulating antibodies can be transferred from one person to another in order to provide immediate artificial passive immunity of short duration.

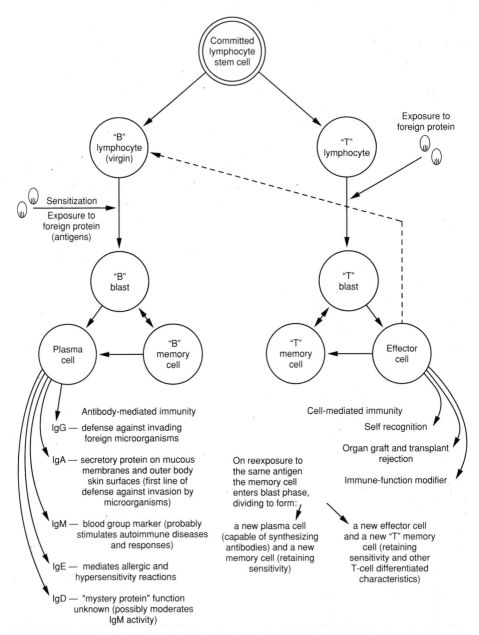

FIGURE 3-3. Differentiated functions of lymphocytes.

Antibody–Antigen Binding

The basic structure of an antibody is a Y-shaped molecule (Fig. 3–4) constructed of two smaller light chains and two larger heavy chains of protein joined together by disulfide bridges. The activity of various parts of this structure has been determined by examining the binding capacity of antibody fragments created through enzyme digestion. The Fc portion of the antibody serves as an anchor for when the antibody is attached to specific self leukocytes. The very ends of the Fab fragments are the areas that actually recognize the specific antigen and bind to it. Because each individual antibody molecule has two Fab fragments, antibody molecules are "bivalent" and can bind either to two separate antigen molecules or to two areas of the same antigen molecule.

Binding of antibody to antigen occurs largely through the noncovalent interactions of hydrogen bonding and other more hydrophobic chemical reactions. These interactions require little energy to form, are thermodynamically favorable, and thus remain very stable through the exclusion of water at the binding site. The binding of antibody to an antigen results in the formation of one type of an "immune complex." In most instances, the actual binding of antibody to the antigen is not a directly lethal action to the antigen. Rather, the presence of the immune complex can stimulate both a permissive and a catalytic role in initiating other actions that ultimately result in the neutralization, elimination, and destruction of the antigen.

Antibody-Binding Reactions

The formation of the immune complex by binding antibody to antigen allows or initiates specific reactions to cause the neutralization, elimination, and/ or destruction of the antigen. The natures of the major reactions are fully described below. Simultaneous execution of all types of major reactions is likely during any one episode of antigen–antibody interactions.

Agglutination

This antibody action is a result of the bivalency of antibody molecules. In this situation, binding multiple antigen molecules to each antibody unit does not directly destroy the antigen. Agglutination permits defensive effects by at least two mechanisms. First, this type of interaction slows the movement of the antigen through the extracellular fluids. Second, the highly irregular shape of the formed antigen–antibody complex enhances the likelihood of nonspecific assaultive and defensive actions by other leukocytes, including macrophages, neutrophils, and cytotoxic T cells. So essentially, agglutination causes the antibody to "hold down" the antigen so that other leukocytes have a chance to come into contact with the antigen and "punch it out."

Complement Fixation

Specific classes of antibodies are able to mediate the neutralization, elimination, or destruction of nonself through activation of the complement cascade and complement fixation. The mechanism by which complement assists in immunity—inflammation is discussed in detail in Chapter 2. The two classes of antibody frequently associated with stimulating the complement system are

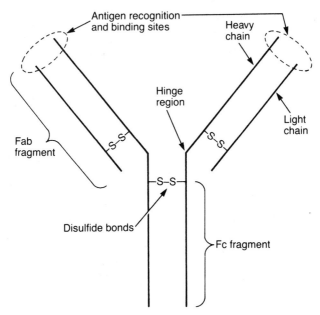

FIGURE 3-4. Basic antibody structure. (From *Medical-Surgical Nursing: A Nursing Process Approach* [p. 543, Fig. 23-8] by D. Ignatavicius and M. Bayne, 1991, Philadelphia: W.B. Saunders.)

IgG and IgM. Binding of antibody from either of these antibody classes to the appropriate antigen provides a recognition/binding site for the first component of complement (C1q) to bind. Once C1q is activated, the other components of the entire complement system are activated as a cascade, which greatly amplifies the effectiveness of opsonization and complement activation. A direct action of complement fixation is membrane lysis. This action occurs wherever the membrane is surrounded by activated complement. This action, also called *complement-mediated lysis, complement-mediated cytolysis,* and the *membrane attack mechanism,* results in a membrane lesion that destroys or neutralizes the antigen (Barrett, 1988). The actual binding causes a disruption of the invading foreign protein's membrane surface. Such disruption permits rapid changes of the intracellular environment of the invader as, in a sense, the invader "spills its guts." Critical substances may be lost from the invader or other harmful substances may gain easy access. The nonself or organisms most susceptible to damage through lysis mediated by the binding of antibody to membrane-surface antigens are bacteria and viruses.

Precipitation

The antibody action of precipitation is similar to agglutination. In this case, antibody closely binds so much antigen that large, insoluble antibody–antigen complexes are formed. These complexes are unable to stay in suspension in the blood. Instead, they form a large, nonmoving precipitate, which can be acted on and cleared by other nonspecific leukocytes.

Inactivation/Neutralization

This antibody action is unique in that it does not result in the immediate destruction of the antigen. Usually, an antigen has a relatively small area that is actually responsible for exerting harmful and unpleasant effects. The rest of the antigen performs duties and activities important to the antigen but not harmful to the host. Binding of antibody can interfere with the function of the active site by directly covering it up (Fig. 3–5) or inducing a change in the active site's physical configuration. Either of these two mechanisms inhibits the activity of the antigen, rendering it harmless without destroying or eliminating it.

Sustained Immunity/Memory

This action of antibody-mediated immunity provides long-lasting or *sustained* immunity to a specific antigen. Sustained immunity is provided through

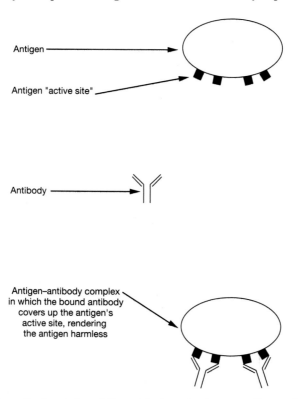

FIGURE 3–5. Schematic description of the antibody action known as "neutralization."

the action of B-lymphocyte *memory cells* generated at the time of antigen sensitization. These memory cells remain sensitized to the specific antigen to which they were originally exposed. On reexposure to the same antigen, these memory lymphocytes are triggered to respond rapidly. First these memory cells divide, forming new sensitized blast cells and new sensitized plasma cells (Fig. 3–3). The blast cells continue to divide and generate even more sensitized plasma cells. The sensitized plasma cells begin to rapidly synthesize and secrete large amounts of antibody.

This response is called a "secondary" or "anamnestic" response because it results in greatly enhanced antibody production on the second (and subsequent) exposure to the same antigen. This secondary response is a rapid and wide-spread immune response to the presence of the antigen. Usually this response completely eliminates the invading antigen before the antigen can replicate in sufficient numbers to make the host ill. It is because of this process that individuals usually do not become ill with many viral diseases more than once even though they are exposed many times to the same causative organisms. Without the process of memory, individuals would remain susceptible to specific diseases every time they were exposed and no sustained immunity would be generated.

GENERAL ANTIBODY CLASSIFICATION

All antibodies are referred to as *immunoglobulins* and *gamma globulins*. These names are based on the structure, location, and function of antibodies. A globulin is a type of secondary protein structure that is "globular," or folds in on itself rather than remaining as a linear three-dimensional structure. Most proteins with a globular secondary structure are insoluble in water-containing fluids. Since antibodies are composed of this type of protein they are globulins. Antibodies deserve the name immunoglobulin because they are globular proteins that assist in immune function. Antibodies are called gamma globulins because when all the proteins in blood plasma are separated out through the process of electrophoresis, different groups of proteins separate out at different times, depending on how they move in response to the electrical charge. The different protein groups are named as they emerge from the process. The first group to emerge (Fig. 3–6) are the plasma albumins, which make up a rather large group. Three smaller groups emerge at specific times after the albumins. The fourth group or protein fraction (gamma fraction) contains all five different types of antibody proteins. For this reason antibodies are called gamma globulins.

Antibodies serve many functions. These functions are optimized by different antibody types or "classes." The five different antibody classifications are determined by differences in antibody structure, molecular weight, and patterns of molecular association. The following narrative describes the composition, concentration, and function of the five different antibody types.

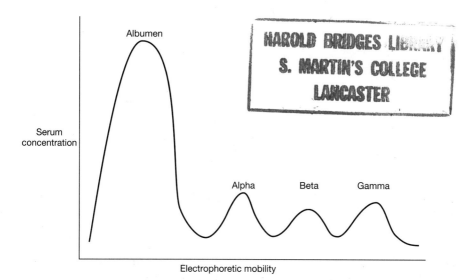

FIGURE 3-6. Electrophoretic separation of serum proteins (immunoglobulins present in gamma fraction).

Immunoglobulin A (IgA)

Immunoglobulin A is also known as the "secretory" immunoglobulin. Although this antibody is made by B lymphocytes found in the intestinal wall, most of the IgA synthesized moves from the blood into other body fluids and secretions such as tears, urine, saliva, milk, and mucus of the respiratory, genitourinary, and gastrointestinal tracts. Because most IgA molecules do not remain in the blood, serum levels of IgA are relatively low, with IgA comprising less than 15 per cent of the serum immunoglobulin pool (Goodman, 1987). The individual molecule of IgA is small (molecular weight, about 155,000); however, in secretory fluids this molecule preferentially associates with itself to form a unit called a dimer or a functional pair (Fig. 3-7).

The purpose of IgA is to participate in actions on the outer body surfaces to prevent antigens (foreign invaders) from entering the actual internal environment. IgA accomplishes this purpose primarily by inhibiting bacteria and viruses (through some unknown mechanism) from adhering to the surfaces of skin and mucous membranes. This inability of foreign invaders to adhere to skin and mucous membranes makes penetration and entry into the body's internal environment more difficult.

Immunoglobulin G (IgG)

Immunoglobulin G is the most abundant type of antibody found in the blood and other extracellular fluids. Usually, IgG accounts for more than 75 per cent

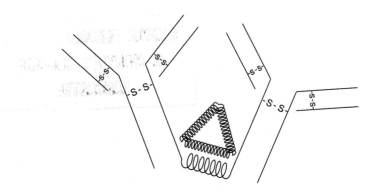

FIGURE 3-7. Schematic representation of IgA dimer.

of all the gamma globulins produced in the blood at any one time. This concentration increases during and immediately following exposure to specific antigens. The IgG molecule is relatively small (molecular weight, about 160,000) and exists in the blood as individual molecules called *monomers*. Because of its size and the fact that it does not tend to self-associate, IgG is the only antibody that freely crosses the placenta in appreciable amounts so that maternal IgG can accumulate in the fetus. Placental transfer of IgG is responsible for natural passive immunity in newborns. Within the IgG class of antibodies, there are at least four major subclasses of IgG. These subclasses vary somewhat from each other in both structure and function.

IgG functions to neutralize toxins and to assist in the destruction or elimination of microorganisms. The binding of IgG to a microorganism allows the microorganism to be more easily phagocytized by neutrophils and macrophages. In addition, the binding of IgG to antigens stimulates the activation of the complement system. Because IgG is the most abundant type of antibody and it has diversified actions, IgG is primarily responsible for providing the most extensive part of acquired natural and acquired artificial sustained immunity.

Immunoglobulin M (IgM)

Although the basic structure of IgM molecules is the same as for IgA and IgG, the individual components of the structure are larger, making IgM a relatively large antibody molecule (molecular weight, approximately 180,000). In addition, IgM preferentially associates with itself in groups of five, forming a unit of five molecules called a *pentamer* (Fig. 3-8). Because of its size and association, IgM is sometimes called a *macroglobulin*. This antibody comprises approximately 10 per cent of the total serum concentration of immunoglobu-

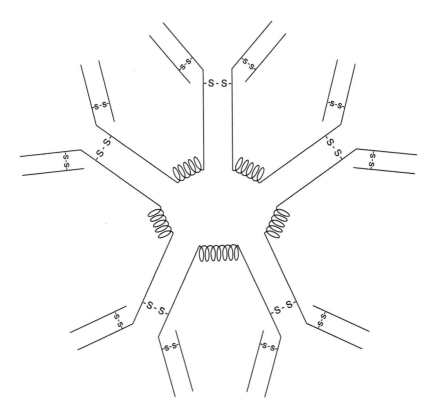

FIGURE 3-8. Pentameric IgM molecule.

lins. Under certain conditions (autoimmune responses) IgM can be found in significant amounts in other extracellular body fluids.

IgM responds to the presence of bacteria in the blood and is especially efficient at the antibody actions of agglutination and precipitation. In addition, the binding of IgM to an antigen stimulates the activation of the complement system. Blood and extracellular fluid levels of IgM are seen to increase significantly during autoimmune responses. In fact, elevation of IgM frequently is a diagnostic indicator for the presence of specific autoimmune diseases such as insulin-dependent diabetes mellitus and rheumatoid arthritis (Theofilopoulos, 1987). IgM is thought to be involved in the initiation of autoimmune responses, although the mechanisms and relationships of IgM to autoimmunity are not clear.

Immunoglobulin E (IgE)

Individual molecules of IgE are relatively large (molecular weight, approximately 180,000), but this antibody class usually is present in blood and body fluids in very low concentrations (less than 1 per cent). The actual serum concentration of IgE varies from individual to individual, and this concentration is determined genetically. The IgE molecule tends to bind to the surface of basophils and mast cells and is responsible for the manifestations of most immediate hypersensitivity reactions. The binding of IgE to antigen results in degranulation of the basophilic and mast-cell membranes. This membrane degranulation allows large amounts of histamine, kinins, serotonin, and other vasoactive amines to be released from basophils and mast cells. These vasoactive amines stimulate an inflammatory response wherever they contact tissues and blood vessels. These responses are responsible for most of the uncomfortable (and sometimes life-threatening) symptoms experienced during allergic reactions.

The actual purpose of IgE is unclear, although this antibody is immunologically very useful during parasitic infestations. Some immunologists suggest that IgE may have had a more important function for humans during the earlier evolutionary periods and now this antibody only has limited beneficial value.

Immunoglobulin D (IgD)

Characterization of the relatively large IgD antibody (molecular weight, approximately 180,000) is not complete. This antibody is found in plasma (but not in serum) in very low concentrations, usually far less than 1 per cent. IgD is rather fragile, and a number of naturally occurring proteolytic enzymes can destroy its antigen-binding activity. The specific function of IgD is not clear. Because IgD frequently is found on the surface of B lymphocytes, usually in close proximity to molecules of IgM, it is thought that perhaps IgD in some way modifies the activity of IgM. Since information regarding the function and features of IgD is limited, this antibody is sometimes called the "mystery" protein.

ACQUIRING ANTIBODY-MEDIATED IMMUNITY

Acquired immunity is the immunity that every individual's body normally makes (or can receive) as an adaptive response to invasion by foreign proteins. Antibody-mediated immunity is one type of acquired immunity. Acquired immunity occurs either naturally or artificially and is either active or passive.

Active Immunity

Active immunity occurs when antigens actually enter the body and the body responds by making specific antibodies against those antigens. This type of immunity is considered to be "active" because the body takes an active part in making the antibodies. Active immunity can occur under conditions that are either natural or artificial.

Natural Active Immunity

Natural active immunity occurs when an antigen enters the body, without human assistance, and the body actively makes antibodies against that antigen (for example, chickenpox virus). Depending on the number of viruses that invade the body and current status of the immune system, usually the first invasion of the body by this chickenpox virus results in the manifestation of signs and symptoms of the disease. However, processes occurring in the body at the same time allow it to learn to make antichickenpox antibodies, thus acquiring immunity to the chickenpox virus antigen. This immune response to invasion by a specific antigen is called the "first" or "primary" response. Upon subsequent exposures to the same antigen the sensitized B lymphocytes and their progeny will rapidly increase the production of antichickenpox antibodies so that enough are present to clear all the viruses and prevent the manifestation of symptoms of the disease. This increased response on reexposure to the same antigen is called the "secondary" or "anamnestic" response. This response increases with each reexposure in the immunocompetent individual. Natural active immunity provides the most complete and long-lasting protection against illness upon reexposure to the same antigen.

Artificial Active Immunity

Artificial active immunity is the type of protection developed against diseases that have the potential for such serious side effects that death or permanent debilitation are more likely to occur before immunity is acquired. For these diseases (such as smallpox, tetanus, and diphtheria) total avoidance of the disease is most desirable. In addition, some diseases (such as measles, mumps, and rubella), while not usually lethal, have the potential for generating serious complications. In these situations, immunity can be acquired by having specific antigens deliberately placed in your body in small numbers so that your body can respond by actively making antibodies against the antigen. Small amounts of antigens that have been specially processed to make them less likely to proliferate within the body are used for this procedure so that this deliberate yet artificial exposure does not in itself cause you to manifest symptoms of the disease. Standard vaccinations against tetanus, diphtheria, measles, smallpox, mumps, rubella, and a wide variety of other diseases are examples of agents used to induce artificially acquired active immunity. Artificial active acquired immunity lasts many years but may require repeated smaller doses of the original antigen as a "booster" to maintain complete protection against the antigen. Toxoids and vaccines are used for stimulating or inducing artificially acquired active immunity.

TOXOIDS. These are substances (toxins) that the infecting organism produces, rather than the infecting organisms themselves. The toxins are first rendered harmless through laboratory denaturation (by heating or exposure to formaldehyde) and are converted into toxoids. These products carry the same universal product code that the infecting organism has so that antibodies generated against the toxoid will be able to bind to and exert specific actions against the infecting organism as well.

KILLED VACCINES. Killed vaccines are composed of the actual virus or organism that causes the disease; however, the organism has been killed so that it is not capable of proliferating once it is injected into the body. Apparently, killing the organism before injecting it sometimes alters the universal product code so that the antibodies generated in response to the presence of the killed organism may not be completely effective against the live, infecting organism.

ATTENUATED VACCINES. Attenuated vaccines are made with live viruses and bacteria that have undergone laboratory manipulation to decrease their abilities to grow in humans.

Passive Immunity

Passive immunity occurs when antibodies against a specific antigen are in the body but the body did not actively participate in the generation of this antibody. Instead, these antibodies are generated in the body of another person or animal and then put into your body. Because these antibodies are "foreign" to you, your body recognizes them as foreign and takes steps to eliminate them relatively quickly. For this reason, passive immunity can provide only immediate, very-short-term protection against a specific antigen.

Natural Passive Immunity

Natural passive immunity occurs when antibodies are passed from mother to fetus through the placenta or to the infant through colostrum and breast milk. These antibodies usually have been cleared from the infant's system within 3 to 6 months.

Artificial Passive Immunity

Artificial passive immunity involves deliberately injecting one person with antibodies produced in another person or animal. Usually, this type of immunity is used in situations in which a person is exposed to a serious disease or illness for which he or she has little or no known actively acquired immunity. The injected antibodies are expected to do the work of inactivating the antigen. This type of immunity provides only temporary protection and has a duration of only days to a few weeks. Another situation in which artificial passive immunity can be used is when the individual is unable to produce sufficient quantities of any antibodies. These conditions include hypogammaglobulinemia and agammaglobulinemia. In order for these individuals to have antibody protection to a variety of pathogenic agents, intravenous infusions of immune globulin (IVIG) pooled from the plasma of at least 1000 different people are used.

IVIG, antitoxins and antivenins, and human hyperimmune sera are used to provide artificially acquired passive immunity.

IVIG. These antibodies are obtained from the serum of a pool of at least 1000 different individuals. IVIG is available as a commercial preparation from a variety of drug companies.

ANTITOXINS AND ANTIVENINS. These agents are antibodies directed against a specific antigen. Usually they are derived from the serum of an animal injected first with a specific toxoid followed by subsequent injections with the specific toxin.

SPECIFIC HUMAN HYPERIMMUNE SERA. These antibodies are obtained from the serum of other humans who have been exposed to a specific antigen and are producing the antibody directed against the specific antigen. Two common specific hyperimmune sera commercially available are HyperTet (antitetanus antibodies) and HypeRab (antirabies antibodies).

NONSPECIFIC HUMAN HYPERIMMUNE SERA. These antibodies are similar to IVIG in that they are obtained from the serum from a large pool of individuals. No one antibody type is guaranteed to be present, but because the pool is large, chances are good that the dose contains some of almost all types of antibodies.

SUMMARY

Antibody-mediated immunity, or the antigen–antibody reaction, is a powerful and important mechanism to provide long-lasting protection against the side effects of invading foreign proteins. However, the effectiveness of this type of immunity is profoundly influenced by a variety of developmental, health, and immune-system–related factors. The degree of effectiveness or activity of the other two components of immunity—inflammation and cell-mediated immunity—profoundly affect antibody-mediated immune function, since B lymphocytes require assistance from other leukocytes for B-lymphocyte proliferation and activation, recognition of self versus nonself, antigen processing, and antibody-dependent cytotoxic actions.

In addition, nonimmune associated factors also influence the general function and effectiveness of antibody-mediated immunity. Major factors include metabolic rate, oxygenation, general nutrition, and protein balance. Active B lymphocytes are metabolically active and require energy-generating substrates such as oxygen, glucose, and adenosine triphosphate. Proteins are needed for synthesis of immunoglobulins and for synthesis of the multitude of enzymes necessary to catalyze immune biochemical reactions.

SELECTED BIBLIOGRAPHY

Abernathy, E. (1987). How the immune system works. *American Journal of Nursing, 87*(4), 456.
Barrett, J. (1988). *Textbook of immunology* (5th ed.). St. Louis: C.V. Mosby.

Colten, H. (1985). Complement biosynthesis. *Clinics in Immunology and Allergy, 5*(2), 287.

Dawson, M. (1988). Specific immunology: 1. *Nursing Times, 84*(18), 73.

Dawson, M. (1988). Specific immunology: 2. *Nursing Times, 84*(19), 69.

Gallucci, B. (1987). The immune system and cancer. *Oncology Nursing Forum, 14*(6, Suppl.), 3.

Goodman, J. (1987). Immunoglobulins I: Structure and function. In D. Stites, J. Stobo, & J. Wells (Eds.), *Basic and clinical immunology* (6th ed.) (p. 27). Norwalk, CT: Appleton & Lange.

Guyton, A. (1991). *Textbook of medical physiology* (8th ed.). Philadelphia: W.B. Saunders.

Ott, M., Senner, A., Esker, S., Knapp, R., & Bolinger, A. (1990). IVIG: Clinical application in pediatric care. *Journal of Pediatric Nursing, 5*(5), 307.

Roitt, I. (1991). *Essential immunology* (7th ed.). Boston: Blackwell Scientific.

Stites, D., Stobo, J., & Wells, J. (1987). *Basic and clinical immunology* (6th ed.). Norwalk, CT: Appleton & Lange.

Taylor, D. (1984). Immune response: Physiology, signs and symptoms. *Nursing 84, 14*(5), 52.

Theofilopoulos, A. (1987). Autoimmunity. In D. Stites, J. Stobo, & J. Wells (Eds.), *Basic and clinical immunology* (6th ed.) (p. 128). Norwalk, CT: Appleton & Lange.

Tizard, I. (1984). *Immunology: An introduction.* Philadelphia: Saunders College Publishing.

Vogler, L., & Lawton, A. (1985). Ontogeny of B cells and humoral immune functions. *Clinics in Immunology and Allergy, 5*(2), 235.

4

CELL-MEDIATED IMMUNITY

Cell-mediated immunity or cellular immunity (CMI) involves a variety of leukocyte actions, reactions, and interactions that range from the simple to the complex. This type of immunity is provided by leukocytes that recognize nonself cells and respond to them either by exerting direct immunologic activities or by inducing the cytotoxic activities of other cells. Some responses and characteristics of CMI are unique to this division of immunity, whereas other responses and characteristics are similar to those expressed in antibody-mediated immunity and inflammation. In addition, certain CMI responses influence and regulate the activities of antibody-mediated immunity and inflammation. Therefore, optimal function of CMI is needed for total immunocompetence. Alterations in CMI function profoundly affect the function of antibody-mediated immunity and inflammation.

CYTOKINES

The inducing and regulatory aspects of cell-mediated immunity are controlled primarily through the selected production and activity of special substances called *cytokines*. Cytokines are low-molecular-weight protein hormones synthesized by the various leukocytes. Cytokines synthesized by the mononuclear phagocytes (macrophages, netrophils, eosinophils, and monocytes) are termed *monokines*, whereas the cytokines produced by T lymphocytes are termed *lymphokines*.

Cytokine activity is similar to the action of any other kind of peptide hormone in that one cell produces and secretes a cytokine that then exerts its effects on other cells of the immune system (Guyton, 1991). The cells responding to the cytokine may be right next to the cytokine-secreting cell or quite remote from the cytokine-secreting cell. The cells that change their activity in response to the presence of a cytokine are known as "responder" cells. In order for a responder cell to be able to react to the presence of a cytokine, the membrane of the responder cell must have a specific receptor to which the cytokine can bind in order to initiate changes in the responder cell's activity.

The purpose of cytokines is to induce or regulate (or both) a wide variety of inflammatory and immune responses. Most cytokines are produced as they are needed and are not stored to any great extent. The actions of some cytokines are *pleiotrophic*, in that the effects are widespread within the immune system, setting into motion a variety of immunomodulating actions. Other cytokines have very specific actions limited to one type of cell. Table 4–1 summarizes the origins and activities of the currently known cytokines.

CELLULAR COMPONENTS

The leukocytes that appear to have the most important roles in cell-mediated immunity include several specific T-lymphocyte subsets along with a special population of cells known as natural killer (NK) cells. T lymphocytes originate from the pluripotent stem cells in the bone marrow. As described in Chapter 1, the pluripotent stem cell is an immature cell that has the potential to mature into any one type of differentiated blood cell depending on which maturational pathway the cell enters. Selection of a specific maturational pathway appears to be determined in part by the presence of specific cytokines that can induce the pluripotent stem cell to commit itself to eventual specific differentiation. Commitment of the pluripotent stem cell to lymphocyte differentiation is thought to be induced by a cytokine known as lymphopoietic factor. Once commitment to a specific maturational pathway has been induced, it is irreversible. The committed lymphocyte stem cell is no longer pluripotent; its maturation potential now is limited to lymphocyte differentiation. The committed lymphocyte stem cells are released from the bone marrow into the blood, where they migrate into a variety of lymphoid tissues. The committed lymphocyte stem cells that migrate into the thymus gland or pericortical areas (or both) of lymph nodes differentiate into T lymphocytes (Fig. 4–1). The committed lymphocyte stem cells that migrate to other lymphoid tissues mature into B lymphocytes (see Chapter 3).

Although B and T lymphocytes have a common origin, their functional characteristics are quite different. Moreover, T lymphocytes further differentiate into a variety of subsets that each have different functions.

One way of identifying different T-lymphocyte subsets is by determining the presence or absence of certain "marker proteins" (antigens) on the cell-membrane surface. Fifty different T-lymphocyte cell-membrane proteins have been identified, and 11 of these (T1 through T11) are commonly used in clinical situations to identify various immune system components. Monoclonal antibodies have been made for each of these 11 proteins. Specific T-lymphocyte

TABLE 4–1. Summary of Cytokine Activity.

Cytokine	Cellular Origin	Inducing Event	Cytokine Action
Interleukin-1 (IL-1)	Macrophage	Contact with gram-negative bacterial products Contact with CD4 cell Presence of TNF	Stimulates increased production of prostaglandins Induces fever Increases proliferation of CD4 cells Stimulates growth and differentiation of B lymphocytes Induces further secretion of IL-1 and IL-6
Interleukin-2 (IL-2)	T helper cells (CD4+) CD8+ T cells	T-cell activation by antigens	Increases the growth and differentiation of T lymphocytes Stimulates increased production of IL-2 from activated lymphocytes
Interleukin-3 (multilineage colony-stimulating factor, IL-3)	T helper cells (CD4+)	Infection or invasion	Stimulates production of immature bone marrow stem cells (pluripotent)
Interleukin-4 (B-cell stimulatory factor, IL-4)	T helper cells (CD4+) Activated mast cells	Presence of anti-Ig antibody	Stimulates growth and proliferation of B lymphocytes Stimulates increased production of IgE Induces further secretion of IL-4, IL-5, and IL-6 Acts as a macrophage-activating factor
Interleukin-5 (B-cell growth factor, IL-5)	T helper cells (CD4+) Activated mast cells	Helminth infections	Stimulates growth and differentiation of eosinophils Stimulates mature B lymphocytes to increase the synthesis of immunoglobulins (especially IgA)

Table continued on following page.

TABLE 4–1. Summary of Cytokine Activity (Continued).

Cytokine	Cellular Origin	Inducing Event	Cytokine Action
Interleukin-6 (IL-6)	Macrophage Vascular endothelial cells Fibroblasts Activated T cells	Infection or inflammation Presence of IL-1 and TNF	Stimulates hepatocytes to make fibrinogen, macroglobulin, and C protein Stimulates the growth of activated B lymphocytes Serves as a cofactor in stimulating production of bone marrow hematopoietic stem cells
Interleukin-7 (IL-7)	Bone marrow stromal cells	Presence of antigen	Stimulates growth and differentiation of committed B-lymphocyte stem cells
Interleukin-8 (monocyte chemotactic factor, IL-8)	Activated T cells, macrophage endothelial cells, platelets, fibroblasts, and epithelial cells	Infection or inflammation Presence of TNF or IL-1	Chemotactic factor for neutrophils, basophils, and eosinophils Neutrophil activation
Tumor necrosis factor (TNF)	LPS-activated macrophage Antigen-stimulated T cells Activated natural killer cells Activated mast cells	Gram-negative bacterial infection	Increases leukocyte adhesion to endothelial cells Induces fever Stimulates fibroblasts and endothelial cells to secrete colony-stimulating factors Enhances cytolysis of virally infected cells Induces coagulation Stimulates macrophages to secrete IL-1 and IL-6 Stimulates metabolic changes that result in cachexia

Factor	Source	Stimulus	Actions
Granulocyte–macrophage colony-stimulating factor (GM-CSF)	Activated T cells Macrophages Vascular endothelial cells Fibroblasts	Infection or inflammation	Increases growth and differentiation of committed myeloid stem cells Minor activator of macrophages
Monocyte–macrophage colony-stimulating factor (M-CSF)	Macrophages Vascular endothelial cells Fibroblasts	Infection or inflammation	Enhances proliferation and maturation of the committed progenitor cells for monocytes–macrophages (CFU-M)
Granulocyte colony-stimulating factor (G-CSF)	Macrophages Vascular endothelial cells Fibroblasts	Infection or inflammation	Enhances neutrophil maturation and release from bone marrow
Interferon (INF) (α, β, γ)	Macrophages (INF-α) Fibroblasts (INF-β) T-helper cells (INF-γ) CD8 + cells (INF-γ) Natural killer cells	Viral infection	Limits viral infection by: inhibiting viral replication increasing NK-mediated lysis increasing cytolytic T lymphocyte recognition of virally infected cells Activates macrophages (INF-γ) Promotes differentiation of T and B lymphocytes (INF-γ) Activates neutrophils (INF-γ) Activates NK cells (INF-γ)

TNF = tumor necrosis factor; Ig = immunoglobulin; LPS = lipopolysaccharide; CFU-M = colony-forming unit–monocyte–macrophage; NK = natural killer.

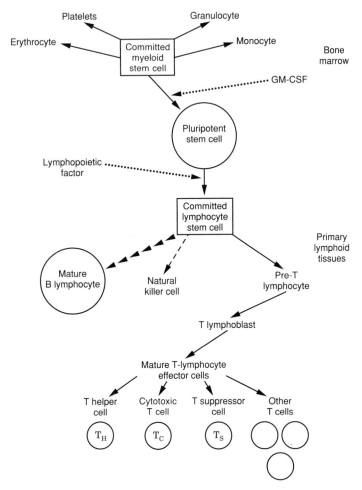

FIGURE 4-1. Maturation pathway of T lymphocytes. GM-CSF = granulocyte–macrophage colony-stimulating factor.

subsets are identified by their varying reactions to exposure to the different monoclonal antibodies. Most T-lymphocyte subsets have more than one antigen on their cell membranes. For example, all mature T lymphocytes contain T1, T3, T10, and T11 proteins. Specific subsets of T lymphocytes have other specific T-lymphocyte membrane antigens.

The nomenclature used to identify specific T-lymphocyte subsets includes the specific antigen present on the T-lymphocyte membrane as well as the overall functional activities of the cells in a subset. The three T-lymphocyte subsets that are critically important for the development and continuation of cell-mediated immunity are helper/inducer T cells, cytotoxic/cytolytic T cells, and suppressor T cells.

RECOGNITION OF ANTIGEN BY T LYMPHOCYTES

In order for T lymphocytes to initiate immunologic actions in response to the presence of antigens, a period of antigen processing must first occur. Without antigen processing, T lymphocytes are unable to recognize antigens and cannot mount an immunologic defense.

Antigen processing for T-lymphocyte recognition must be accomplished through the actions of cells that share major histocompatibility complex (MHC) proteins in common with the T lymphocytes (see Chapter 1). The cell type most responsible for antigen processing is the macrophage, although other leukocytes and some other nucleated body cells can also participate in this activity (Grey, Sette, & Buus, 1989; Abbas, Lichtman, & Pober, 1991). Cells that process antigens for T-lymphocyte recognition are termed *antigen-processing cells* (APCs).

Essentially, the APC comes into contact with a foreign protein or body cell expressing a previously unknown antigen on its surface. The APC determines that the protein or antigen is nonself and engulfs the antigen or the cell containing the antigen. Enzymes in the cytoplasm, endosomes, or both of the APC partially degrade ("process") the antigen. The processed antigen is moved from the interior of the APC to its membrane at the site where the MHC proteins are located. X-ray analysis of processed antigens indicates that the processed antigens are placed within the MHC proteins on the APC's surface, forming an antigen–MHC complex.

After the antigen is processed and attached to the APC's MHC proteins, the APC presents the antigen–MHC complex to the T lymphocyte. Each T lymphocyte within an individual's body has a membrane receptor for cells containing that individual's MHC proteins. It appears that T lymphocytes are restricted to binding to and being activated by processed antigens present in the antigen–MHC complex formed by the APC. In addition, the T lymphocyte can recognize the antigen–MHC complex only if at least some of the proteins within the MHC are identical to the T lymphocyte's MHC proteins. Therefore, T-lymphocyte recognition of antigen is MHC-restricted in that the T lymphocyte and the processing/presenting cell must share some identical MHC cell-surface proteins. Cytotoxic/cytolytic T lymphocytes are restricted to recognizing antigens processed and presented by cells sharing the same Class I MHC proteins. T helper/inducer lymphocytes are restricted to recognizing antigens processed and presented by cells sharing the same Class II MHC proteins. All nucleated body cells have Class I MHC proteins on their membranes. Class II MHC proteins are present on lymphocytes, tissue macrophages, and dendritic cells.

MECHANISMS OF ACTION

Helper/Inducer T Cells

The cell membranes of helper/inducer T cells contain the T4 protein and most commonly these cells are called *T4 cells* or T_H *cells*. An additional newer name for helper/inducer T cells is CD4 (short for cluster of differentiation 4). Several different companies have made monoclonal antibody to the T4 cell membrane protein. These monoclonal antibodies include OKT4 and Leu-3, thus the helper/inducer T cells may also be referred to as the cells that are OKT4-positive or Leu-3-positive.

Helper/inducer T cells are very efficient at the recognition of self versus nonself after antigen processing. Although helper/inducer T cells contain cytoplasmic lysosomes and presumably can act as phagocytes, the use of phagocytosis against nonself cells is not an important function of helper/inducer T cells (Abbas, Lichtman, & Pober, 1991). Rather, helper/inducer T cells indirectly participate in cell-mediated immunity by stimulating the activity of many other leukocytes. In response to the recognition of nonself (antigen), helper/inducer T cells secrete lymphokines that are able to induce and regulate the activity of other leukocytes (see Table 4–1).

Generally, the lymphokines secreted by the helper/inducer T lymphocytes have overall stimulatory effects on immune function. These lymphokines increase bone marrow production of stem cells and enhance the maturation of myeloid- and lymphoid-origin cells. More specific lymphokines enhance the activity of one type of leukocyte. Some of these lymphokines have "autokine" activity in that the presence of the specific lymphokine stimulates the cell secreting the lymphokine to increase the secretion of that same lymphokine. In effect, the helper/inducer T lymphocyte acts as an organizer in calling to arms the various squads of leukocytes involved in inflammatory, antibody, and cellular defensive actions to destroy, eliminate, or neutralize antigens.

Cytotoxic/Cytolytic T Cells

These special T lymphocytes also are called T_C *cells* and *CTL cells*. They may be a subset of suppressor cells, as they are positive for the presence of CD8 protein on their membrane surfaces. Cytotoxic/cytolytic T cells function in cell-mediated immunity by lysing or destroying cells that contain a processed antigen–MHC complex. This activity is most effective against host cells infected by parasitic organisms such as viruses or protozoa.

Parasite-infected host cells express some parasitic proteins on the cell-membrane surface, serving as antigens to the host's immune system cells. In addition, because these infected cells are host cells, their universal product codes or Class I MHC proteins are identical to those of the host's leukocytes. Thus, when the cytotoxic/cytolytic T lymphocyte is exposed to the processed antigen–MHC complex on the surface of a parasite-infected host cell, the cytotoxic/cytolytic T lymphocyte can bind to the MHC portion of the complex through the T lymphocyte's Class I MHC protein receptor and can modify the receptor so that it will also bind specifically to the processed antigen in the antigen–MHC complex. Modification of the receptor so that it will bind specifically to the antigen in the antigen–MHC complex requires prior exposure to the same processed antigen. This specificity appears to be irreversible for the cytotoxic/cytolytic T lymphocyte.

The binding of the cytotoxic/cytolytic T lymphocyte to the infected cell's antigen–MHC complex stimulates activities that result in the death of the infected cell. The close contact of the cytotoxic/cytolytic T lymphocyte with the infected cell as a result of binding allows enzymes and protein toxins to be released from the T lymphocyte and to bore a hole or pore in the membrane of the infected cell. This pore allows a "lethal hit" of proteolytic enzymes from the cytotoxic/cytolytic T lymphocyte to enter the infected cell, causing osmotic lysis and destruction (Abbas, Lichtman, & Pober, 1991). Once the lethal hit has been administered to the bound infected cell, the cytotoxic/cytolytic T lymphocyte releases the dying infected cell and can go on to attack and destroy other infected cells that carry the same antigen–MHC complex.

Suppressor T Cells

The cell membranes of suppressor T lymphocytes contain the T8 lymphocyte antigen, and these cells are commonly called *T8 cells, T_8 cells,* or *CD8 cells.* Suppressor T cells participate in the regulation of cell-mediated immunity. The primary function of these cells is to prevent the occurrence of continuous overreactions in response to exposure to nonself cells or antigens. This function may be especially important in preventing the formation of auto-antibodies directed against normal, healthy self cells, the basis for many autoimmune diseases.

The suppressive or immune inhibitory action of suppressor T lymphocytes appears to have two different mechanisms (Abbas, Lichtman, & Pober, 1991). The first mechanism is suppressor T-lymphocyte production of cytokines that inhibit the proliferation and activity of other leukocytes. This inhibition may be mediated through competitive inhibition at cytokine receptor sites. If inhibitory cytokines resemble the enhancing cytokines closely enough, then inhibitory cytokines can occupy the receptor sites and prevent enhancing cytokines from binding to the receptor, thus inhibiting the enhancing cytokines from exerting their enhancing activities on responsive immune system cells.

A second proposed mechanism of suppression indicates that suppressor T lymphocytes may actually absorb (and possibly degrade) the growth- and differentiation-promoting lymphokines secreted by the helper/inducer T lymphocytes.

In general, suppressor T cells directly oppose the activity of helper T cells. Therefore, optimal function of cell-mediated immunity requires that a balance between helper-T-cell activity and suppressor-T-cell activity be maintained. Usually this balance is provided when the helper T cells outnumber the suppressor T cells by a ratio of 2 to 1. When this ratio increases, overreactions can be expected to occur (some of these overreactions are tissue-damaging as well as unpleasant). When the helper-to-suppressor ratio decreases, immune function is suppressed profoundly and the individual is much more vulnerable to invasion and infections of all types.

Natural Killer Cells

This interesting leukocyte population is extremely important in providing cell-mediated immunity. The actual site of differentiation and maturation of natural killer (NK) cells is unknown and currently the subject of much controversy. Although this cell population has some T-lymphocyte characteristics, it is not considered to be a true T-lymphocyte subset (Abbas, Lichtman, & Pober, 1991).

The primary function of NK cells is the exertion of direct cytotoxic/cytolytic effects on target nonself cells. Unlike cytotoxic T cells, the NK cells are able to exert these cytotoxic effects without first undergoing a period of sensitization to nonself membrane antigens. In addition, NK cells do not need to share any of the major histocompatibility proteins with the nonself cell in order to initiate defensive actions against the nonself cell. The defensive actions of NK cells appear to be totally unrelated to either antigen sensitivity or the interactions of other leukocytes.

Natural killer cells appear to be most effective in destroying unhealthy or abnormal self cells. The nonself cells most susceptible to defensive actions of NK cells are the self cells infected by organisms that live within host cells (virally infected cells) and the self cells that have been mutated at the DNA level and are no longer totally normal, such as cancer cells.

Two mechanisms of action have been suggested to explain how NK cells destroy target nonself cells. Both mechanisms require that on recognition of a target nonself cell, the NK cell must bind directly and very tightly to the membrane of the target nonself cell. The first proposed mechanism of action suggests that after binding to the target cell, the NK cell extrudes a series of special lysosomal enzymes through its membrane directly into the target cell (Fig. 4–2). At this point the NK cell releases the target nonself cell. The enzymes placed inside the nonself cell then literally digest critical components of the

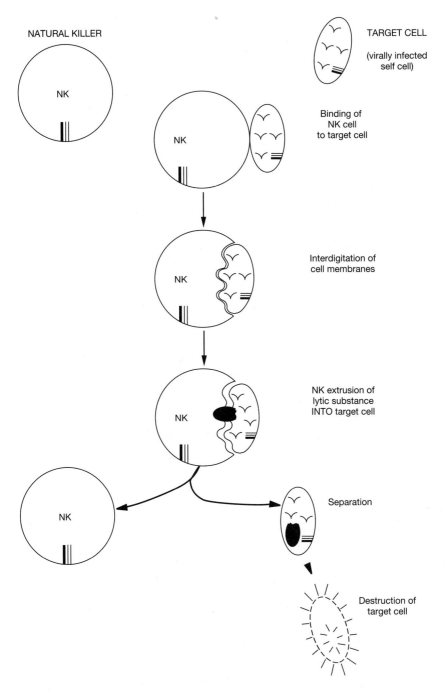

FIGURE 4–2. Proposed mechanism of natural killer (NK) cell action.

nonself cell, forcing it to self-destruct quickly. The NK cell is not harmed by this activity and is capable of more seek-and-destroy missions on other targeted nonself cells. A second postulated mechanism of action for the NK cell is through the secretion of a special substance called natural killer cytotoxic factor (NKCF). This factor seems to be specifically attracted to the same target nonself cells that NK cells recognize and attack. NKCF itself appears to be directly cytotoxic to target cells, and it also appears to enhance the cytotoxic/cytolytic effects of NK cells. Experimental evidence supports both postulated mechanisms of action, and it is possible that NK cells use both mechanisms simultaneously to destroy and eliminate nonself cells.

PROTECTION PROVIDED

Specific components of CMI assist in providing protection by their highly developed abilities to distinguish self from nonself. The nonself cells most easily recognized by CMI are the self cells infected by organisms that live within host cells and the self cells that have been mutated at the DNA level and are no longer normal. CMI provides a surveillance system for ridding the body of self cells that could potentially harm the body. Through these mechanisms CMI is critically important in the prevention of cancer development and metastasis after exposure to carcinogenic agents.

Another action of NK cells and cytotoxic T cells is the destruction of cells from other individuals or animals. While this action is generally helpful, it also is responsible for rejection of grafts and transplanted organs. Therefore, CMI must be suppressed deliberately in individuals who receive grafts or organ transplants in order to prevent the destruction of these lifesaving transplanted tissues.

SUMMARY

Cell-mediated immunity regulates and works with antibody-mediated immunity and the inflammatory response to provide full immunity or immunocompetence. Although some of the CMI characteristics resemble a combination of the characteristics of both inflammation and antibody-mediated immunity, most of the CMI functions are unique to this division of immunity. The actions of CMI are different in two ways from the nonspecific responses that comprise the inflammatory responses. First, phagocytosis, the critical feature of inflammation, is not a function of T lymphocytes but (mediated through macrophages) is an important step for cell-mediated antigen recognition. Second, some of the T lymphocytes involved in CMI reactions require sensitization to the nonself cells before being able to exert cytotoxic effects. This process is specific and is an adaptive response rather than a general nonspecific response.

Because certain cells and aspects of CMI actually regulate the activity of the other two divisions of immunity, whenever cell-mediated immunity is less than optimal, the functions of inflammation and antibody-mediated immunity also will be less than optimal.

SELECTED BIBLIOGRAPHY

Abbas, A., Lichtman, A., & Pober, J. (1991). *Cellular and molecular immunology.* Philadelphia: W.B. Saunders.

Balkwill, F., & Burke, F. (1989). The cytokine network. *Immunology Today, 10,* 299.

Gallucci, B. (1987). The immune system and cancer. *Oncology Nursing Forum, 14*(6, Suppl.), 3.

Grady, C. (1988). Host defense mechanisms: An overview. *Seminars in Oncology Nursing, 4*(2), 86.

Grey, H., Sette, A., & Buus, S. (1989). How T cells see antigen. *Scientific American, 261*(5), 56.

Guyton, A. (1991). *Textbook of medical physiology* (8th ed.). Philadelphia: W.B. Saunders.

Henkart, P. (1986). Mechanisms of NK-cell mediated cytotoxicity. In R. Herberman (Ed.), *Cancer immunology: Innovative approaches to therapy* (p. 123). Boston: Martinus Nijhoff.

Herberman, R., & Holdon, H. (1978). Natural cell mediated immunity. *Advances in Cancer Research, 27,* 305.

Nicola, N. (1989). Hematopoietic cell growth factors and their receptors. *Annual Review of Biochemistry, 58,* 45.

North, R. (1985). Down-regulation of the antitumor response. *Advances in Cancer Research, 45,* 1.

Oppenheim, J., Ruscetti, F., & Faltynek, C. (1987). Interleukins and interferons. In D. Stites, J. Stobo, & J. Wells (Eds.), *Basic and clinical immunology* (6th ed.) (p. 82). Norwalk, CT: Appleton & Lange.

Roitt, I. (1991). *Essential immunology* (7th ed.). London: Blackwell Scientific.

Roitt, I., Brostoff, J., & Male, D. (1989). *Immunology* (2nd ed.). St. Louis: C.V. Mosby.

Rosenberg, S. (1990). Adoptive immunotherapy for cancer. *Scientific American, 262*(5), 62.

Smith, K. (1990). Interleukin-2. *Scientific American, 262*(3), 50.

Stobo, J. (1987). Lymphocytes. In D. Stites, J. Stobo, & J. Wells (Eds.), *Basic and clinical immunology* (6th ed.) (p. 65). Norwalk, CT: Appleton & Lange.

Stutman, O. (1985). Ontogeny of T cells. *Clinics in Immunology and Allergy, 5*(2), 191.

Tami, J., Parr, M., & Thompson, J. (1986). The immune system. *American Journal of Hospital Pharmacy, 43,* 2483.

Tizard, I. (1984). *Immunology: An introduction.* Philadelphia: Saunders College Publishing.

Van Snick, J. (1990). Interleukin-6: An overview. *Annual Review of Immunology, 8,* 253.

UNIT II

CONDITIONS CAUSING IMMUNOSUPPRESSION

Syndromes of Immunodeficiency

5

PRIMARY IMMUNODEFICIENCY SYNDROMES

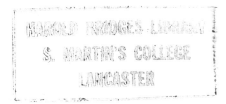
Syndromes of immunodeficiency are usually considered primary when they are caused by a congenital problem present at birth. Some of these conditions are heritable, usually as a recessive trait. Other primary immunodeficiency syndromes have no identified inheritance pattern and are considered immune system malformations. Even though the pathologic condition may be present at birth, the associated signs and symptoms may not be apparent until some time after birth.

The more severe immunodeficiency syndromes are relatively rare, whereas the more mild syndromes are relatively common. Some of the more mild immunodeficiencies may be present in adults who have remained nonsymptomatic or in whom the symptoms are so very minor in nature that the actual disorder is never diagnosed. Primary immunodeficiencies are categorized on the basis of which immune functions are impaired.

B-LYMPHOCYTE DISORDERS

The primary syndromes of immunodeficiency that have B-lymphocyte disorders as their pathologic basis are more common than syndromes that have T-lymphocyte disorders as their pathologic basis. Although the syndromes associated with B-lymphocyte disorders vary considerably in the degree to which immunosuppression is present, all B-lymphocyte disorders have more mild signs and symptoms and a better prognosis for longevity than do T-lymphocyte disorders.

Bruton's Agammaglobulinemia

This disorder was first described in 1952 by Bruton. Individuals with Bruton's agammaglobulinemia have no circulating B-lymphocyte plasma cells and no antibodies. All classes of antibodies are absent. Because these individuals do have pre-B lymphocytes in their bone marrow, it is assumed that the pathologic defect for this disorder lies in the ability of the individual to mature the pre-B lymphocytes into functional B-lymphocyte plasma cells. In addition, these individuals do not have active lymphoid tissue in the normal sites of B-lymphocyte maturation, including germinal centers of lymph nodes, tonsils, or white pulp of the spleen. The inflammatory response and cell-mediated immunity are not impaired in these individuals.

Etiology

Bruton's agammaglobulinemia is an X-linked recessive disorder. Usually only males are affected through inheritance of an abnormal X chromosome from their mothers. Thus, females are carriers but do not manifest any signs or symptoms of this disorder. Because affected males are now living into adulthood as a result of improved medical management of the condition, it is theoretically possible for an affected male who marries a female carrier to transmit this disorder to female offspring.

Clinical Manifestations

Children with Bruton's agammaglobulinemia appear normal at birth and are not generally any more susceptible to infection than are other children during the first 4 to 5 months of life. This is because at birth the infant has a large load of maternal antibodies (almost exclusively IgG) circulating in the plasma and other extracellular fluids as a result of placental transfer during pregnancy. The infant's circulating levels of these maternal antibodies gradually decline over the first 4 to 6 months after birth. As the levels of maternal antibodies decline, the infant is not able to synthesize his or her own antibodies and becomes increasingly susceptible to infection, especially bacterial infections. The most common infections among these infants include dermatitis, conjunctivitis, otitis media, pharyngitis, bronchitis, and pneumonia. Common causative organisms are Staphylococcus and Haemophilus.

The typical pattern of recurring bacterial infections usually begins between 6 and 8 months of age. The infections become progressively more severe and have a "continuous" pattern, in that with antibiotic treatment the infection improves but never completely clears. The infant fails to grow at an appropriate rate and may begin to lose weight. In addition, continuous skin irritations and infections are present.

Diagnosis

Diagnosis is made on the basis of clinical presentation along with laboratory indicators of impaired immune function. Specifically, these indicators are a total lack of circulating antibodies (determined by either immunoelectrophoresis or specific quantitation of serum immunoglobulins) and the failure of the infant to produce antibodies in response to administration of a killed vaccine.

Treatment

Treatment regimens for Bruton's agammaglobulinemia are aimed at (1) prevention of infection and (2) prevention of complications. Typical maintenance treatment includes continuous prophylaxis with maintenance doses of a broad-spectrum antibiotic in conjunction with regularly scheduled infusions of intravenous immunoglobulins (see Chapter 3). When the individual is known to be exposed to a specific disease, prophylaxis can include treatment with hyperimmune gamma globulin specific for that disease. Acute bacterial infections are managed with appropriate antibiotics.

Although fungal and viral infections generally do not appear to be exceptionally problematic for the individual with agammaglobulinemia (inflammation and cell-mediated immunity eliminate most of these organisms), vaccination with live-virus vaccines can cause life-threatening complications. Therefore, individuals with Bruton's agammaglobulinemia should never be immunized with live-virus vaccines.

Prognosis

Many individuals diagnosed with Bruton's agammaglobulinemia survive into early adulthood. With intravenous immunoglobulin (IVIG) therapy more readily available, it is expected that survival time will increase. The major complication increasing morbidity and mortality among individuals who do not succumb to acute bacterial infections is chronic lung disease secondary to persistent pulmonary infections with resultant fibrosis and scarring (Ammann, 1987). Early intervention for all pulmonary infections is critically important for these individuals.

Although individuals with Bruton's agammaglobulinemia are immunosuppressed with regard to antibody-mediated immunity, autoimmune disease develops in approximately 20 per cent of those who survive to adulthood (Cotran, Kumar, & Robbins, 1989). The most common disorders are systemic lupus erythematosus, hemolytic anemia, and rheumatoid arthritis. The etiology and pathologic mechanism(s) for the associated development of autoimmune disease are not known.

Common Variable Immune Deficiency

This immunodeficiency closely resembles Bruton's agammaglobulinemia in that affected individuals produce little or no antibodies and are considered to have hypogammaglobulinemia. However, the disorder has no specific pattern of inheritance and males and females are affected equally. There appear to be two types of common variable immune deficiency. One type is clearly congenital, with symptoms manifesting during infancy. A second type is less clear, with individuals not expressing symptoms of the disorder until late adolescence or early adulthood. It is not known whether this type is a separate and acquired disorder or if it is a late onset of the congenital disorder.

Etiology

Although the clinical picture of common variable immune deficiency is extremely similar to Bruton's agammaglobulinemia, the basic defect is quite different. Individuals with common variable immune deficiency usually have hypogammaglobulinemia or agammaglobulinemia even though the number of circulating B lymphocytes is normal. In addition, their secondary lymphoid tissues associated with B-lymphocyte maturation show hyperplasia (white pulp of the spleen, tonsils, germinal centers of lymph nodes). The circulating B lymphocytes are unable to complete terminal differentiation into antibody-producing plasma cells even though they are capable of recognizing antigen (Cotran, Kumar & Robbins, 1989).

Clinical Manifestations

The clinical manifestations associated with common variable immune deficiency are very similar to those of Bruton's agammaglobulinemia. Manifestations in the form of recurrent bacterial infections begin to appear after 6 months of age. For the later-onset type of disorder, the recurrent bacterial infections begin in late childhood or early adulthood (Abbas, Lichtman, & Pober, 1991). These individuals frequently have problems with infestation by the intestinal parasite *Giardia lamblia*. This infestation causes profound chronic diarrhea and malabsorption, resulting in growth impairment and electrolyte disturbances.

Diagnosis

The diagnostic indicators for this disorder are the clinical presentation in conjunction with extremely low or absent plasma immunoglobulins. The differentiating characteristic of common variable immune deficiency from Bruton's agammaglobulinemia is the presence of normal circulating levels of B lymphocytes.

Treatment

Current treatment regimens for common variable immune deficiency are identical to those for Bruton's agammaglobulinemia. Treatment is started as soon as a positive diagnosis is made.

Prognosis

Although the risk of succumbing to overwhelming infection at any age is always present, many individuals with common variable immune deficiency live into the sixth or seventh decade (Ammann, 1987). Affected individuals have a relatively high risk for autoimmune diseases developing, especially hemolytic anemia and rheumatoid arthritis (Cotran, Kumar, & Robbins, 1989). Recurrent pulmonary infections resulting in pulmonary scarring and fibrosis limit functional capacity and lead to early death.

IgA Deficiency

Primary IgA deficiency is a familial disorder in which the affected individual has neither circulating nor secretory levels of IgA. In most individuals, production of all other antibodies is normal, although a small percentage of affected individuals do experience a concurrent decrease in the production of IgG.

Etiology

IgA deficiency is the most common of the primary immune deficiency syndromes, occurring in 1 of every 600 individuals. Although most people with IgA deficiency have this disorder from birth, some acquire it later in life. The two factors associated with acquiring IgA deficiency are infections and complications of drug therapy. IgA deficiency has been known to occur as an aftermath of measles infection and toxoplasmosis infection (Cotran, Kumar, & Robbins, 1989). Long-term use of phenytoin, other anticonvulsants, and penicillamine have resulted in acquired IgA deficiency in some people. Discontinuing the drug therapy results in a return to normal IgA production.

Individuals with IgA deficiency have normal numbers of circulating B lymphocytes and B-lymphocyte plasma cells, including B lymphocytes with surface IgA. This finding, consistent among most individuals with the disorder, suggests that the primary defect for this immune deficiency is either decreased synthesis of IgA or an inability of the plasma cell to release the IgA it synthesizes (Ammann, 1987).

Clinical Manifestations

The signs and symptoms of IgA deficiency revolve around chronic infections of organ systems or tracts leading from the external environment to the internal environment through a mucous membrane pathway. Patients most commonly present with recurrent or chronic sinopulmonary infections, urinary tract infections, or genitourinary tract infections. Many of the affected individuals also have significant respiratory allergies. Autoimmune disorders of systemic lupus erythematosus and rheumatoid arthritis are not uncommon among individuals with primary IgA deficiency.

Diagnosis

Definitive diagnosis of IgA deficiency is not always possible in young children. A tentative diagnosis is made based on deficiency to absence of plasma and secretory IgA along with indications of normal cellular immune function. In addition, approximately 40 per cent of all individuals with this disorder have circulating antibodies against IgA (Ammann, 1987).

Treatment

The main mode of treatment for this disorder is "watchful waiting." When persistent or chronic infections become problematic, a regimen of antibiotic prophylaxis is instituted. Gamma globulin administration is not recommended for these individuals for two reasons. First, the exogenous gamma globulin would contain only a relatively small amount of IgA, mostly in monomeric form, and it does not appear that this monomeric IgA can become dimeric secretory IgA in individuals with IgA deficiency. A second reason for not administering exogenous gamma globulin is that IgA-deficient individuals do produce normal amounts of all other classes of antibodies; thus, they are at relatively high risk for the development of severe allergic reactions to the exogenous gamma globulin.

Prognosis

Many individuals with primary IgA deficiency survive into their seventh or eighth decade. The most common complication of this disorder that has a negative impact on longevity is the development of pulmonary scarring and fibrosis as a result of chronic pulmonary inflammation and infection. Prevention of pulmonary infection and avoidance of occupations or habits that increase the exposure to inhalational irritants should be a major teaching focus for these individuals.

T-LYMPHOCYTE DISORDERS

DiGeorge's Syndrome

Individuals with DiGeorge's syndrome have a deficiency in cell-mediated immunity, although their inflammatory responses and antibody-mediated immunity appear unimpaired. In this respect, DiGeorge's syndrome closely resembles another condition, Nezelof's syndrome, in which the affected individual does not have a thymus gland. However, the problems associated with DiGeorge's syndrome extend far beyond impaired immune function.

Etiology

DiGeorge's syndrome is actually a birth defect resulting from incomplete embryonic development of the third and fourth pharyngeal pouches (Cotran, Kumar, & Robbins, 1989). Affected individuals have an absent or very rudimentary thymus gland and no parathyroid glands. Cardiac malformations are frequently present in these individuals, as are a variety of other structural anomalies. This syndrome does not have a specific pattern of inheritance and appears to be the result of a random mutational event. No single, specific, causative agent has been implicated in this developmental disruption.

Clinical Manifestations

Children with DiGeorge's syndrome are usually diagnosed shortly after birth because of the structural and functional birth defects. Tetany frequently develops within 24 to 48 hours after birth as a result of hypocalcemia secondary to the absence of parathyroid glands. These children have no defenses against fungal and viral infection and oral candidiasis may develop before they are 1 month old. Secondary lymphoid tissues dependent on thymic hormones for development are absent or very underdeveloped, especially the lymph nodes. It is interesting to note that among the individuals with DiGeorge's syndrome, those who have any functioning thymic tissue have completely normal antibody-mediated immunity. This finding indicates that although thymic function is essential for complete B-lymphocyte activity, even small levels of thymic function are sufficient for this purpose.

Diagnosis

The primary diagnostic indicators for DiGeorge's syndrome are immunologic and radiographic. Chest x-ray is negative for the thymic shadow. The child has a total lack of circulating T lymphocytes and normal or near-normal circulating levels of plasma cells and antibodies. Differentiation of DiGeorge's syndrome from Nezelof's syndrome is made by the presence of other birth defects, specifically, the cardiac anomalies and the lack of functional parathyroid glands.

Treatment

Symptomatic treatment for DiGeorge's syndrome includes therapy to correct the hypocalcemia. Oral calcium supplement with vitamin D can help control the hypocalcemia. In some instances, exogenous parathyroid hormone is administered. Fungal and viral infections are treated as they occur with appropriate antibiologic agents. Corrective treatment for the immune function problems associated with DiGeorge's syndrome has included fetal thymus transplant. Although this is not currently a common surgery, when it is successful this type of transplantation has resulted in what appears to be permanent remission of immune function impairment.

Prognosis

Without successful transplantation of thymic tissue, individuals with DiGeorge's syndrome have a life expectancy of less than 5 years. Thymus transplantation dramatically improves immune function and is presumed to improve longevity.

T AND B LYMPHOCYTE DISORDERS

Wiskott–Aldrich Syndrome

Individuals diagnosed with Wiskott–Aldrich syndrome are thrombocytopenic and experience a progressive loss of cell-mediated immunity as evidenced by a lack of circulating lymphocytes. Children initially have a normal thymus with normal levels of all lymphocytes, although their platelet counts are abnormal from birth. As the circulating lymphocytes gradually become depleted, the child begins expressing signs and symptoms of immune deficiency.

Etiology

This disorder has an X-linked recessive pattern of inheritance and affects only males. The molecular error responsible for the disorder has not yet been identified.

Clinical Manifestations

The typical pattern of clinical manifestations begins in the neonatal period with petechiae and other indications of impaired clotting ability. As the lymphocytes become depleted, the child experiences recurrent infections and an associated persistent eczema.

Diagnosis

A diagnosis of Wiskott–Aldrich syndrome is tentatively made in the early neonatal period because of the obvious thrombocytopenia. Although most individuals demonstrate low levels of circulating lymphocytes and bone marrow hypoplasia in infancy, some individuals maintain nearly normal lymphocyte levels for many years (Cotran, Kumar, & Robbins, 1989). This variability in expression of immune system impairment suggests multiple mechanisms of pathogenesis.

Treatment

Symptomatic treatment for Wiskott–Aldrich syndrome includes antibiotic prophylaxis together with platelet infusions and intravenous immunoglobulin therapy. The only curative treatment is allogeneic bone marrow transplantation.

Prognosis

Without transplantation, most individuals with Wiskott–Aldrich syndrome die within the first 5 years of life. Bone marrow transplantation for this disorder has been most successful when donor marrow is T-cell depleted and haploidentical to the recipient. The best donors are parents and siblings. Because bone marrow transplantation as therapy for this disorder is relatively new, its ultimate impact on long-term survival is not known.

Severe Combined Immune Deficiency Syndrome

Severe combined immune deficiency syndrome (SCIDS) is a type of inherited disorder resulting in generalized impairment of immunity and inflammation. Individuals with this disorder produce no antibodies and do not have functional circulating lymphocytes. They are at extreme risk for the development of life-threatening infections.

Etiology

This rare inherited disorder appears to have two different patterns of inheritance, suggesting that multiple separate genes control immune function. One type is X-linked recessive and another has an autosomal recessive pattern of inheritance (Cotran, Kumar, & Robbins, 1989; Stiehm, 1989). One basic mechanism for this disorder is thought to be a deficiency of one or more of the class of enzymes called "recombinase enzymes" (Roitt, 1991). Another mechanism is a deficiency of adenosine deaminase (ADA) that converts deoxyadenosine triphosphate into inosine and the useful high-energy compound adenosine triphosphate (ATP). Without sufficient amounts of this enzyme, intracellular levels of deoxy-ATP build up and this substance is highly toxic to lymphocytes. Some forms of SCIDS do not fit these patterns and their basic etiologies have yet to be elucidated.

Clinical Manifestations

Recurrent, severe infections plague these individuals right from the neonatal period. Common causative organisms include Pseudomonas, Candida, Pneumocystis, Cytomegalovirus, and Herpes simplex virus. Some neonates even experience graft-versus-host disease (GVHD) in the early neonatal period as a result of placental transfer of maternal T lymphocytes (see Chapter 12).

Diagnosis

Diagnosis is made on the basis of presenting clinical manifestations. In addition, these individuals do not have circulating levels of their own antibodies (only maternal antibodies) and no hypersensitivities. T cells, when present, show no response to test antigens on second exposure.

Treatment

Symptomatic treatment for this disorder is not very effective, and sepsis is common. Thymus transplantation has improved immune function for these individuals, although it does not result in a total cure. Successful allogeneic bone marrow transplantation has resulted in good immune function. A new experimental approach for cure using the genetic engineering technique of inserting a fully functional version of the defective or missing gene into the affected individual's own bone marrow stem cells has had some success but is still in the very early stages of development.

Prognosis

The prognosis for individuals with SCIDS is very poor without aggressive therapy. Most children die before reaching their first birthday. One child lived 12 years in a plastic bubble, which maintained a sterile environment, before acquiring a lethal infection. Current data show that some individuals with SCIDS have survived 10 years after a successful bone marrow transplant (Ammann, 1987). Gene therapy, with the insertion of the missing gene, shows promise as a cure for this disorder (Kantoff, Freeman, & Anderson, 1988; Verma, 1990).

CASE PRESENTATION

Danny is a 12-month-old white male admitted to the hospital with a diagnosis of failure to thrive and a history of recurrent infections. He is the first child of a 30-year-old accountant father and a 27-year-old mother who teaches language arts at the junior high level. The pregnancy was uncomplicated, and Danny was born by normal vaginal delivery after a 9-hour labor. He weighed 8 lb 3 oz at birth and was 21 in. long. He was breast-fed for 6 months, starting on solid foods at 5 months and on infant formula at 6 months. At 6 months, Danny's growth rate was normal, and he had reached all developmental milestones slightly ahead of the expected average.

At 6 months Danny was placed in day care when his mother returned to work. During the first week in day care, Danny developed a cold with conjunctivitis and otitis media. He was started on oral antibiotic therapy and the infections appeared to clear. During the next 3 months Danny had seven episodes of otitis media and three bouts of diarrhea lasting over 48 hours each. Antibiotic agents were changed, as was the infant formula.

Over the next 3 months Danny had otitis media continuously when he was not on the antibiotics. He continued to have intermittent diarrhea with a generalized skin eruption, although the lesions were worse in the diaper area. The skin eruption was diagnosed as a staphylococcal infection. At 11 months he was hospitalized with pneumonia; he responded to intravenous antibiotic therapy and came home.

On admission, Danny weighs 15 lb (his weight at 6 months) and is 27 in. long. He is on a maintenance dose of oral Augmentin. Developmentally, Danny does not stand alone. He can crawl, but his mother states that he seems more content to sit in an infant seat or lie in his crib. She states that he seems less bright and happy than at an earlier age. He eats well when fed, but he makes no attempt to feed himself. His mother asks if there is any chance the antibiotics are retarding his development or if her working away from home has caused Danny's health problems.

Danny's blood work shows a total white-cell count of 15,000/cu mm. The differential cell count is segs, 60 per cent (9000); band forms, 25 per cent (3750); lymphocytes, 10 per cent (1500); monocytes, 3 per cent (450); eosinophils, <1 per cent; and basophils <1 per cent. Electrophoresis of Danny's serum proteins indicates a complete absence of all gamma globulins. This finding is significant in view of the fact that Danny had received DPT (diphtheria–pertussis–tetanus) immunizations at 2, 4, and 6 months (normal infants should have circulating antibodies to these organisms after three immunizations). In addition, Danny's peripheral-blood lymphocytes react only to T-cell antibodies, indicating a total lack of circulating B lymphocytes.

Danny is diagnosed as having Bruton's agammaglobulinemia and is started on IVIG therapy. His condition rapidly improves on the prescribed regimen. Danny's parents are referred to a genetics counsellor because of the known inheritance pattern associated with this disorder. Please refer to the care plan in Chapter 15 for suggested interventions appropriate for the nursing care of immunocompromised patients.

SELECTED BIBLIOGRAPHY

Abbas, A., Lichtman, A., & Pober, J. (1991). *Cellular and molecular immunology.* Philadelphia: W.B. Saunders.

Ammann, A. (1987). Immunodeficiency diseases. In D. Stites, J. Stobo, & J. Wells (Eds.), *Basic and clinical immunology* (6th ed.) (p. 317). Norwalk, CT: Appleton & Lange.

Cotran, R., Kumar, V., & Robbins, S. (1989). *Robbins pathologic basis of disease* (4th ed.). Philadelphia: W.B. Saunders.

Kantoff, P., Freeman, S., & Anderson, W. (1988). Prospects for gene therapy for immunodeficiency diseases. *Annual Review of Immunology, 6,* 581.

McCance, K., & Huether, S. (1990). *Pathophysiology: The biologic basis for disease in adults and children.* St. Louis: C.V. Mosby.

Ott, M., Senner, A., Esther, S., Knapp, R., & Bolinger, A. (1990). IVIG clinical applications in pediatric care. *Journal of Pediatric Nursing, 5*(5), 307.

Rapaport, S. (1987). *Introduction to hematology* (2nd ed.). Philadelphia: J.B. Lippincott.

Roitt, I. (1991). *Essential immunology* (7th ed.). Boston: Blackwell Scientific.

Roitt, I., Brostoff, J., & Male, D. (1989). *Immunology* (2nd ed.). St. Louis: C.V. Mosby.

Stiehm, E. (1989). *Immunologic disorders in infants and children* (3rd ed.). Philadelphia: W.B. Saunders.

Verma, I. (1990). Gene therapy. *Scientific American, 263*(5), 68.

Vickers, P. (1990). SCID syndrome. *Nursing, 4*(23), 32.

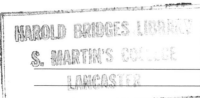
6

ACQUIRED IMMUNODEFICIENCY SYNDROME

Acquired immunodeficiency syndrome (AIDS) is a pathologic condition resulting from chronic infection with the human immunodeficiency virus (HIV). Because this virus selectively infects specific immune system cells (in addition to other body cells), the infection results in a progressive and profound general immunosuppression. At present, treatment of the infection does not result in cure, and the disease is considered to be uniformly fatal. The primary causes of death among patients with AIDS are related to failure of the immune system to recognize nonself cells and to mount an effective defense against them.

AIDS was first defined as a specific disease entity in 1981. By 1990 more than 100,000 people in the United States had contracted it. Over 50 per cent of the patients diagnosed with AIDS had already died, including 75 per cent of those who were diagnosed before 1986.

The incidence of AIDS in the United States and the rest of the world is increasing at an alarming rate. The Centers for Disease Control predict the number of patients diagnosed with AIDS in the United States to increase to 500,000 by 1994. Because of the rapidly increasing incidence, the excessive mortality rate, and the fact that this disease entity is relatively new, with a brief known natural history, this chapter includes in-depth discussion of etiology, modes of transmission, course of the disease, and pathophysiology.

ETIOLOGY

The causative agent for AIDS is the virus identified as the human immunodeficiency virus (HIV). This same virus is also known by other names, including human T-cell lymphotrophic virus type III (HTLV-III), lymphadenopathy virus (LAV), and the AIDS virus (Melbye, 1986). This virus belongs to a special class of viruses known as *retroviruses*. While retroviruses have many characteristics in common with "ordinary" viruses, they also have special characteristics that make them more efficient at the process of infection and they are difficult to stop replicating once infection has occurred. The following paragraphs provide explanations and comparisons between ordinary viruses and retroviruses.

Ordinary Viruses

Humans are subject to infection by thousands, perhaps millions, of ordinary viruses (nonretroviruses). Some of these ordinary viruses are pathogenic and cause specific illnesses and diseases. Other viruses appear to live in peaceful coexistence with their human host and cause few if any overt manifestations of their presence. Most nonretroviruses share similar characteristics for anatomy, infection, and modes of transmission.

Anatomy

All viruses are very small living "creatures" that act as cellular parasites. Viruses are so small that they cannot be seen with standard microscopic techniques. Viruses do resemble (to a limited extent) other single-cell organisms, in that viral genetic material is either DNA or RNA and in order to reproduce the virus must duplicate some or all of this material. However, viruses are unable to reproduce by themselves. Instead, viruses must enter (infect) other living cells and use the energy and resources of the infected cell to make new viruses and viral particles. Some viruses can infect only bacterial cells, other viruses can infect only plant cells, and still other viruses can infect only animal cells. Of the viruses capable of infecting human cells, not all viruses are equally efficient at carrying out the infection process.

Infection

Viruses infect human cells only after they have gained entry into the body. In order for true infection to occur, either the whole virus or a special part of the virus, which contains the genetic material (virion), breaks through the membrane of a human cell. Once inside the human cell the virus or virion must enter the area of the human cell where the DNA is located, the nucleus. The action of some viruses in the nucleus is to break a strand of the cell's DNA and "splice" all or part of the viral genetic material into the human cellular DNA (see Fig. 6–1). When this action is successfully carried out, every time the human cell replicates or makes RNA from the DNA in the area where the viral genetic material is located, the human cell will make new viral particles (and sometimes even whole viruses) (Bishop, 1985).

After many rounds of replication, in which hundreds to thousands of new

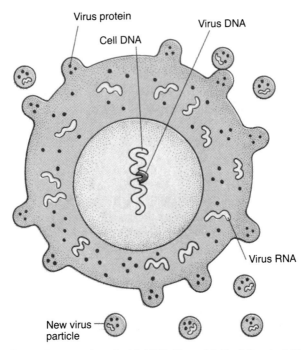

Virus protein

Virus DNA

Cell DNA

Virus RNA

New virus particle

FIGURE 6–1. A T lymphocyte infected with HIV. (From *Medical-Surgical Nursing: A Nursing Process Approach* [p. 632, Fig. 27-1] by D. Ignatavicius and M. Bayne, 1991, Philadelphia: W.B. Saunders.)

viruses or viral particles are produced, these viruses/viral particles leave the human cell in one of three ways:

1. Budding off the cell
2. Lysing the cell
3. Moving through the cell membrane

Once the viruses or viral particles have left the cell and are in the host's body fluids, they can infect other cells and continue the viral replication process.

The DNA "splicing" process appears to be a random event for most viruses and it is not always successful, for a variety of reasons, including incomplete inclusion of genetic material, DNA inactivation, and improper positioning. The actual splicing may be incomplete, leaving out critical components of viral genetic material. The actual splicing or incorporation may inactivate the normal cellular DNA or disrupt the reading sequence. Splicing may occur in an area of the DNA that is either repressed or normally not active. In addition, even when the splicing in process occurs correctly and viral DNA is incorporated into human cellular DNA, the cell may recognize the viral genetic material as foreign or at least incorrect and not be able to read it properly for replication or RNA synthesis.

Mode of Transmission

Viruses vary in their abilities to transmit infection from one person to another and to survive outside the host body. Most viruses are sensitive to temperature changes and do not survive when environmental temperatures are significantly below normal body temperature. The chance of infection increases in direct proportion to the amount of contact an uninfected individual has with the cells or body fluids from an infected individual.

Many viruses remain alive in nasal secretions, on skin surfaces, and in the feces of the infected individual as well as in the blood, blood cells, and tissues that contain blood or blood cells. With viruses that are present (alive and virile) in all these body fluids, transmission followed by infection can occur with relatively casual or slight direct contact with the infected individual. For some viruses, the ability of the virus to enter a cell and then successfully splice into that cell's DNA is so low that virtually millions of viruses must enter the body before the person has any symptoms of infection. Also important in this process is how well the individual's immune system is functioning and whether or not the individual has previously acquired an immunity to the specific virus. Transmission of infection with these viruses is most efficient if contact with live virus or body cells and tissues infected with the live virus is direct, prolonged, or frequent.

Retroviruses

Retroviruses make up only a very small percentage of all the known types of viruses. Retroviruses differ from "ordinary" viruses in their functional anatomy, genetic makeup, and efficiency of infection. The majority of the identified retroviruses have the additional special ability to cause cancer in some animals and, possibly, in humans (Varmus, 1985).

Anatomy

Retroviruses have only RNA as their genetic material. Frequently, this RNA has at least one gene sequence more than does the genetic material of ordinary viruses. The most important difference between retroviruses and nonretroviruses is the presence of a special complex of enzymes within the retrovirus. This special complex of enzymes is called *reverse transcriptase.* The purpose of this enzyme complex is to increase the efficiency of viral replication once the retrovirus enters a host cell (Haseltine & Wong-Staal, 1988; Varmus, 1985).

Retroviruses, including HIV, are not particularly more virile or stronger than nonretroviruses. The retroviruses appear to be at least as susceptible to temperature changes and other changes in the chemical and ionic environments as are nonretroviruses. Outside the body, retroviruses can be destroyed as easily as nonretroviruses.

Infection

Once retroviruses gain entry into the body and infect host cells, the reverse transcriptase enzyme complex greatly enhances the efficiency of successful infection and viral replication. When both reverse transcriptase and viral RNA are in the host's cell, the reverse transcriptase forces the host's DNA synthesis machinery to use the viral RNA as a template or pattern and to synthesize a new piece of human DNA exactly complementary to the viral RNA. This new human DNA is incorporated successfully into the host's cellular DNA, where it can remain for a long time. In some cells, the new DNA is dormant or inactive for months to years. When this new DNA is actively transcribed or replicated the result is the synthesis of huge numbers of viral particles. These viral particles appear to leave the infected cell by the same mechanisms that nonretroviral particles leave infected cells.

Unlike nonretroviruses, the incorporation of this new DNA into the host's cellular DNA is a relatively efficient process. Because the new piece of DNA is human rather than viral, although it carries the codes for viral proteins, the new DNA is more likely to be correctly incorporated into the cellular DNA without damaging the normal reading sequence or activity. In addition, because the new DNA is technically human, it does not arouse some host defenses.

Modes of Transmission

In order for AIDS actually to develop, the HIV retrovirus must gain access to the blood in large enough numbers to infect specific immune system cells. Many body fluids and secretions from patients with AIDS do contain HIV. These fluids include blood, breast milk, mucus, perspiration, saliva, semen, stool, tears, and urine. However, only blood, semen, and breast milk appear to contain the active HIV in large enough quantities to transmit the virus to another individual and infect that individual's cells.

Successful transmission of HIV is dependent on the virus penetrating into the internal environment and entering the blood or extracellular fluid of the uninfected individual. Casual contact cannot result in transmission to the blood or extracellular fluid. The modes of transmission for HIV to cause AIDS are sexual, perinatal, and blood.

1. Sexual transmission—This mode of transmission is currently the most common cause of HIV infection. Transmission is not necessarily successful with every sexual encounter. This mode is most successful when the sexual contact involves the exchange or contact of semen or blood from an infected person to the blood of an uninfected individual. Rate of transmission varies with the type of sexual encounter and the sex of the partners. The rate of

transmission is always enhanced when the integrity of the mucous membranes of the uninfected individual is disrupted.

   a. Sexual encounters involving seminal fluid from an infected male coming into contact with mucous membranes of an uninfected male have a high rate of transmission.

   b. Transmission rate is relatively high for sexual encounters involving seminal fluid from an infected male coming into contact with mucous membranes of an uninfected female.

   c. Transmission rate is relatively low for sexual encounters involving an infected female and an uninfected male.

2. Perinatal transmission—This type of HIV transmission occurs from mother to child during pregnancy and at or near the time of birth. Perinatal transmission includes transplacental processes, direct processes, and indirect processes.

   a. Prenatal transmission—Because viruses are so small, they easily cross the placenta from the mother's blood into the fetus. Although the success of the transmission is dependent on the mother's blood levels of the active virus, transmission during the third trimester appears more likely to result in the eventual development of AIDS in the baby. This type of transmission is currently the most common cause of HIV infection among children.

   b. Transmission during birth—This mode of transmission is suspected as a potential route but has not yet been demonstrated as a primary cause of HIV infection among children. During vaginal delivery the infant comes into prolonged direct skin and mucous membrane contact with mother's blood in the vaginal tract. The opportunity exists at this time for virus in the mother's blood to enter the infant's internal environment.

   c. Postnatal transmission—This mode of transmission has been documented as a result of an infected mother's transmitting HIV to the infant through colostrum and breast milk. The amount of virus in breast milk is reported to be relatively low. However, even this low concentration can result in transmission because the frequency of exposure is very high.

3. Blood transmission—Because the blood and blood cells (leukocytes) of an infected individual contain the highest concentrations of HIV, contact with infected blood constitutes a very effective mode of transmission. However, many factors, such as the amount of blood, how much contact, and how many viruses (antigens) are present in the infected blood all influence the infection process. Blood transmission can occur through direct and indirect contact (Henderson, Saah, Zak, et al., 1986; Hierholzer, 1987; Marcus, 1988).

   a. Direct blood contact—This mode of transmission requires that the blood of the HIV-infected person come into direct contact with the blood of an uninfected person. The most effective type of transmission occurs with transfusion of blood or blood products from infected individuals. In addition, transmission can occur when an uninfected person experiences subcutaneous (or deeper) exposure to sharp objects (e.g., needles) that contain the blood of infected individuals.

b. Indirect blood contact—This mode of transmission involves the blood of an infected person coming into direct contact with the skin or mucous membranes of an uninfected individual. While this mode can and has resulted in the transmission of HIV to uninfected individuals, the overall efficiency of indirect blood contact is low. The efficiency is greater when blood comes into contact with broken skin or mucous membranes. Transmission also has been reported when infected blood has come into prolonged contact with intact but highly vascular skin and mucous membranes.

PATHOPHYSIOLOGY

Upon penetration into the internal environment, HIV preferentially infects body cells that express a cell-surface protein (antigen) known as the CD4 molecule. The immune system cells that express the greatest concentration of the CD4 molecule are the T helper/inducer lymphocytes, although macrophages also express some levels of this protein (see Chapters 2 and 4). Additional cells known to be susceptible to infection by HIV include lymph node cells, cells of the thymus gland, bone marrow, glial cells of the brain, and chromaffin cells of the colon, duodenum, and rectum (Weber & Weiss, 1988). As a result, manifestations of HIV infection include symptoms of cerebral dysfunction and gastrointestinal irritation in addition to problems associated with major immune system failure.

Immune System Manifestations of HIV Infection

HIV-infected macrophages appear able to continue to perform their normal differentiated functions. Because mature macrophages have a relatively long lifespan and do not divide frequently, when HIV infects these cells the incorporated new viral-coded DNA can remain dormant for years. It is thought that the virally infected macrophages serve as reservoirs and sanctuaries for HIV. While incorporated into macrophage cellular DNA the viral genes are protected from detection and destruction by other immune system cells. As a result of protecting incorporated viral genes, macrophages appear to be responsible for the relatively long latency period between initial HIV infection and the manifestation of any immune function abnormalities or other symptoms of overt AIDS.

When HIV infects the T helper/inducer cells the virus is able to force the cell to assist in viral replication within a short time after infection. Eventually, enough virions are replicated to destroy the cell and escape into the blood, where infection of other cells can occur. The result is a diminishing population of T helper/inducer cells. When the number of T helper/inducer cells falls below a critical level (200/cu mm), cell-mediated immune function is profoundly altered. Because both inflammation and antibody-mediated immunity also are dependent on the activity of T helper cells, the functions of these two divisions of immunity become less effective. The following specific alterations in immune system function are frequently found among patients with AIDS.

Abnormal B-Lymphocyte Function (Antigen–Antibody Reaction)

With the presence of HIV in the blood and the T helper/inducer cell population severely depleted, sensitized B lymphocytes (plasma cells) are constantly stimulated to produce their preprogrammed antibodies. Thus, the total serum level of antibodies (gamma globulins) is high. However, these antibody levels represent relatively small quantities of many different specific antibodies. As a result no single specific antibody is present in high enough concentrations to be very beneficial. In addition, this system appears not to be able to generate new antibodies on exposure to new foreign invaders.

The clinical problems associated with this HIV-related immune system dysfunction vary with the stage of illness. When symptoms of HIV infection are first apparent the individual still has some antibody protection and immunity acquired from previous antigen exposure, such as chickenpox and rubella. Therefore, repeated exposure to these antigens does not result in overt expression of the illness. However, immune impairment at this point is such that the individual is not able to generate new antibodies in response to exposure to new antigens. Thus, repeated exposures to this same new antigen result in repeated bouts of the same illness.

With progression of the disease, the plasma cells become unable to generate sufficient quantities of specific antibodies to protect the patient even from infections to which he or she has previously acquired an immunity. The most outstanding example of this problem is the low antibody production to varicella–zoster, the virus responsible for chickenpox and shingles. Individuals who have had chickenpox always harbor the virus in the dorsal-root ganglia, where the virus is relatively safe from immune system cells. Some viruses leave this sanctuary periodically and are attacked and eliminated by the antichickenpox antibodies circulating in the patient's blood. When the serum levels of the antichickenpox antibodies are low, they may be insufficient to eliminate viruses escaping from the dorsal-root ganglia, and the patient develops shingles. If the serum levels of antichickenpox antibody and the number of chickenpox-sensitized plasma cells are very low, the individual has little if any acquired protection to the varicella virus and is highly susceptible to the development of chickenpox on exposure to the varicella virus. It is even possible for chickenpox and shingles to develop in this person at the same time.

Loss of the Ability to Differentiate Foreign Invaders from Self

Because the immune system cells that are most efficient at distinguishing self from nonself are either no longer present in normal amounts or are not as functionally efficient, the natural killer cells, neutrophils, and the phagocytes of the immune system are no longer able to seek and destroy the foreign invaders constantly present in our environment. Without this part of the immune system working properly to keep these invaders under control, the individual with AIDS is susceptible to all sorts of opportunistic infections and diseases. Many of these infections are caused by so-called normal flora, or microorganisms with which humans usually live in harmony and which are not considered pathogenic. However, without the continuous surveillance and protection by the natural killer cells, the neutrophils, and the macrophages, these normal flora overgrow in specific body areas and then gain access to other areas where they can proliferate and lead to serious infections and actual sepsis. Such organisms include candida, monilia, *Escherichia coli,* and *Pneumocystis carinii.*

Loss of the Ability to Differentiate Abnormal Self Cells from Normal Healthy Self Cells

Some of the cells involved in cell-mediated immunity have the capacity to attack and destroy self cells that have been identified as either altered in some way (such as cancer cells) or infected with a virus. These cells are the natural killer cells and the cytotoxic/cytolytic T cells. Because both of these cell types are highly dependent on the activity of T helper/inducer cells to remain functional, patients with AIDS have very diminished natural killer and cytotoxic/ cytolytic-T-cell functional activity. As a result, the cancer surveillance system is ineffective. Cells that have been transformed by some carcinogenic event are not recognized by the immune system as abnormal, and little if any attempt is made to eliminate the transformed cells. This situation allows any cells that have become malignant to gain a strong foothold without immune system interference. As a result, patients with AIDS are very prone to the development of specific malignancies (Donehower, 1987). Kaposi's sarcoma develops in many patients with AIDS. Although this disease is a low-grade malignancy, it is still a cancer and can cause severe impairment of respiratory function if the lesions are present on pulmonary epithelium. Other malignancies associated with AIDS include Hodgkin's lymphoma and non-Hodgkin's lymphoma.

Neural Manifestations of HIV Infection

Neurologic changes are associated with the development and progression of AIDS. In addition to the macrophages and T helper/inducer cells, HIV appears to have a special affinity to infect cells within the central nervous system (CNS). HIV in the blood crosses the blood–brain barrier and the blood–cerebrospinal fluid barrier. When HIV infects central nervous system cells, neural manifestations are present.

One of the first symptoms of HIV infection, present within 10 days to 3 weeks after exposure to HIV, is an acute febrile syndrome resembling other viral infections (Redfield & Burke, 1988). Patients present with intermittent general muscle aches, a rash, and low-grade fever. When neural infection accompanies the initial infection patients also have headaches, temperatures above 102°F, nuchal rigidity, and other symptoms of meningeal irritation. These symptoms usually subside within a few weeks but are clear indicators that HIV is present in the CNS.

Many drugs are unable to penetrate the blood–brain barrier, so even drugs that have some efficacy in controlling the replication of HIV do not reach the sanctuary of the CNS. As a result, HIV in the CNS proliferates and slowly damages or destroys cells within the CNS. The actual CNS target cells of HIV are currently unknown, but since the manifestations of damage are so insidious, it is thought that the probable targets include the macrophages of the CNS (microglia) and possibly the actual nondividing neuronal cells.

Infection of these cells results in the eventual development of encephalopathy usually confined to the subcortical brain areas. This HIV encephalopathy has a very slow onset and is also referred to as AIDS encephalopathy and AIDS dementia (McArthur & Palenicek, 1988). The problem is characterized by a progressive loss of cognitive, motor, and behavioral function. The early symptoms are mild, usually consisting of minor memory loss and a diminished capacity to concentrate. Some individuals experience depression at this early stage.

As the encephalopathy progresses alterations in motor function become apparent, and commonly include ataxia and spastic muscle weakness in the extremities, which may progress to paraplegia and hyperreflexia. The cognitive functions deteriorate, and memory loss includes recent and remote events. Speech patterns may be disrupted because of an inability to retrieve and articulate language. Behavioral manifestations range from depression to inappropriate behavior, organic psychosis, hallucinations, and coma.

Even though HIV infection may result in the associated CNS pathologies listed above, actual diagnosis of HIV encephalopathy is difficult and may be delayed, since many of the signs and symptoms are identical to other problems that result from systemic HIV infection and impaired immune function. Many of the behavioral alterations are attributed to psychogenic origin as a result of the diagnosis of AIDS. The cognitive and motor manifestations of HIV encephalopathy are similar to those associated with opportunistic CNS infections frequently accompanying AIDS.

Gastrointestinal Manifestations of HIV Infection

HIV has been found to infect directly specific cells within the gastrointestinal system. The result of this infection is a chronic irritation manifested by diarrhea and a malabsorption-like syndrome. These manifestations are associated with abdominal cramping and pain, along with multiple watery stools that can lead to dehydration and other imbalances of fluid and electrolytes. Treatment for this condition is aimed at ameliorating the symptoms and preventing complications.

Unfortunately, the pathophysiologic sequelae of HIV infection causing immunosuppression results in a greatly increased susceptibility to opportunistic infections. Many of the organisms responsible for opportunistic infections overgrow in the intestinal tract, causing diarrhea and abdominal discomfort. This problem makes difficult the distinction between HIV-induced and opportunistic-infection–induced gastrointestinal alteration in function. Because the latter can be successfully treated directly along with symptomatic management and support, the etiology of diarrhea in patients with HIV infection must be established.

DIAGNOSIS AND PROGRESSION

The diagnosis of AIDS is a complex process involving laboratory tests and the documentation of the presence or absence of various accompanying clinical manifestations and alterations of immune function. The Walter Reed classification system for AIDS has been used to establish the stage of progression and to determine the stability of the disease in a given patient. Table 6–1 presents and defines the Walter Reed classification system. In addition, the following paragraphs provide an explanation of current terminology.

HIV-Antibody-Positive

The presence of antibodies to HIV in the blood is an indication that the person has been exposed to HIV and has taken the virus into the blood long enough for B lymphocytes to become sensitized to it and make antibodies against it. Current tests used to determine whether an individual has HIV

TABLE 6–I. Walter Reed Classification System for AIDS.

Stage	HIV Antibody and/or Virus	Chronic Lymphad- enopathy	T Helper Cells/cu mm	Delayed Hyper- sensitivity	Thrush	Opportunistic Infections
WR0	–	–	>400	Normal	–	–
WR1	+	–	>400	Normal	–	–
WR2	+	+	>400	Normal	–	–
WR3	+	±	<400	Normal	–	–
WR4	+	±	<400	P	–	–
WR5	+	±	<400	C and/or thrush		–
WR6	+	±	<400	P/C	±	+

P = partial defect; C = complete failure to respond to skin test.
(Adapted from Illustration by Ian Worpole in HIV Infection: The Clinical Picture, by R. Redfield and D. Burke, October, 1988, *Scientific American, 259* (4), p. 93. Copyright ©1988 by Scientific American, Inc. All rights reserved.)

antibodies include the ELISA (enzyme-linked immunosorbent assay), the Western blot (examines whether or not antibodies have bound to HIV proteins separated by gel electrophoresis), and IFA (immunofluorescence assay). Usually individuals are tested first by ELISA. If the blood is positive by the ELISA method for detecting antibodies to HIV, it is then tested by Western blot. Western blot tends to yield fewer false positive results but is still not completely specific. In addition, individuals who are infected with HIV but whose B lymphocytes have not yet made anti-HIV antibodies in large quantities may have negative test results. The IFA is the most sensitive test and the one least likely to yield either false positive or false negative results. However, this test is not in widespread use because of the high cost and the fact that many third-party reimbursement agencies will not pay for this test.

HIV-antibody-positive means that at some point the individual has had HIV in the blood. It does not mean that HIV is still in the blood, neither does it mean that the individual will go on to have AIDS. The individual who is only HIV-antibody-positive does not express laboratory manifestations or clinical symptoms of AIDS. It is not known whether the individual who is only antibody-positive to HIV is able to transmit the infection to another individual.

HIV-Culture-Positive

An individual who is HIV-culture-positive is also HIV-antibody-positive. This individual has live HIV in the blood, where it has infected some cells and has stimulated some B lymphocytes to make anti-HIV antibodies. At this point the individual does not have any subtle or overt symptoms of AIDS and may be referred to as HIV-asymptomatic. Laboratory analysis of how well various components of the immune system are functioning does not show any functional impairment. However, because live virus is present in the blood, making the individual *antigenemic,* transmission of the infection to another person is possible at this time. Transmission appears to depend on

1. how antigenemic the infected individual is (how many live viruses are present in the body fluid to which the uninfected individual is exposed);
2. the susceptibility of the uninfected individual;
3. the route of exposure;
4. the degree of exposure.

At the current state of knowledge, it is not known if all individuals who are HIV-culture-positive will eventually have symptoms of AIDS. AIDS will definitely develop in some individuals, but how long this process takes appears to vary with the individual and subsequent exposure to a precipitating event(s). Events thought possibly to permit or enhance the expression of AIDS include coinfection with other viruses (such as cytomegalovirus or hepatitis), the presence of other health problems that impair immune function, or subsequent reinfection with HIV.

AIDS-Related Complex (HIV, Symptomatic)

Individuals diagnosed with AIDS-related complex (ARC) are defined as being HIV-culture-positive and having immune system abnormalities demonstrated on laboratory tests. Such individuals are also said to be "HIV symptomatic." The immune function abnormalities include a diminished ratio of T helper/inducer to T suppressor cells. Usually individuals with ARC express two or more physical symptoms of AIDS. Blood, semen, spinal fluid, and breast milk from these individuals definitely contain live HIV and are capable of transmitting the virus to another individual. Physical changes at this point usually include generalized lymph node enlargement.

AIDS

Individuals actually diagnosed with AIDS have positive cultures for HIV and express the immune system changes described in the pathophysiology section of this chapter. The accompanying physical signs and symptoms vary with the degree of immune function impairment and the location of HIV infection. Typical signs and symptoms are listed in the pathophysiology and case presentation sections of this chapter.

TREATMENT

There is currently no treatment for HIV infection that results in cure. The focus of treatment is to slow the progress of the disease and improve both the long-term survival and quality of life for patients with AIDS. Treatments are aimed both at HIV directly and at the side effects of HIV infection.

Therapy for AIDS

Although many attempts have been made to reconstitute the immune system of patients with AIDS, none have been successful (Lane & Fauci, 1985). Therapy for AIDS is aimed primarily at eliminating or controlling replication of HIV. The agents described below are currently used for this purpose.

Azidothymidine

Azidothymidine (AZT) is chemically similar to the nucleoside thymidine in human DNA. In viral culture studies this drug prevents the replication of many viruses, including HIV. The exact mechanism of action of AZT is not clear, but the drug is thought to inhibit the enzyme complex reverse transcriptase competitively and prevent retroviral replication rather than to exert direct killing actions on the virus. In addition, this drug appears to cause premature termination of viral DNA synthesis, before the new DNA strand is complete. This drug is able to cross the blood–brain barrier.

AZT for treatment of AIDS is administered orally, 100 to 200 mg every 4 hours. The drug has profound and sometimes toxic side effects that limit the dosage (Richman, Fischl, Grieco, et al., 1987). The 2 major side effects are fever and bone marrow suppression, leading to anemia, thrombocytopenia and leukopenia.

Antiviral Agents

Antiviral agents that have specific as well as nonspecific viral killing or proliferation-limiting activities also have been used in the treatment of HIV (Robertson, 1989). These agents, unproven for their effectiveness in AIDS, include *acyclovir* (an approved drug successful in treating systemic herpes) and *ribavirin* (a nucleoside analogue somewhat successful in treating respiratory syncytial virus).

Interferons

Subcutaneous injections of interferon appear useful in the treatment of AIDS. Interferon, a biologic-response modifier, has a variety of mechanisms of action. The most-well-characterized activity is the ability of interferon to induce resistance to viral replication among non-virus-infected leukocytes. In addition, interferon appears to have some direct antiviral action as well as an ability to improve the overall immune response.

Biologic-Response Modifiers

Other agents that have known activities to enhance immune function are currently being used in early-phase clinical trials for patients with AIDS. These agents include interleukin-2, and granulocyte–macrophage colony-stimulating factor (Lynch, Yanes, & Todd, 1988). The focus of the biologic-response modifiers is to improve the immune function of patients with HIV infection. The efficacy of these agents in improving length of survival among patients with AIDS has yet to be established.

Therapy for Opportunistic Infections

The most common causes of death among patients with AIDS are side effects of the opportunistic infections associated with immunosuppression. The causative organisms for opportunistic infections include protozoa, fungi, bacteria, and viruses.

Common protozoal infections associated with AIDS are *Pneumocystis carinii, Toxoplasma gondii,* Isospora, and Cryptosporidium (Mills & Masur, 1990). Infection with *P. carinii* is primarily pulmonary and usually results in pneumonia. Patients present with fever, nonproductive cough, and difficulty with pulmonary gaseous exchange. Infection with *Toxoplasma gondii* usually is confined to the central nervous system. Presenting symptoms include fever, change in mental status, and seizures. Most of the symptoms are associated with the presence of cerebral edema. Infections with Isospora and Cryptosporidium occur in the gastrointestinal tract. These infections lead to an almost uncontrollable and painful diarrhea, with complications of malnutrition and severe imbalances of fluid and electrolytes.

Common fungal infections associated with AIDS are caused by the organisms Candida, Cryptococcus, and *Histoplasma capsulatum*. Infections with Candida usually are found in the upper digestive tract, especially the mouth and esophagus. Presenting symptoms include a thick coating on the oral mucous membranes and altered taste sensations. Esophageal candidiasis can cause dysphagia. This infection can extend further into the gastrointestinal system and cause diarrhea. Pulmonary infection with Candida also is seen among patients with AIDS and is treated systemically.

Cryptococcal infections among AIDS patients usually are found in the central nervous system, and the associated symptoms are induced by meningeal irritation and cerebral edema. These symptoms include fever, altered mental status, and headache. Some patients experience respiratory symptoms, along with central nervous system symptoms, but respiratory effects are assumed to be from alterations in the function of the central respiratory centers rather than from actual pulmonary infection with Cryptococcus.

Viral infections commonly associated with AIDS include herpes simplex and cytomegalovirus (CMV). The effects of herpes simplex largely are confined to the specific tissue or site of eruption, although pulmonary problems and even systemic herpes have been reported. Infection with CMV can have widespread and devastating side effects in patients with AIDS. Not only is this infection also somewhat immunosuppressive, it is associated with the following pathologic manifestations: retinitis, pneumonitis, colitis, and systemic infection.

Antiprotozoal Agents

There are few agents specifically categorized as antiprotozoals. One such drug is pentamidine. This drug is helpful in combating *P. carinii* infections but has many serious and dose-limiting side effects. Other drugs that demonstrate effectiveness in treating protozoal infections in patients with AIDS include the antibiotic trimethoprim–sulfamethoxazole (Septra, Bactrim) and the sulfonamide antibacterial agent, dapsone. These drugs have been highly successful in the treatment of *P. carinii* pneumonia but cannot be used in individuals with a demonstrated sulfa sensitivity.

Antifungal Agents

Two primary antifungal agents have emerged as the most effective first-line treatment for most of the systemic fungal infections common to patients with AIDS. These agents are ketoconazole and amphotericin B. Both agents have many serious and sometimes toxic side effects.

Antiviral Agents

In addition to the antiviral agents used for their potential efficacy against HIV, two other antiviral agents are widely used to treat viral-origin opportunistic infections among patients with AIDS. These agents are acyclovir (Zovirax) and ganciclovir. Acyclovir is effective at controlling herpes simplex infections and ganciclovir is used in the treatment of CMV.

CASE PRESENTATION

Brian is a 33-year-old white male stockbroker who was diagnosed with AIDS 2 years ago, after having experienced three successive episodes of viral pneumonia. He is a homosexual who went through a 6-month period of promiscuity 5 years ago, when his long-term, live-in companion moved to another state. During the promiscuous period Brian had sexual encounters with approximately 25 different men. Brian currently lives with his sister and is sexually abstinent.

For the past 2 years Brian has been seen through an outpatient treatment center for AIDS. He is classified at the WR6 stage of AIDS. During the past year he has had pneumocystis pneumonia twice and oral thrush five times. He has eight Kaposi's sarcoma lesions well controlled by x-ray treatment. He was brought to the AIDS clinic by his sister with complaints of fever and diarrhea. A complete physical was done. Results were as follows:

Height: 5'10"
Weight: 128 lb
Vital signs: Temperature, 102°F; Pulse, 98 beats per minute;
    Respirations, 28 per minute; Blood pressure, 90/56 mm Hg
Ear, nose, throat: Oral mucous membranes, pale and dry
Hands/skin: Pale, warm, dry, and flaky; skin turgor poor; eight Kaposi's
    sarcoma lesions noted on back
Head/eyes: Within normal limits
Chest: Lungs clear
Cardiovascular: Pulse thready; normal sinus rhythm.
Abdomen: Soft, tender, bowel sounds hyperactive; complains of painful,
    watery, foul-smelling stools for 2 days
Rectal: Negative for blood or Kaposi's sarcoma lesions; perirectal area
    erythematous and tender
Musculoskeletal/extremities: Within normal limits
Neurologic: Alert, but unable to give the date or name the current
    president. Affect flat. Had difficulty walking a straight line. Sister

states he has been increasingly forgetful. She related an episode when she found Brian lying on the bedroom floor; he was difficult to arouse and was unable to recall what had occurred.

Because of his fever, diarrhea, and physical examination results, Brian was admitted for further testing and treatment. On admittance to his room, his primary nurse Susan helped him settle in. She admitted Brian and explained that he would be having some laboratory tests done and would need to give both a urine sample and a sample of his stool. A complete blood count (CBC) with a differential cell count; renal, bone, and hepatic samples; and bacterial and fungal cultures times 2 were drawn, and a chest x-ray film was obtained. An intravenous (IV) infusion of 5 per cent dextrose normal saline was started at 150 ml per hour. After Brian gave Susan his urine and stool samples, he was sent for a computed tomographic (CT) scan of the brain.

His CBC results were as follows: white cells, 5000/cu mm; hemoglobin, 13.5; hematocrit, 34; platelets, 150,000/cu mm; differential cell count: Segs, 20 per cent; band forms, 10 per cent; monocytes, 5 per cent; and lymphocytes, 60 per cent. His renal profile was normal except for a serum potassium level of 3.0. His bone/hepatic profiles were within normal limits. The chest x-ray film was negative. His CT scan showed some suspicious lesions and mild cerebral edema.

Noting Brian's hypokalemia, Susan notified his physician, who added 30 mEq of potassium (K^+) to the IV fluids. A clear liquid diet was ordered in order to rest Brian's bowels. Susan explained to Brian the importance of an adequate fluid intake and encouraged him to drink a glass of water or fruit juice every 1 to 2 hours. An antidiarrheal medication was given to slow the diarrhea. Because of the abnormal CT scan results and his altered neurologic status, Brian's physician did a spinal tap and sent a sample of Brian's cerebrospinal fluid for study. Brian's symptoms and abnormal CT scan results, coupled with the fact that he had four cats, suggested a toxoplasmosis infection. Consequently, he was started on sulfadiazine 2 gm by mouth every 4 hours and a loading dose of 200 mg of pyrimethamine, then 75 mg/day by mouth.

Susan instructed him to take the pyrimethamine with meals to reduce gastrointestinal upset and reiterated the need for adequate fluid intake so that no crystallization would occur from the sulfadiazine. She also watched Brian's daily CBC to monitor for pyrimethamine-induced bone marrow depression, and she monitored his K^+ level closely. Because of the probable seizure he had at home, Susan provided for his safety by padding the side rails of the bed and keeping them up at all times. Brian was reminded frequently to call for assistance in getting to the bathroom. He was placed in a room close to the nurses' station so other nurses could monitor him. Susan also had a lighter caseload in order to monitor Brian more closely. Neurologic checks were done every 2 hours for the first 24 hours, and every 4 hours thereafter. For his fevers, acetaminophen 650 mg every 4 hours as needed was given.

Three days into his hospitalization, Susan noted some large vesicles filled with red fluid on his upper left chest and back. These were cultured. Acyclovir,

500 mg IVPB (administered by intravenous piggy-back infusion) every 12 hours was started prophylactically for herpes zoster. Brian's stool cultures grew *Cryptosporidium*. Susan explained to Brian that there is currently no approved treatment for this, although there is an agent called spiramycin that is under investigation. Brian's treatment would deal with the symptoms only.

Brian's sister and Susan both noted dramatic improvements in Brian's mental status and gross motor skills by the end of his first week of hospitalization. He did not have any seizures, was no longer forgetful, and he slowly became more alert and cheerful. Although his diarrhea had slowed, he needed to be hospitalized for 2 weeks in order to replace the fluids and electrolytes lost. The shingles on his left upper trunk became dry and crusty, and the acyclovir was discontinued after 7 days of treatment.

Before Brian returned home, Susan spent time teaching him about self-care. Because it is believed at present that treatment for toxoplasmosis in an AIDS patient should be indefinite, Brian will continue to take sulfadiazine and pyrimethamine at home. Susan emphasized the importance of continuing adequate fluid intake, both to prevent drug crystallization and to replace diarrhea-induced fluid loss. He was placed on an oral potassium supplement, and Susan gave him a list of foods that contain high amounts of potassium. He was scheduled to come to the clinic every 2 weeks for a CBC with a differential count and a renal profile. Susan taught Brian and his sister signs and symptoms of bone marrow depression. Because of his high-pressure job, Susan and Brian discussed stress and worked on a plan to help him cope effectively. Although he is not currently sexually active, Susan discussed safe sex issues with Brian, gave him informational pamphlets, and answered his questions.

SELECTED BIBLIOGRAPHY

Barrick, B. (1988). Caring for A.I.D.S. patients: A challenge you can meet. *Nursing 88, 18*(11), 50.
Beckhan, M., & Rudy, E. (1986). Acquired immunodeficiency syndrome: Impact and implication for the neurological system. *Journal of Neuroscience Nursing, 18,* 5.
Bennett, J. (1986). What we know about AIDS. *American Journal of Nursing, 86,* 1016.
Bennett, J. (1988). Helping people with AIDS live well at home. *Nursing Clinics of North America, 23*(4), 731.
Bishop, J. (1985). Viruses, genes, and cancer: Retroviruses and cancer genes. *Cancer, 55*(10), 2329.
Blanchet, K. (1988). *AIDS: A health care management response.* Rockville, MD: Aspen.
Donehower, M. (1987). Malignant complications of AIDS. *Oncology Nursing Forum, 14*(1), 57.
Edwards, K. (1989). Training today's health professionals about AIDS. *Ohio Medicine,* February, 130.
Facts about AIDS (1987). Atlanta: Centers for Disease Control.
Fauci, A. (1985). The acquired immunodeficiency syndrome: An update. *Annals of Internal Medicine, 102,* 800.
Fischl, M., Richman, D., Grieco, M., et al. (1987). The efficacy of azidothymidine (AZT) in the treatment of patients with AIDS and AIDS-related complex. *New England Journal of Medicine, 317,* 185.
Flaskerud, J., & Ungvarski. (1992). *HIV/AIDS: A guide to nursing care.* Philadelphia: W.B. Saunders.

Folks, T., Kelly, J., Benn, S., et al. (1986). Susceptibility of normal human lymphocytes to infection with HTLV-III/LAV. *Journal of Immunology, 136,* 4049.

Fowler, M. (1988). Acquired immunodeficiency syndrome and refusal to provide care. *Heart and Lung, 17*(2), 213.

Friedman-Kein, A. (1989). *A color atlas of AIDS.* Philadelphia: W.B. Saunders.

Gallo, R. (1986). HTLV-III: Untangling the retroviral origin of the AIDS pandemic. *Advances in Oncology, 2,* 3.

Gallo, R., & Montagnier, L. (1988). AIDS in 1988. *Scientific American, 259*(4), 41.

Grady, C. (1989). The immune system and AIDS/HIV infection. In J. Flaskerud (Ed.), *AIDS/ HIV infection: A reference guide for nursing professionals* (p. 37). Philadelphia: W.B. Saunders.

Grady, C. (1992). HIV disease: Pathogenesis and treatment. In J. Flaskerud & P. Ungvarski (Eds.), *HIV/AIDS: A guide to nursing care* (p. 30). Philadelphia: W.B. Saunders.

Haseltine, W., & Wong-Staal, F. (1988). The molecular biology of AIDS. *Scientific American, 259*(4), 52.

Henderson, D., Saah, A., Zak, B., et al. (1986). Risk of nosocomial infection with human T-cell lymphotrophic virus type III/lymphadenopathy-associated virus in a large cohort of intensely exposed health care workers. *Annals of Internal Medicine, 104,* 644.

Henochowicz, S., & Hoth, D. (1988). Unproven agents in the treatment of human immunodeficiency virus (HIV) infection. *AIDS Updates, 1*(2), 1.

Heyward, W., & Curran, J. (1988). The epidemiology of AIDS in the U.S. *Scientific American, 259*(4), 72.

Hierholzer, W. (1987). AIDS and the health-care worker: Reducing the risk. *Mediguide to Infectious Diseases, 7*(4), 1.

Kennedy, M. (1987). AIDS: Coping with the fear. *Nursing 87, 17*(4), 45.

Lane, H., & Fauci, A. (1985). Immunologic abnormalities in the acquired immunodeficiency syndrome. *Annual Review of Immunology, 3,* 477.

Lane, H., & Fauci, A. (1985). Immunologic reconstitution in the acquired immunodeficiency syndrome. *Annals of Internal Medicine, 103,* 714.

Lovejoy, N. (1988). The pathophysiology of AIDS. *Oncology Nursing Forum, 15*(5), 563.

Lynch, M., Yanes, L., & Todd, K. (1988). Nursing care of AIDS patients participating in a phase I/II trial of recombinant human granulocyte-macrophage colony stimulating factor. *Oncology Nursing Forum, 15*(4), 463.

Marcus, R., & The CDC Cooperative Needlestick Surveillance Group. (1988). Surveillance of health care workers exposed to blood from patients infected with the human immunodeficiency virus. *New England Journal of Medicine, 319,* 1118.

McArthur, J., & Palenicek, J. (1988). Human immunodeficiency virus and the nervous system. *Nursing Clinics of North America, 23*(4), 823.

Melbye, M. (1986). The natural history of human T-lymphotrophic virus-3 infection: The cause of AIDS. *British Medical Journal, 295,* 5.

Meredith, T., & Acierna, L. (1988). Pulmonary complications of acquired immunodeficiency syndrome. *Heart and Lung, 17,* 173.

Mills, J., & Masur, H. (1990). AIDS-related infections. *Scientific American, 263*(2), 50.

Moran, T., Lovejoy, N., Viele, C., et al. (1988). Informational needs of homosexual men diagnosed with AIDS or AIDS-related complex. *Oncology Nursing Forum, 15*(3), 311.

Nakamura, S., Salahuddin, S., Biberfeld, P., et al. (1989). Kaposi's sarcoma cells: Long-term culture with growth factor from retrovirus-infected from CD4 + T cells. *Science, 242,* 426.

Parris, N. (1992). Infection control. In J. Flaskerud & P. Ungvarski (Eds.), *HIV/AIDS: A guide to nursing care* (p. 397). Philadelphia: W.B. Saunders.

Pickersgill, F. (1987). Care of critically ill patients suffering from HIV infection. *Intensive Care Nursing, 3,* 106.

Pratt, R. (1986). *AIDS: A strategy for nursing care.* London: Edward Arnold.

Quarterly report to the domestic policy council on the prevalence and rate of spread of HIV and AIDS—United States (1988). *Mortality and Morbidity Weekly Report, 37*(36), 551.

Quinnan, G., Masur, H., Rook, A., et al. (1984). Herpes virus infections in the acquired immunodeficiency syndrome. *Journal of the American Medical Association, 252,* 72.

Quinnan, G., Siegel, J., Epstein, J., et al. (1985). Mechanisms of T-cell functional deficiency in the acquired immunodeficiency syndrome. *Annals of Internal Medicine, 103,* 710.

Redfield, R., & Burke, D. (1988). HIV infection: The clinical picture. *Scientific American, 259*(4), 90.

Richman, D., Fischl, M., Grieco, M., et al. (1987). The toxicity of azidothymidine (AZT) in the treatment of patients with AIDS and AIDS-related complex. *New England Journal of Medicine, 317,* 192.

Robertson, S. (1989). Drugs that keep AIDS patients alive. *RN,* February, 35.

Rosenthal, Y., & Haneiwich, S. (1988). Nursing management of adults in the hospital. *Nursing Clinics of North America, 23*(4), 707.

Sande, M., & Volberding, P. (1990). *The medical management of AIDS* (2nd ed.). Philadelphia: W.B. Saunders.

Shiramizu, B., & McGrath, M. (1991). Molecular pathogenesis of AIDS-associated non-Hodgkin's lymphoma. *Hematology/Oncology Clinics of North America, 5*(2), 323.

Surgeon General's report on acquired immune deficiency syndrome (1987). Washington, DC: U.S. Public Health Service.

Tami, J., & Parr, M. (1986). The immune system. *American Journal of Hospital Pharmacy, 43,* 2483.

Tizard, I. (1984). *Immunology: An introduction.* Philadelphia: Saunders College Publishing.

Touchette, N. (1992). Tracking HIV transmission and pathogenicity. *Journal of NIH Research, 4,* 25.

Turner, J., & Williamson, K. (1986). AIDS: A challenge for contemporary nursing, Part I. *Focus on Critical Care, 13*(3), 53.

Turner, J., & Williamson, K. (1987). AIDS: A challenge for contemporary nursing, Part II. *Focus on Critical Care, 13*(4), 41.

Ungvarski, P. (1988). Assessment: The key to nursing an AIDS patient. *RN,* September, 28.

Ungvarski, P. (1989). Nursing management of the adult client. In J. Flaskerud (Ed.), *AIDS/ HIV infection: A reference guide for nursing professionals* (p. 74). Philadelphia: W.B. Saunders.

U.S. Department of Health and Human Services. (1986). AIDS in the workplace: How to prevent transmission of the infection. *International Nursing Review, 33*(4), 117.

Varmus, H. (1985). Viruses, genes, and cancer. *Cancer, 55*(10), 2324.

Weber, J., & Weiss, R. (1988). HIV infection: The cellular picture. *Scientific American, 259*(4), 101.

Wolfe, P. (1989). Clinical manifestations and treatment. In J. Flaskerud (Ed.), *AIDS/HIV infection: A reference guide for nursing professionals* (p. 58). Philadelphia: W.B. Saunders.

Yarchoan, R., Mitsuya, H., & Broder, S. (1988). AIDS therapies. *Scientific American, 259*(4), 110.

Zunich, K., & Lane, H. C. (1991). Immunologic abnormalities in HIV infection. *Hematology/ Oncology Clinics of North America, 5*(2), 215.

Immunodeficiency Secondary to Disease

7

THE LEUKEMIAS: ACUTE AND CHRONIC

As described in Chapters 1 and 4, the immune system provides some protection against the development of cancer. However some types of cancer occur in the immune system cells. When this happens, the immune system cells are not able to perform their specific differentiated functions and the person becomes immunocompromised. This chapter briefly discusses mechanisms of general cancer development and the characteristics of specific malignancies of immune system cells.

CARCINOGENESIS/ONCOGENESIS

Malignant disorders of the hematopoietic and lymphopoietic organs cause immunosuppression. Malignant cells (cancer cells) are not foreign invaders of the body. Every malignancy arises from one cell or one group of cells that started life as normal cells. These normal cells were altered, changed, or *transformed* by some event so that they lost some or all of their normal characteristics and expressed abnormal, malignant characteristics. The concept that groups of cancer cells can arise from a single transformed cell is called the *monoclonal origin of cancer.*

The key to cancer development is in the genes of a cell. Genes are specific segments of DNA that code for specific cell products or actions. Some genes are actually the pattern for making certain cell proteins used in that cell or others, and other genes regulate cell activity. The regulatory genes may control cell activity either at the DNA level by changing the expression of some genes, or at the level of the cell by causing the cell to make a regulatory protein. In normal cells, these genes are "turned on" and "turned off" as needed for normal cell functions.

Early in embryonic development, many specific genes are turned on and are actively involved in making the small organism behave in the way that is normal for early embryos. At a certain point in development, early embryonic behavior stops and differentiation must occur. To ensure normal development, the early embryonic genes must be turned off forever. This turning off of early embryonic genes is accomplished through the activity of special "repressor" genes, which repress the activity of the early embryonic genes so that they can no longer be freely expressed. As long as these early embryonic genes remain repressed, the cell behaves in the expected, normal way for its specific differentiated type. It contributes to the overall effort necessary for healthy human function.

Exposure of cells to events that can damage the genes within the DNA can cause the exposed cells to stop normal functions and take on the appearance and activity of malignant cells. This process of changing from a normal cell to a cancer cell is called *malignant transformation* and occurs through *carcinogenesis,* which is a sequential process beginning with the exposure of a normal cell to a carcinogenic substance that causes DNA breaks and rearrangements. Carcinogenic agents include ionizing radiation, ultraviolet radiation, chemicals, and viruses. When a normal cell is exposed to any of these substances, the normal cell's DNA can be damaged or mutated. The mutations can cause the early embryonic genes, which should be repressed forever, to be turned on again at an inappropriate time. When these genes are turned on they can cause the cell to change from normal to malignant.

The early embryonic genes capable of causing cancer if turned on again after development is complete are called *oncogenes.* About 50 different oncogenes have been identified so far, and scientists estimate that at least 50 more probably exist. These oncogenes are not abnormal genes. They are all part of every cell's normal makeup and were critically important in early development. Oncogenes become a problem only if they are activated (derepressed) after development is complete by exposure to anything capable of damaging the DNA. Therefore, part of the process of carcinogenesis is oncogene activation. Activation of some specific oncogenes is known to cause specific malignancies. For example, activation of the c-*myc* oncogene, located on chromosome 8, can cause Burkitt's lymphoma. Figure 7–1 summarizes the action of carcinogens in oncogene activation.

OVERVIEW OF LEUKEMIA

Leukemia is a malignancy of the hematopoietic or lymphopoietic system, or both, characterized by excessive cellular growth and incomplete cellular maturation. Commonly thought of as a cancer of the leukocytes, leukemia of

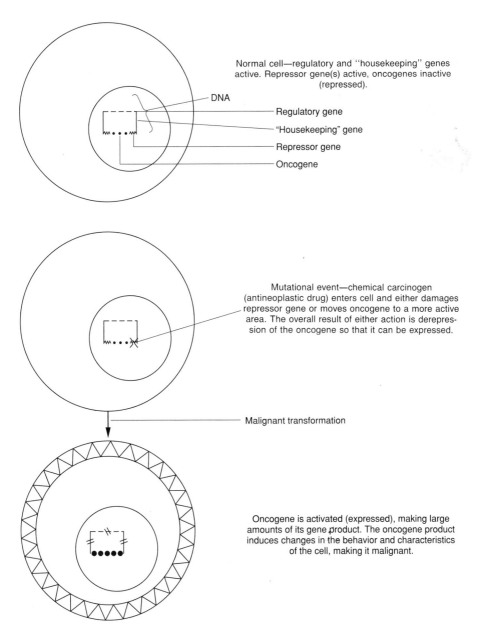

FIGURE 7–1. Theoretical model of carcinogenesis related to genetic mutation events.

the erythrocytes and the platelets can also occur. Classification of leukemia is by (1) the point at which the cell's maturation ends and malignant changes occur (see Fig. 1–3 for stem-cell differentiation and maturation pathways) and (2) the time of onset and duration of the disease. Therefore, leukemia is classified as either myeloid or lymphoid and as either acute or chronic (Wujcik, 1990). Although many subcategories of leukemia do exist, this chapter will address the pathologies and disease courses of the four major classes of leukemia: acute myelogenous leukemia (AML), acute lymphocytic leukemia (ALL), chronic myelogenous leukemia (CML), and chronic lymphocytic leukemia (CLL). Although the course and treatment of each disease is different, the end result is immunosuppression in varying degrees.

INCIDENCE AND ETIOLOGY

The incidence and frequency of leukemia depends on many factors: the morphologic type, age, sex, race, and locale (Mitus & Rosenthal, 1991). AML occurs with a similar frequency at all ages. ALL is more commonly a childhood disease, although it does occur in adults. According to the American Cancer Society's *Cancer Facts and Figures—1991,* the leukemias account for 3 per cent of all newly diagnosed cases, and they are responsible for 4 per cent of all cancer deaths. The estimated incidence of CLL is approximately 8000 new cases each year, 28 per cent of all the leukemias diagnosed (American Cancer Society, 1991). Its incidence is higher in men than in women. It is usually seen in the population between the ages of 50 and 80 (Rowe, 1983; American Cancer Society, 1991). Some clustering in families has been observed. Although this clustering is relatively rare, it supports the theory that persons with CLL may have a genetic predisposition for the disease. CML accounts for 20 to 30 per cent of adult leukemias (Campbell, Preston, & Smith, 1983; Collins, 1990). It generally occurs between the ages of 25 and 60, and there seems to be a male predominance (Campbell et al., 1983; Collins, 1990).

Epidemiologic studies have found that many different genetic and environmental factors are involved in the development of leukemia. Only a very few of these factors have been identified as having a definite role in leukemia development. The following list of risk factors has been summarized from Mitus & Rosenthal (1991).

Risk Factors

1. Ionizing radiation: Exposure to large quantities of radiation appears to be a major risk factor for the development of leukemia. Exposures ranging from therapeutic irradiation for diseases such as ankylosing spondylitis and Hodgkin's disease to major radiation exposure from the atomic bomb at Hiroshima or from the Chernobyl accident increase the incidence of AML and CML. Radiation remains the most conclusively identified leukemogenic factor in human beings (Wujcik, 1990).

2. Chemicals and drugs: Many different chemicals and drugs have been associated with the development of leukemia. Of these chemicals, benzene exposure is the most closely associated with development of leukemia (Cotran, Kumar, & Robbins, 1989). Phenylbutazone, arsenic, and chloramphenicol also

have been related to later development of leukemia. Unfortunately, antineoplastic drugs, especially alkylating agents, used as treatment for other malignant conditions, have also been linked to leukemia development (Fraser & Tucker, 1989; Workman, 1989).

3. Marrow hypoplasia: A reduction or alteration in production of hemopoietic cells may cause a predisposition to leukemia. Examples of such associations with later development of leukemia include Fanconi's anemia, paroxysmal nocturnal hemoglobinuria during its aplastic phase, and myelodysplastic syndromes (Yeomans & Harle, 1990).

4. Environmental interactions: Environmental factors that cause a predisposition to leukemia are difficult to identify, as they can be multiple and interactive. A child exposed to many risk factors or who had prenatal exposure with subsequent development of leukemia is an example of someone exposed to multifactorial influences on cancer development. Such exposures include in utero irradiation, maternal irradiation, maternal history of fetal wastage, and early childhood viral disease.

5. Genetal factors: An increase in frequency of leukemia in the following has suggested genetic involvement: the identical twin of a leukemic patient, Down's syndrome, Bloom's syndrome, Fanconi's anemia, and Klinefelter's syndrome. Chromosomal aberration may be an important factor in the development of leukemia in these syndromes.

6. Viral factors: Infection with the RNA viruses has been implicated in the causation of leukemia. Retroviruses that carry the gene for reverse transcriptase are also suspect (Bishop, 1985; Varmus, 1985). One virus confirmed to cause leukemia is human T-cell leukemia virus type I (HTLV-I).

7. Immunologic factors: Deficiency in the immune system may favor the development of leukemia. It has not yet been determined whether leukemia is a result of immunosurveillance failure or if the pathologic mechanisms that cause the immune deficiency also trigger malignant transformation of leukopoietic cells. Because CLL tends to be a disease of older people, immune system incompetence may be a factor in its development.

8. Interactive factors: The interaction of multiple host and environmental factors may result in leukemia. The interaction of these factors is tolerated differently by every person, frequently making it difficult to determine the etiology of any specific leukemia. Some of the personal variables that appear to influence the ability of environmental carcinogens to induce leukemia in any one person are age, sex, degree of immunocompetence, genetic predisposition, effectiveness of DNA repair mechanisms, amount of carcinogenic exposure, and the timing of the carcinogenic exposure.

PATHOPHYSIOLOGY

In Chapter 2, an explanation was given of the regulatory mechanisms that control cell reproduction and maturation. In the leukemias, these regulatory

mechanisms are absent or have gone awry. Major differentiating characteristics of these disorders are presented in Table 7–1. A brief explanation of the
four leukemias follows.

AML

Acute myelogenous leukemia, as the name would indicate, orginates from
the myeloid stem-cell line. Different types of myelogenous leukemia are myelocytic, monocytic, erythrocytic, and megakaryocytic; the most common type
is acute myelocytic leukemia. In AML an error occurs in the normal maturational pathway of myeloid cells. Usually there is a failure of the myeloid cells
to progress in the maturational pathway. As a result, the bone marrow continuously produces an immature myeloid cell that is incapable of any normal
immune function. These cells accumulate in the marrow and are also released
into circulation, where they are unable to perform any useful function. The
error in bone marrow cell maturation may also cause the marrow to overpro-
duce only these immature cells so that few other types of blood cells are synthesized. Most symptomatic patients present with severe bone marrow depression: anemia, thrombocytopenia, and neutropenia. If untreated, patients with
AML will die within a few months from uncontrollable bleeding, infection, or
both. Median survival with treatment is 1 year (Wujcik, 1990).

ALL

Malignant changes occurring in the lympoid stem-cell line result in ALL.
These malignant cells infiltrate organs such as the spleen and lymph nodes,
and they take sanctuary in the central nervous system (CNS) and the testes.
The CNS offers safe harbor to the leukemic cells from the toxic effects of most
chemotherapeutic agents, thus allowing them to continue to reproduce and
eventually overcome the patient. For adults with ALL, median survival with
treatment is 2 years (Wujcik, 1990).

CLL

In CLL, the malignant changes occur in the lymphocytes, including the
cells that produce immunoglobulins. The B cell is most often involved. Because
the CLL cell is malignant, it is immature and incapable of performing its normal functions of changing into plasma cells and secreting immunoglobulins.
Instead of a rapid proliferative or growing state, these malignant lymphocytes
grow very slowly and live a long time, hence the name, chronic lymphocytic
leukemia. Median survival with treatment is 4 to 6 years (Wujcik, 1990).

CML

In CML, the malignant changes occur in the hemopoietic system at the
stem-cell level. Ninety to ninety-five per cent of these patients have a chromosomal abnormality (the Philadelphia chromosome) in the cancerous bone
marrow cells (Rowe, 1983; Cork, 1983; Collins, 1990; Champlin, Gale, Foon, &
Golde, 1986). The chromosomal abnormality is composed of a broken area of

TABLE 7–I. Differential Features of the Four Major Types of Leukemia.

Leukemia Type	Age at Onset (Yr)	Sex	Race	Cell of Origin	Specific Markers	Comments
ALL	<15	M	Caucasian	B cell	CALLA+	Prognosis poorer for adults than for children
					Hyperdiploidy	Prognosis better than in AML
					TDT+	Curable in children
AML	15–39	Equal incidence		Myeloblast	TDT−	Prognosis generally poor
				Myelocyte	t(9;22)	Heterogeneous tumor-cell populations
				Promyelocyte	t(15;17)	Best prognosis with bone marrow transplant
				Myelomonocyte		
CML	>50	M		Myeloid cell	Ph¹ chromosome	Prognosis generally poor; worse if no Ph¹ chromosome
						No blockage of maturation of nonmalignant leukocytes
						Blastic crisis indicative of more acute disease
CLL	>50	M	Caucasian	B cell	Trisomy 12	Prognosis poor
						Long (4–10 yr) course with rare conversion to acute form
						Only leukemia with a possible genetic predisposition

CALLA = common acute lymphocytic leukemia antigen; TDT = terminal deoxyribonucleotidyl transferase; Ph¹ = Philadelphia chromosome.
(From *Medical-Surgical Nursing: A Nursing Process Approach* [p. 2261] by D. Ignatavicius and M. Bayne, 1991, Philadelphia: W.B. Saunders.)

the long arms of chromosome 22 being translocated to the end of the long arms of another chromosome (usually 8 or 9). It is thought that exposure to a carcinogenic agent or event damaged the DNA of these bone marrow cells and caused the chromosomal abnormality. The abnormality may "turn on" an oncogene (see Fig. 7–1).

The activated or turned-on oncogene causes the stem cell to become malignant. This malignant stem cell results in the formation and proliferation of malignant granulocytes (especially neutrophils), which only partially mature and differentiate. Because these immature, nonfunctional cells are overproduced to the exclusion of normal immune system cells, the patient's ability to fight infection decreases drastically as the disease progresses.

There are two stages of CML. The first is the chronic stage, in which clinical manifestations are confined to the hemopoietic system. This stage may be controlled for a few years by drug therapy. Inevitably, this chronic stage progresses to the terminal stage, which has two distinctive phases: *accelerated* and *blastic*. In the accelerated phase (which precedes the blast phase), drug therapy is no longer effective, and the patient's signs and symptoms extend beyond the hemopoietic system. The patient may present at this time with fever, malaise, and splenomegaly. This phase may last weeks to months. In the blast phase, the white-cell count and the differential count show increasing numbers of immature, or "blast," cells. The blast cells rapidly proliferate and interfere with the bone marrow's production of other hemopoietic cells. This condition is called *blastic crisis* and actually represents the progression of the disease from a chronic state to acute leukemia. This results in anemia and thrombocytopenia. At this point, the patient's symptoms resemble those of acute leukemia. Median survival with treatment is 3 to 6 years (Wujcik, 1990).

Specific Immune Function Alteration

Although patients with leukemia have many more white blood cells than normal, they are immunodeficient and at great risk of infection. This apparent contradiction may be confusing to patients and their families. The explanation for this problem starts with determining at what point malignant changes occur, making things go wrong with the normal process of creating white blood cells. In the process of normal hemopoiesis or growth process of white blood cells, it is believed that the malignant changes occur in the pluripotent or the hemopoietic (lymphopoietic) stem-cell pool. Basically, precursor or immature white blood cells undergo malignant changes, which can have at least one of three possible results:

1. These immature white blood cells or blast cells may become sterile, incapable of dividing, and die.

2. Another path that may be taken by the blast cells is a resting period. They may stop dividing but have the potential to return to the cell cycle.

3. The blast cells can divide and go through various stages of differentiation.

As discussed earlier, normal leukocyte maturation occurs as a series of regulated steps. In the leukemias, one or all of these regulated steps are no longer controlled (Mitus & Rosenthal, 1991).

The proliferation or "out-of-control" growth of these blast cells is what initially predisposes this patient population to immunosuppression. First of all, remember these blast cells are immature and therefore incapable of performing their normally assigned duties of fighting infection. Secondly, the rapid growth of these blast cells literally "crowds out" the normal white blood cells and prevents them from maturing. This is why when many patients are diagnosed with leukemia they often have normal or below normal peripheral white-cell counts.

Interpretation of the Data

It is extremely important that anyone caring for a patient with leukemia have a thorough understanding of the white-cell count and its differential count. As described in Chapters 1 and 2, the white-cell count is measured in terms of the total number of white blood cells in a milliliter of blood. The differential count is actually the percentage of a particular type of blood cell, or leukocyte, in the total white-cell count.

The importance of looking at the white-cell count and its differential count in the patient with leukemia is to determine the patient's absolute granulocyte count (AGC). Although the classification or terminology of *granulocytes* includes eosinophils and basophils, as discussed in Chapter 2, these cells are not critical to the functions of phagocytosis and the immediate protection of the patient from the side effects of invasion by microorganisms. Therefore, the AGC includes only cells capable of immediate phagocytic function, the mature neutrophils, and the soon-to-be-mature segmented neutrophils, the "band" neutrophils (Table 7–2).

Why is the AGC important? It gives the health care professional an idea of the patient's ability to fight infection. If the patient's AGC is less than 500 neutrophils per microliter, she or he is at a severe risk of infection. Moderate risk of infections is seen if the AGC is between 500 and 1000 neutrophils per microliter. With an AGC less than 500 neutrophils per microliter, the patient is seriously immunosuppressed and requires specialized nursing care to protect her or him from harmful effects of invasion by microorganisms.

Signs and Symptoms

The pathologic defect in leukemia is an abnormal accumulation of immature leukocytes (Wujcik, 1990). Most of the clinical signs and symptoms noted

**TABLE 7-2. Normal White-Cell Count and Differential Count
(White-Cell Count, 5000–10,000 per Microliter).**

Differential
Segmented leukocytes 55–70%
Band forms 2–5%
Eosinophils 1–4%
Basophils 0.5–1%
Monocytes 2–8%
Lymphocytes 20–40%

are a direct result of bone marrow depression; anemia, fatigue, malaise, dyspnea, and pallor are often seen. Easy bruising, characterized by petechiae (small pinpoint bruises) or ecchymoses (large bruises), epistaxis (nosebleeds), hematuria (blood in urine), hematemesis (coffee-ground emesis), melena (tarry, black stools), and gingival bleeding (easy bleeding of gums) are a result of a decreased total number of platelets and circulating red blood cells. Many patients with leukemia present with symptoms of an infection, including fevers and chills. Often the presenting symptoms are those associated with an acute infection, such as a pneumonia or an abscess. Other physical findings may include an enlarged spleen, bone pain, headaches, nausea and vomiting, and swollen glands.

Skin and Mucous Membranes

Skin and mucous membranes may manifest abnormalities associated with leukemia. The skin may be pale and cool to the touch as a result of the accompanying anemia. Pallor is especially evident on the face, around the mouth, and in the nailbeds. The conjunctiva of the eye is pale, as are the creases on the palmar surface of the hand (most evident when the skin over the palm of the hand is stretched). Petechiae may be present on any area of skin surface, especially the lower extremities. The petechiae may be unrelated to any obvious trauma. Careful inspection of the skin for the presence of skin infections or traumatized areas that have failed to heal is important. Always inspect the mouth for evidence of gingival hyperplasia, bleeding from the gums, and the presence of any sore or lesion of the oral cavity indicating infection. Care should be taken to examine both sides of the tongue. Another area of mucous membranes to examine closely for the presence of fissures and abscesses is the rectal mucosa. Loss of skin integrity in this area may result in abscess formation and may lead to sepsis in the patient with leukemia.

Cardiovascular

Cardiovascular manifestations of leukemia generally are related to anemia. Heart rate may be increased, with blood pressure decreased (especially systolic). Murmurs and bruits may be present. Capillary filling time is increased. When leukemia is very severe, leukemic cells can infiltrate organs and tissues. Leukemic-cell infiltration can occur in the myocardium, valves, and electrical conduction pathways of the heart. Thus, the patient with leukemia may present with dysrhythmias, symptoms of congestive heart failure, and other nonspecific symptoms of cardiac impairment.

Respiratory

Respiratory manifestations of leukemia are primarily associated with anemia and complications of gram-negative or fungal infections. Respiratory rate is increased in proportion to the degree of anemia present. If respiratory infections are present, the patient may experience shortness of breath with abnormal breath sounds present on auscultation.

Gastrointestinal

Gastrointestinal manifestations may be related to the increased bleeding tendency and to the fatigue. Weight loss, nausea, and anorexia are common. The nurse should examine the rectal area for fissures and test the stool for the presence of occult blood. Many patients with leukemia have diminished bowel sounds and constipation. Hepatosplenomegaly and abdominal tenderness also may be present as the result of leukemic infiltration of abdominal viscera.

Central Nervous System

CNS manifestations include possible cranial nerve disturbances, headache, and papilledema as a result of leukemic infiltration of the meninges or deeper areas of the CNS. Although fever is commonly present, this manifestation appears to be more a response to the presence of infection rather than to malignancy-related changes in the hypothalamic temperature-regulating center.

Miscellaneous

Other manifestations of leukemia include bone and joint tenderness as a result of marrow involvement and bone resorption. Leukemic-cell growth or infiltration may produce enlarged lymph nodes or masses.

AML/ALL

In patients with AML/ALL, presenting symptoms such as fever, fatigue, and malaise are usually indeterminate. These symptoms are often of recent onset and relate directly to the leukemic-cell infiltration and resulting depression of the bone marrow. Consequently, symptoms such as bladder infections, sore throats, pneumonia, heavy menstrual bleeding, easy bruising, shortness of breath, anorexia, headaches, and bone pain are commonly seen.

CLL

Patients may have CLL for years before they become symptomatic. The symptoms with which they do present depend on how far the CLL has progressed. An abnormally high white-cell count (lymphocytosis) may be found during a routine physical examination in early-stage CLL, along with swollen glands and an enlarged spleen. In late-stage CLL, the patient may present with signs and symptoms of thrombocytopenia and anemia.

CML

In CML, an abnormally high white-cell count may be found during a routine physical examination, but most patients seek medical help because of signs and symptoms of bone marrow depression. Symptoms related to the increased metabolism (hypermetabolic state) are weight loss and increased levels of uric acid in the urine and blood. These patients may also present with an enlarged spleen.

Overview of Medical Management

Purpose

The ultimate goal of medical management is to destroy as many of the leukemic cells as possible. Ideally, all the leukemic cells would be destroyed. Unfortunately, this is rarely the case. Because complete obliteration of the leukemic cells cannot be ensured, more than one treatment phase usually is necessary.

AML

A typical treatment regime for ALL involves three distinct phases. The first phase is usually called the *induction phase* (Jedlow, 1991). Chemotherapeutic agents commonly used in this phase are daunorubicin, cytosine arabinoside cytarabine (Ara-C), and 6-thioguanine (6-TG). The goal of this treatment is to achieve a remission. A remission usually is defined clinically as an absence of leukemic cells in the bone marrow.

The second phase is called the *consolidation phase*. This phase is defined as chemotherapy given in the same intensity as the induction program in the period immediately after the patient enters remission (Champlin et al., 1986). This phase of treatment uses the same chemotherapeutic agents as in the induction phase and is intense so as to destroy any residual leukemic cells.

The next phase of treatment is called the *maintenance phase*. In this phase, a lower dose of chemotherapy is given in a series of cycles from months to years. Different combinations of daunorubicin, cytarabine, and 6-TG may be used.

ALL

There are also three phases of medical management in ALL. Induction therapy is the first phase of treatment; its goal is to achieve a remission. Whereas complete remission is possible to achieve in children, remission rates among adults are significantly lower. Chemotherapeutic agents commonly used are vincristine, prednisone, L-asparaginase, and daunorubicin. The next treatment phase is CNS prophylaxis. As noted earlier, the ALL cells find sanctuary in the CNS. Prophylactic CNS treatment usually begins a few weeks after induction therapy and may consist of intracranial radiation and intrathecal administration of methotrexate (Jedlow, 1991). The maintenance phase follows, and as in AML treatment, a lower dose of chemotherapy is given in a series of cycles from months to years. These drugs might be combinations of methotrexate, vincristine, 6-mercaptopurine, and prednisone.

CML

In the chronic phase of CML, symptoms are treated with chemotherapy, such as with bulsulfan or hydroxyurea. The spleen may be irradiated or removed surgically to relieve symptoms of splenomegaly. Leukapheresis can be used to reduce abnormally high levels of white blood cells. In the blast phase, medical treatment becomes similar to that of acute leukemia, using drugs such as cytarabine and daunorubicin (Adriamycin). Autologous bone marrow transplantation (patients receiving their own bone marrow) after high-dose chemotherapy and radiotherapy has been attempted to achieve permanent remission of the leukemia. However, with CML this treatment has had little success.

The goal of the medical management of CML is primarily symptom management. During the blast-crisis phase, treatment is similar to that of acute leukemia.

CLL

The goal of medical management for CLL is symptom management. Early stages of CLL may not require any medical intervention. In later stages, there are many different medical interventions available, depending on the symptoms.

For patients with CLL, little therapy is done during the protracted early stages marked by moderate elevations of lymphocytes (Carson & Callaghan, 1991). Later treatment with chemotherapy (such as with chlorambucil, cytoxan, prednisone, or combination therapy) may control the abnormally high white-cell count, which often causes enlarged lymph glands and an enlarged spleen. Reduction of extremely high levels of white blood cells may be done by leukapheresis. Surgical removal of the spleen may be necessary, or local radiation to the spleen may be used to relieve symptoms of an enlarged spleen. Other symptom control treatments might involve the use of gamma globulin, interferon, and colony-stimulating factors (Collins, 1990). The purpose of using these agents is to reconstitute the immune system.

Immunosuppression

Risks and Complications

The most obvious risk/complication of immunosuppression is infection, or sepsis. Before chemotherapy, the patient with acute leukemia has immunologic deficiency. The deficit is most severe with neutrophil function and antibody production. Cell-mediated immunity is moderately impaired. With chemotherapy, all three types of immunity are severely compromised, leaving these patients at extreme risk for infection. These patients commonly contract pneumonia, cellulitis, otitis media/sinusitis, skin and perirectal abscesses, gastrointestinal viral and parasitic infections, meningitis, and septicemia. The most common pathogenic organisms causing these infections are Pseudomonas, *Staphylococcus aureus,* gram-negative and gram-positive organisms, and Klebsiella. Viral organisms are Cytomegalovirus (CMV) and Herpes simplex virus (HSV). Other opportunistic organisms are Pneumocystis, Toxoplasma, Candida, and Aspergillus (Gurevich & Tafuro, 1986).

Ironically, most of the infections these patients have are caused by the patient's own (endogenous) flora (Gurevich & Tafuro, 1986). There are other opportunistic organisms that come from outside sources. Aspergillus can be found whenever construction is in progress. *Pseudomonas aeruginosa* grows in stagnant water. Essentially, the patient with leukemia is at risk for anything and everything. It is the nurse's responsibility to maintain a protective environment for these patients, to minimize risk of nosocomial infections. Nurses working with patients with leukemia must have a strong knowledge base of the immune system and management of immune system incompetence.

CASE HISTORY: ACUTE MYELOGENOUS LEUKEMIA

Mr. Young, a 28-year-old white male mechanical engineer, presented to his family doctor complaining of extreme fatigue, malaise, and small bruises on his lower extremities. A complete physical examination was performed and a complete blood count with differential was drawn. The patient was pale, fatigued-looking, and had multiple petechiae on his lower extremities. The following parameters are the findings of his examinations:

Ear, nose, throat: Within normal limits
Hands/skin: Pale and warm, pale nailbeds, multiple petechiae on lower
  extremities
Head/eyes: Within normal limits
Neck/nodes: Within normal limits
Chest: Lungs clear
Cardiovascular: Peripheral pulses palpable, normal sinus rhythm
Abdomen: Soft, nontender, bowel sounds positive
Nervous system: Within normal limits
Rectal: Membranes intact, no abnormalities noted
Musculoskeletal/extremities: Within normal limits, no peripheral edema
  noted

Mr. Young denies fever, chills, cough, shortness of breath, hemoptysis, hematemesis, diarrhea, melena, joint pain, and areas of erythema or tenderness. His complete blood count results were as follows: white-cell count, 4000 per microliter; hemoglobin, 10.5; hematocrit, 30; platelets, 55,000 per microliter; differential count—segmented leukocytes, 20 per cent; band forms, 10 per cent; monocytes, 5 per cent; lymphocytes, 60 per cent. Noting Mr. Young's pancytopenia and shift to the left, his doctor referred him to a hematology/oncology specialist, Dr. Thomas.

The following day, Dr. Thomas did a bone marrow aspiration (BMA) and biopsy and explained what the possible causes of Mr. Young's low counts might be. The initial smear showed blast cells, and the pathology report confirmed Dr. Thomas' suspicion of leukemia. Mr. Young was told that he had acute myelogenous leukemia (AML). After hearing his options, Mr. Young chose aggressive therapy. He was admitted that afternoon to University Hospital on the hematology-oncology unit.

His primary nurse, Alex, introduced himself and helped Mr. Young settle in. He admitted Mr. Young and explained that he would be having some laboratory work done and would need to give a urine specimen for culture. A complete blood count with differential; renal, bone, and hepatic profiles; type and cross match; and bacterial/fungal cultures times two were drawn. A chest x-ray film was also obtained. An intravenous infusion was started, and 2 units of packed red blood cells (PRBC) were given. Alex gave Mr. Young pamphlets on AML, chemotherapy, and on the Hickman catheter. He spent time teaching Mr. Young about the triple-lumen Hickman catheter that would be placed the next day. A consent form was signed, and Mr. Young was given a sleeping pill so he would rest well.

The Hickman catheter is one type of large-bore central venous access line that involves surgical placement. The venous end of the catheter is placed in the central venous system (inferior vena cava, innominate vein, or right atrium). The midportion of the catheter extends from the central venous site, under the skin, to an exit site 3 to 8 in. from the venous site. Several inches of tubing protrude from the skin at the exit site. A triple-lumen catheter would have three access ports and flow controls at the exterior end of the tubing. The purpose of this type of intravenous catheter is to provide continuous, multiple access to large, high-flow veins.

The next day a hydration line was begun and 8 units of random donor platelets (RDP) were given prior to surgery. While Mr. Young was in surgery, Dr. Thomas wrote the chemotherapy prescription to begin that evening: cytarabine, 200 mg per square meter of body-surface area per day by continuous intravenous infusion for 7 days and daunorubicin 60 mg per square meter of body-surface area per day administered by intravenous push (IVP) on days 1 to 3. Lorazepam 2 mg IVP was to be given one-half hour prior to the daunorubicin on days 1 to 3. An antiemetic was also ordered to be administered as needed. Daily medications ordered were nystatin 5 ml to swish and swallow (S&S) 5 times per day and a multivitamin every day.

Mr. Young tolerated the Hickman placement well. Prior to initiation of chemotherapy, Alex taught Mr. Young about the two drugs and their side effects. Mr. Young knew to expect his urine would be orangish while receiving daunorubicin; he would lose his hair; he might have some nausea; and his counts would drop. He tolerated the chemotherapy well, with mild nausea that was controlled with antiemetics.

Mr. Young was also started on a meticulous oral care regimen. He was encouraged to drink plenty of fluids and to walk at least twice a day. A dietician visited with him to determine his food preferences, explained what the low-bacteria diet was, and initiated a calorie count. Alex also taught Mr. Young what his white-cell/absolute granulocyte count (AGC) means, signs and symptoms of infection, and how to protect himself with good handwashing and personal hygiene.

Mr. Young was able to maintain an adequate caloric intake and walked twice a day. He did his oral care faithfully. He became quick to calculate his AGC, verbalized understanding of signs and symptoms of infection, and began showing interest in the care of his Hickman catheter.

Each morning, a complete blood count with differential and renal panel were drawn, and a type and cross match was done every other day. If Mr. Young's hematocrit/hemoglobin (H/H) was less than 25/9, he received 2 units of PRBCs, and he received 8 units of RDP if his platelets were less than 20,000. Each day nurses assessed his oral mucosa, breath sounds, gastrointestinal function, urinary system, and skin for signs and symptoms of infection or bleeding.

On day 12, Mr. Young's AGC fell below 500, and he was placed in reverse isolation. On day 15, his temperature rose to 101.2°F. Dr. Thomas was notified. Bacterial/fungal cultures were drawn peripherally and from his central line; cultures of the Hickman catheter exit sites were obtained, urine and stool cultures were sent, and an immediate portable chest x-ray was performed. After the cultures and chest x-ray films were obtained, he was started immediately on ticarcillin 3 g administered by intravenous infusion piggy-back (IVPB) every 4 hours and tobramycin 100 mg IVPB every 8 hours. A maintenance intravenous infusion with supplemental potassium (K^+) also was started.

On day 17, Alex noted several small white patches in Mr. Young's mouth and an ulcer on his lip. Both were cultured. The white patches were positive for Candida. The lip ulcer was positive for herpes simplex virus (HSV). Consequently, acyclovir 500 mg IVPB every 12 hours was begun. Mr. Young suffered mouth pain and had difficulty eating. Alex taught him to avoid extreme temperatures in food or fluids and to avoid mechanically irritating foods. He began doing his oral care every 2 hours. A soft diet was ordered. Viscous xylocaine was kept at the bedside to swish before meals. This provided only temporary relief, so acetaminophen with codeine was ordered every 4 hours as needed. He took the acetaminophen 3 to 4 times a day. Because his oral intake was poor, docusate (Colace) 100 mg by mouth twice a day was also begun to avoid constipation.

Mr. Young's AGC began to rise slowly. His mouth healed and his renal profile remained stable. By day 24, his AGC was above 500, and he was removed from reverse isolation. His antibiotics were discontinued, and he was monitored closely. Another bone marrow aspiration and biopsy were done with no signs of leukemia. When his AGC reached 1000, he was allowed to go home.

During his hospitalization, Alex and other nurses taught him how to care for his Hickman catheter and how to care for himself at home. He learned to recognize signs and symptoms of infection and how to monitor his temperature.

Because he chose to go with aggressive therapy, Mr. Young returned 1 month later and underwent the same treatment. This time because of his previous episode of HSV, he was also started on acyclovir prophylactically.

This course was similar to the first course, except he developed a fever earlier. He was started again on ticarcillin and tobramycin. A few days later, Mr. Young complained of tenderness around his Hickman catheter. Erythema and tenderness were noted for approximately 2 in. superior to the exit site. Vancomycin 1 g IVPB every 12 hours was begun for prophylaxis against *Staphylococcus aureus*. After 48 hours of vancomycin, Mr. Young remained febrile. Although all cultures remained negative, amphotericin was begun for fungal coverage. After a test dose, which he tolerated well, he was titrated daily up to 50 mg every other day. Acetaminophen 650 mg, diphenhydramine (Benadryl) 50 mg IVP, and hydrocortisone 100 mg IVP were given prior to the amphotericin, and meperidine (Demerol) 25 to 50 mg IVP was ordered as needed for chills and rigors. His renal profile was monitored daily. He was heavily supplemented with intravenous K^+. His creatinine and blood urea nitrogen remained stable. Mr. Young remained on antibiotics and amphotericin until his AGC rose above 500. His AGC was over 1000 by day 30, and he returned home.

After consolidation treatment, he continues to see Dr. Thomas monthly. Mr. Young's bone marrow remains negative and he continues on low-dose methotrexate and prednisone as maintenance therapy. He has been able to return to work and his Hickman catheter was removed 8 months after treatment. A general care plan for immunocompromised patients, including patients in blast-crisis stage of acute leukemia, is presented in Chapter 15.

SELECTED BIBLIOGRAPHY

American Cancer Society (1991). *Cancer facts and figures—1991.* Atlanta: American Cancer Society.

Barry, S. (1989). Septic shock: Special needs of patients with cancer. *Oncology Nursing Forum, 16*(1), 31.

Bishop, J. (1985). Viruses, genes, and cancer: Retroviruses and cancer genes. *Cancer, 55*(10), 2329.

Brandt, B. (1984). A nursing protocol for the client with neutropenia. *Oncology Nursing Forum, 11*(2), 24.

Campbell, J., Preston, R., & Smith, K. (1983). The leukemias: Definition, treatment and nursing care. *Nursing Clinics of North America, 18*(3), 523.

Carlson, A. (1985). Infection prophylaxis in the patient with cancer. *Oncology Nursing Forum, 12*(3), 56.

Carson, C., & Callaghan, M. (1991). Hematopoietic and immunologic cancers. In S. Baird, R. McCorkle, & M. Grant (Eds.), *Cancer nursing* (p. 536). Philadelphia: W.B. Saunders.

Champlin, R., Gale, R., Foon, K. & Golde, D. (1986). Chronic leukemias: Oncogenes, chromosomes, and advances in therapy. *Annals of Internal Medicine, 104*(5), 671.

Collins, P. (1990). Diagnosis and treatment of chronic leukemia. *Seminars in Oncology Nursing, 6*(1), 31.

Cork, A. (1983). Chromosomal abnormalities in leukemia. *American Journal of Medical Technology, 49*(10), 703.

Cotran, R., Kumar, V., & Robbins, S. (1989). *Robbins pathologic basis of disease* (4th ed.). Philadelphia: W.B. Saunders.

Fraser, M., & Tucker, M. (1989). Second malignancies following cancer therapy. *Seminars in Oncology Nursing, 5*(1), 43.

Gurevich, I., & Tafuro, P. (1986). The compromised host: Deficit-specific infection and the spectrum of infection. *Cancer Nursing, 9*(5), 263.

Henschel, L. (1985). Fever patterns in the neutropenic patient. *Cancer Nursing, 8*(6), 301.

Hughes, C. (1985). Interpreting the white blood cell count in the cancer chemotherapy patient: Nursing responsibilities. *National Intravenous Therapy Association, 8,* 279.

Jedlow, C. (1991). Leukemia. In S. Baird (Ed.), *A cancer source book for nurses* (6th ed) (p. 276). Atlanta: American Cancer Society.

Lamb, L. (1982). Think you know septic shock? *Nursing 82, 12*(1), 34.

Littleton, M. (1988). Pathophysiology and assessment of sepsis and septic shock. *Critical Care Nursing Quarterly, 11*(1), 30.

Mitus, A., & Rosenthal, D. (1991) Adult leukemias. In A. Holleb, D. Fink, & G. Murphy (Eds.), *American Cancer Society textbook of clinical oncology*. Atlanta: American Cancer Society.

Newman, K. (1985). The leukemias. *Nursing Clinics of North America, 20*(1), 227.

Rowe, J. (1983). Clinical and laboratory features of the myeloid and lymphocytic leukemias. *American Journal of Medical Technology, 49*(2), 103.

Rubin, P. (1983). Clinical oncology: A multidisciplinary approach (6th ed.). New York: American Cancer Society.

Somerville, E. (1986). Special diets for neutropenic patients: Do they make a difference? *Seminars in Oncology Nursing, 2*(1), 55.

Varmus, H. (1985). Viruses, genes, and cancer. *Cancer, 55*(10), 2324.

Workman, M. (1989). Immunologic late effects in children and adults. *Seminars in Oncology Nursing, 5*(1), 36.

Wujcik, D. (1990). Leukemia. In S. Groenwald, M. Frogge, & M. Goodman (Eds.), *Cancer nursing: Principles and practice* (2nd ed.) (p. 931). Boston: Jones & Bartlett.

Yeomans, A., & Harle, M. (1990). Myelodysplastic syndromes. *Seminars in Oncology Nursing, 6*(1), 9.

Ziegfeld, C. (1987). *Core curriculum for oncology nursing*. Philadelphia: W.B. Saunders.

8

THE MYELOPROLIFERATIVE DISORDERS

ETIOLOGY AND INCIDENCE

The myeloproliferative disorders are diseases that result from abnormal proliferation of all or part of the cell types derived from the committed myeloid stem cell (see Fig. 2–1). These diseases include chronic myelogenous leukemia (discussed in Chapter 7), polycythemia vera, myeloid metaplasia with myelofibrosis, and essential thrombocythemia (Robbins & Kumar, 1987; Rapaport, 1987). The basic error that underlies all the myeloproliferative disorders is the loss of regulation for growth and differentiation in the myeloid stem cells produced in the bone marrow. An interesting characteristic of the myeloproliferative disorders is the tendency of one disorder, involving the abnormal production of a specific cell type, to change and become a disorder of abnormal production of a different specific cell type. In addition, the myeloproliferative disorders are sometimes called *preleukemic disorders* because of the propensity of the diseases to progress to acute leukemia among individuals who do not succumb to direct and indirect complications of the disorder (Yeomans & Harle, 1990).

In general, all the myeloproliferative disorders are more rare than are the lymphoproliferative disorders. Of the four types of myeloproliferative disorders, chronic myelogenous leukemia occurs most frequently and essential thrombocythemia occurs most rarely. All of these disorders occur more frequently among individuals over age 50, with men being affected slightly more frequently than women. Factors implicated in causing the myeloproliferative disorders include exposure to mutagenic substances, especially radiation and chemical carcinogens. Such exposures leading to development of myeloproliferative disorders include previous treatment with radiation therapy, chemotherapeutic agents, or both. Because chronic myelogenous leukemia is discussed in Chapter 7, and because essential thrombocythemia does not significantly interfere with immune function, this discussion of the myeloproliferative disorders is limited to myeloid metaplasia with myelofibrosis and polycythemia vera.

MYELOID METAPLASIA WITH MYELOFIBROSIS

Pathophysiology

This neoplastic condition is characterized by a failing bone marrow, resulting in decreased hematopoiesis and hypocellularity. Because hematopoiesis is essential for life, the bone marrow failure of myeloid metaplasia with myelofibrosis stimulates "extramedullary" hematopoiesis. This phenomenon is the synthesis of cellular blood components in sites where hematopoiesis does not normally occur after fetal life. The major site of abnormal extramedullary hematopoiesis among individuals with myeloid metaplasia is the spleen, although some hematopoietic activity may be found in the liver.

Myeloid metaplasia has its origin in the bone marrow. In response to an unknown triggering event or agent, the bone marrow begins to synthesize excessive numbers of platelets. In addition to the platelets being too plentiful, they also appear to function abnormally. This abnormal function includes the synthesis and release of extremely large amounts of a substance called *platelet-derived growth factor* (PDGF). PDGF stimulates the growth and differentiation of precursor cells into fibroblasts. Although fibroblast precursors are most commonly found in endothelial tissues and basal layers of skin, undifferentiated bone marrow cells, if persistently exposed to PDGF can be induced to differentiate into fibroblasts. Fibroblasts are a major component of scar tissue. Under the influence of PDGF, huge numbers of fibroblasts replace the active red marrow of the bone marrow with proliferating fibroblasts. These cells scar the bone marrow, making it nonfunctional and unable to participate in normal hematopoiesis.

In response to diminished bone marrow activity, the red pulp of the spleen engages in hematopoietic activity. As the areas of splenic hematopoiesis increase, the spleen greatly increases in size and becomes firm to hard in texture. In some individuals the liver also is stimulated to participate in hematopoiesis and becomes moderately enlarged. Interestingly, the lymph nodes are not enlarged in these individuals.

The course of progression for this disease can take 4 to 5 years. The extramedullary sites of hematopoiesis are not under the same regulatory constraints as is normal bone marrow and have no feedback mechanisms for stimulating and repressing hematopoiesis. Therefore, blood cell synthesis in individuals who have myeloid metaplasia with myelofibrosis lacks orderly control.

In the early stages of the disorder the number of leukocytes may be normal, elevated, or decreased. In the later stages the blood level of leukocytes is enormously increased, but as these leukocytes are immature and nonfunctional, the patient is at extreme risk for infection.

As the disorder progresses and more myeloid leukocytes are produced by the extramedullary hematopoietic sites, production of platelets and erythrocytes dramatically decreases to the point that the patient is thrombocytopenic and anemic. In addition, the few platelets and erythrocytes being produced are abnormal in appearance and function. The patient has severe bleeding tendencies.

The clinical manifestations of myeloid metaplasia with fibrosis closely resemble the acute leukemias. In fact about 10 per cent of the patients with myeloid metaplasia and myelofibrosis develop a blastic crisis similar to that seen with acute myelogenous leukemia (AML).

POLYCYTHEMIA VERA

Pathophysiology

Polycythemia vera (PV) is a malignant condition with a slow, insidious onset. The disorder is characterized by an abnormal increase in the actual number of circulating red blood cells (erythrocytes). Normally, the rate of red-cell production is regulated by circulating levels of erythropoietin, a specific growth factor secreted by kidney cells in response to hypoxia. It is interesting to note that polycythemia vera is not correlated with an increase in the circulating levels of erythropoietin. In fact, blood levels of erythropoietin among individuals with PV is actually lower than normal. One mechanism suggested for this observation is the idea that the precursor red blood cells in individuals with PV have abnormal membranes, which are extremely sensitive to the presence of erythropoietin. Thus, even low levels of erythropoietin overstimulate red-cell production.

Examination of the bone marrow from individuals with PV shows a "hypercellular" condition. Essentially all myeloid cells (erythrocytes, platelets, neutrophils, monocytes) are being overproduced to some degree, and the rate of erythrocyte production is enormously increased. This abnormal overproduction either results in or is a result of changes of the functional areas of bone marrow. Not only are myeloid-origin cells being produced in the normal active areas of red marrow, but the areas of inactive, yellow (fatty) marrow are replaced with active red marrow so that total bone marrow production is increased, even in areas that are normally nonfunctional. The hypercellularity of the bone marrow is reflected in a concurrent hypercellularity of the peripheral blood. The white-cell count is elevated (in early stage disease the total white-cell counts usually range from 11,000 to 20,000; in late stage disease the counts may be greater than 80,000 cells/cu mm) with few lymphocytes present.

The total red-cell count ranges between 6 million and 20 million cells/cu mm. The number of circulating platelets also is increased, ranging from 400,000 to 1 million/cu mm.

The clinical manifestations of an individual with PV are associated at first with the extreme hypercellularity of the peripheral blood. The skin, especially of the face, and mucous membranes have a dark, flushed (plethoric) appearance. These areas may appear purplish or cyanotic as the blood in these tissues is incompletely oxygenated. Most patients experience intense itching sensations thought to be related to vasodilation and variation in tissue oxygenation. The viscosity ("thickness") of the blood is greatly increased, causing a corresponding increase in vascular friction and peripheral resistance. Superficial veins are visibly distended. Blood moves more slowly through all tissues and places increased demands on the pumping action of the heart, resulting in hypertension. In some highly vascular areas, blood flow may become so slow that vascular stasis occurs. Vascular stasis causes thrombosis within the smaller vessels to the extent that the vessels are occluded and the surrounding tissues experience hypoxia progressing to anoxia and then to infarction and necrosis. Tissues most prone to this complication are the heart, spleen, and kidneys, although infarction with loss of tissue and organ function can occur in any organ or tissue.

Because the actual number of cells in the blood is greatly increased and the cells are not completely normal, lifespans of individual cells are shorter. The shorter lifespans, coupled with increased cell production, result in a rapid turnover of peripheral cells. This rapid turnover increases the amount of intracellular products (released when cells die) in the blood, adding to the general "sludging" of the blood. These products include uric acid and potassium and are responsible for the associated symptoms of gout and hyperkalemia.

Most individuals with PV are underweight for height and body build. This condition is thought to be related to the extremely increased rate of caloric consumption required by the hypermetabolism occurring in the bone marrow.

Later clinical manifestations of PV include those related to abnormal blood cells, in addition to hypercellularity and hypermetabolism. Even though the number of circulating erythrocytes is greatly increased, oxygen-binding capacity of these cells is impaired, and the individual may experience severe generalized hypoxia. In spite of having so many erythrocytes and platelets, individuals with PV have a tendency to bleed. The actual mechanism behind the bleeding tendency is not well understood and may be related to (1) abnormal platelet membranes that don't "stick together" well to form stable platelet plugs; or (2) insufficient amounts of fibrin present in formed clots as compared with the number of red blood cells, causing the clot to be unstable and easily lysed (Rapaport, 1987).

Polycythemia vera is a malignant disease that progresses in severity over time. If left untreated, few people with PV live longer than 2 years. Death is usually a consequence of either infarction of essential organs or severe hemorrhage. In the past, treatment has been directed toward increasing mean survival time but not curing the disorder. Conservative management with repeated phlebotomies (two to five times per week) can prolong life for 5 to 10 years. As the disease progresses, more intensive therapies that suppress bone marrow activity are indicated. These therapies include administration of oral alkylating agents and irradiation with injections of radioactive phosphorus. An experimental treatment aimed at cure for PV is allogeneic bone marrow transplantation. This treatment is promising, but the results are too limited at present to generalize its application to polycythemia vera.

Immune Function Alteration

The chronically rising peripheral white-cell count causes the individual with PV to experience immune function alterations. In spite of the leukocytosis, general immune function is depressed. Circulating lymphocytes are greatly decreased. While the individual may remain immune to diseases and substances to which antibodies have already been generated, the individual's capacity to develop immunities to new antigens is severely impaired. The granulocytic leukocytes in the peripheral blood, although greatly increased in number, are largely immature and nonfunctional. Thus, even though many neutrophils are present, because they are not functionally mature the individual experiences the same immune consequences as someone with profound neutropenia.

Case Presentation

Larry is a 55-year-old man who was seen by his company's physician for a routine annual physical. At that time his face was purplish red with suffused, cyanotic lips. His blood pressure was 188/110 mm Hg with a full, bounding pulse. Larry's spleen was three times normal size and was palpable below the left costal margin. His liver was also moderately enlarged, palpable 4 cm below the right costal margin. He was found to have lost 22 lb over the past year, which put him slightly below normal for his height and body build.

Larry stated that he had not noticed any major change in his activity level over the past year but that he felt tired more quickly. He also stated that he felt thirsty much of the time and was being "driven crazy" by intense skin itching, especially at night. His hemorrhoids, which had been present for a number of years and had been treated with over-the-counter external preparations, recently seemed larger and tended to bleed very easily.

Larry's complete blood count was abnormal. His red-cell count was 8 million/cu mm, with a hematocrit of 62 per cent and a hemoglobin of 18.5 gm/dl. His platelets were 500,000/cu mm. His white-cell count showed a total of 14,000 leukocytes/cu mm. The differential count showed 10 per cent lymphocytes, 1 per cent eosinophils, 1 per cent monocytes, 25 per cent band forms, and 60 per cent segmented neutrophils. A bone marrow aspiration showed marked hypercellularity, with increased numbers of proerythroblasts and megakaryoblasts (precursors of mature red blood cells and platelets).

At this time Larry was diagnosed with polycythemia vera. His treatment regimen consisted of phlebotomy two to three times per week. He remained stable with this treatment for 5 years, at which time he was hospitalized for a posterior-wall myocardial infarction. His complete blood count and bone marrow smear indicated progression of the disease. Larry's total red-cell count was 16 million/cu mm, with a hematocrit of 77 per cent and a platelet count of 800,000/cu mm. His white-cell count showed a total of 50,000 leukocytes/cu mm. The differential count showed 2 per cent lymphocytes, 1 per cent eosinophils, 1 per cent monocytes, 22 per cent band forms, 3 per cent segmented neutrophils, and 62 per cent metamyelocytes. (Please refer to Chapter 15 for a detailed plan of care for immunocompromised patients.)

SELECTED BIBLIOGRAPHY

Alkire, K., & Collingwood, J. (1990). Physiology of blood and bone marrow. *Seminars in Oncology Nursing, 6*(2), 99.
Collins, P. (1990). Diagnosis and treatment of chronic leukemia. *Seminars in Oncology Nursing, 6*(1), 31.
Hays, K. (1990). Physiology of normal bone marrow. *Seminars in Oncology Nursing, 6*(1), 3.
Oniboni, A. (1990). Infection in the neutropenic patient. *Seminars in Oncology Nursing, 6*(1), 50.
Pitot, H. (1986). *Fundamentals of oncology* (3rd ed.). New York: Marcel Dekker.
Rapaport, S. (1987). *Introduction to hematology* (2nd ed.). Philadelphia: J.B. Lippincott.
Robbins, S., & Kumar, V. (1987). *Basic pathology* (4th ed.). Philadelphia: W.B. Saunders.
Yeomans, A., & Harle, M. (1990). Myelodysplastic syndromes. *Seminars in Oncology Nursing, 6*(1), 9.

9

MULTIPLE MYELOMA

The disease multiple myeloma is the most common malignant condition of B-lymphocyte plasma cells. The malignancy is characterized by the unbalanced proliferation of a single clone of plasma cells. The neoplastic or malignant plasma cells continue their normal differentiated functions of synthesis and secretion of immunoglobulins, most commonly either IgG or IgA. Although these immunoglobulins are essentially normal, their disproportionate synthesis, along with the synthesis of free light chains (known as Bence Jones proteins), leads to a disproportion or unbalancing of other immune system actions. Multiple myeloma and its variants usually have two distinctly different phases, both of which disrupt normal immune function to some degree and can cause the patient to express signs and symptoms of immunosuppression. Primary complications of the disease include skeletal involvement, renal failure, and infection (Fig. 9-1).

INCIDENCE

The annual incidence of multiple myeloma is 3 per 100,000 population (Osserman, Merlini, & Butler, 1987), with new cases in 1990 estimated at 11,800 (Silverberg, Boring, & Squires, 1990). The disease is slightly more common in males than in females. Blacks are at higher risk than whites, with multiple myeloma comprising 2.1 per cent of malignancies, compared with 1.1 per cent for whites. Median age of onset is about 70 years (Salmon & Cassady, 1989), with a peak incidence between 75 and 80 (Blattner, 1980).

There is evidence to suggest an occasional familial relationship for certain cases of multiple myeloma (Blattner, 1980; Alexander & Benninghoff, 1965). In addition, a number of studies have noted an increase in polyclonal immu-

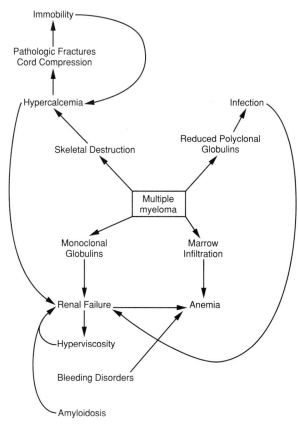

FIGURE 9-1. Complications of multiple myeloma.

noglobulin levels in relatives of individuals with multiple myeloma (Blattner, 1980; Maldonado & Kyle, 1974). These findings may indicate the presence of an inherited impairment in immunoregulation.

There has also been reported a familial aggregation of multiple myeloma and other lymphoreticular disorders with degenerative or demyelinating diseases of the central nervous system, such as Parkinson's disease and Alzheimer's disease (Grufferman, Cohen, Delzell, Morrison, Schold, & Moore, 1989). The researchers suggest that the phenomenon discovered in their review of 439 myeloma cases may be indicative of a group of "protean diseases," which are characterized by a common genetic predisposition and variable disease expression. Further study is needed to determine the relationship between the two disease processes.

Cytogenetic studies have revealed chromosomal abnormalities associated with multiple myeloma. The most commonly reported alteration, 14q +, involves translocation of chromosomal fragments to the terminal region of the long arm on chromosome 14. This site is the locus for the gene responsible for immunoglobulin heavy-chain proteins (Nishida et al., 1989a). Other translocations at this site have been associated with a variety of B-cell malignancies (Nishida, Tanikawi, Misawa, & Abe, 1989b).

Ionizing radiation exposure also has been implicated in the development of multiple myeloma. Excess numbers of cases have been noted among radiologists, workers at nuclear processing plants, and atomic bomb survivors in Japan (Cuzick, 1981; Ichimaru, Ishmaru, Mikami, & Matsunaga, 1979; Gilbert, Petersen, & Buchanan, 1989). A twofold to sixfold increase in incidence is noted only after a follow-up period of 15 to 25 years (Oken, 1984).

Other possible occupational exposures that may be linked to multiple myeloma include asbestos, arsenic, lead vapors, plastics, petrochemicals, and wood or leather working (Oken, 1984). The data to date are not strong enough to support conclusively an association between these occupational exposures and the development of myeloma. However, it is possible that an inadequate follow-up period for workers in high-risk industries does not identify myeloma cases that develop late in life.

PATHOPHYSIOLOGY

Antibody-Mediated Immunity

As a B-cell neoplasm, immunodeficiency secondary to multiple myeloma involves primarily antibody-mediated immunity. The proliferation of malignant plasma cells results in the production of a monoclonal immunoglobulin or paraprotein. The monoclonal immunoglobulin is referred to as an M protein with the "M" referring to monoclonal. In contrast, a normal immune response will evoke a heterogeneous mixture of immunoglobulins from multiple clones (polyclonal). In some cases, paraproteins will be nearly identical to their normal counterpart, with extreme homogeneity due to monoclonal origin as their only distinguished characteristic (Broder & Waldman, 1985).

Multiple myeloma results in a profound depression of antibody-mediated immunity through decreased production of normal immunoglobulin and antibody. Research using a mouse model has demonstrated a feedback mechanism that may explain the process through which the immunodeficiency develops.

In reporting the findings of a series of studies, Kennard and Zolla-Paznur (1980) described two factors that mediated immunosuppression in mice with myeloma. The first, plasmacytoma (PC) factor, is a protein produced by the myeloma cells. PC factor has no direct immunosuppressive properties. However, it stimulates macrophages to produce the second factor, plasmacytoma-induced macrophage substance (PIMS). PIMS acts by converting normal macrophages to become suppressor macrophages, which inhibit antibody production. The researchers postulated that normal plasma cells produce a negative regulatory signal that suppresses the production of antibodies once an adequate humoral response has been accomplished. The phenomenon demonstrated in their research would, therefore, represent a pathologic exaggeration of normal plasma-cell and macrophage functions.

Whereas decreased antibody synthesis is probably the primary factor in the reduction of polyclonal immunoglobulin, an increase in the rate of IgG catabolism further complicates the antibody immune status in patients with IgG paraproteins (Broder & Waldman, 1980). The rate of IgG catabolism varies in direct proportion to IgG concentration. As the IgG level increases, so will the rate of IgG catabolism. In some myeloma patients, the survival half-time of IgG may decline from the normal 20 days to as low as 11 days (Waldman & Strober, 1969). IgG survival is not affected by concentrations of other immunoglobulins.

Cell-Mediated Immunity

While the defects of antibody-mediated immunity are well documented in multiple myeloma, interference with cell-mediated immunity is less clear. In general, it appears that although the capacity for response to a new antigen may be impaired, expression of a previously developed response is less severely affected. Depression of cellular immunity, when present, has not been demonstrated at the same level of magnitude seen with humoral immunity.

Certain T-cell subsets may have a role in the decreased polyclonal immunoglobulin production associated with myeloma. Elevated numbers of T suppressor/cytotoxic cells (OKT8) have been measured in myeloma patients, while the numbers of T helper/inducer cells (OKT4) have been decreased. The OKT4 demonstrated normal activity; however, the activity of OKT8 cells was significantly enhanced. It has been suggested that the increased T-cell suppressor function may represent one factor contributing to immunoglobulin deficiency (Oken & Kay, 1981).

Inflammation and Nonspecific Immune Function

Research using a variety of techniques has demonstrated several defects in nonspecific immunity among patients with multiple myeloma. Granulocyte migration was impaired in 15 of 25 patients studied by Ziegler, Hansen, & Penny (1975). Two studies have reported a defect in granulocyte adhesiveness (Penny & Galton, 1966; Spitler et al., 1975). Inhibition of phagocytic activity has been observed, along with a decrease in intracellular lysozyme concentration in circulating granulocytes (Karle, Hansen, & Plesner, 1976).

Furthermore, patients with multiple myeloma may have defects in certain components of the complement system. Decreased levels of components C1q, C2, and C4 may compromise activation of C3, which has a critical role in granulocyte phagocytosis (Broder & Waldman, 1985; Spitler et al., 1975).

CLINICAL EVALUATION

Diagnosis

Diagnosis of multiple myeloma is usually established by the presence of an increase in abnormal, atypical, or immature plasma cells in the bone marrow. In addition, either serum/urine electrophoresis, revealing a monoclonal protein, or x-ray films, demonstrating osteolytic lesions characteristic of myeloma, are required to confirm the diagnosis (Oken, 1984). Clinical studies commonly used to establish the diagnosis and the extent of the disease are listed in Table 9–1.

Alteration in Immunoglobulin Production

Serum protein electrophoresis and immunoelectrophoresis will often reveal substantial quantities of a homogeneous gamma globulin, usually IgG or IgA, in 80 per cent of the patients with multiple myeloma. Most of the remaining 20 per cent will not demonstrate the abnormal serum protein, but will excrete large amounts of monoclonal light chains (Bence Jones proteins) in their urine. Bence Jones protein excretion in the latter group averages 4 gm/day and may be as high as 40 gm/day. In contrast, only 25 per cent of patients with myeloma and complete serum monoclonal immunoglobulins excrete Bence Jones proteins at levels greater than 1 gm/day (Alexanian, 1985).

TABLE 9–1. Tests to Diagnose the Presence and Extent of Multiple Myeloma.

Blood components	Hematocrit, hemoglobin, white-cell count, platelets bone marrow aspiration
Blood chemistry	Total protein, blood urea nitrogen, uric acid, calcium, aklaline phosphatase
Differentiation of serum proteins	Albumin level, M protein, quantitate immunoglobulins
24-hour urine components	Creatinine clearance, albumin, quantitate immunoglobulins and Bence Jones proteins
Skeletal	Radiographic examination of skull and long bones, analysis of joint effusions for presence of amyloid
Neurologic	Myelogram, lumbar puncture, cerebrospinal fluid analysis for concentrations of cells, proteins, glucose, and chloride

(Adapted from Plasma cell neoplasms by D. Bergsagel and W. Rider, 1985. In V. Devita, S. Hellman, and S. Rosenberg [Eds.], *Cancer: Principles and practice of oncology* [2nd ed.] [p. 1753]. Philadelphia: J.B. Lippincott. Copyright 1985 by J.B. Lippincott. Reprinted by permission.)

The reduced capacity of patients with myeloma to produce functional im-munoglobulin places them at high risk for the development of life-threatening infection. Infection remains a common presenting symptom in cases of mye-loma and is the cause of death in at least 50 per cent of patients with myeloma (Broder & Waldman, 1985; Oken, 1984). Pathogens most frequently involved are *Streptococcus pneumoniae* and *Staphylococcus aureus,* causing recurrent bouts of pneumonia, and *Escherichia coli* and Pseudomonas, Proteus, and Kleb-siella species, responsible for urinary tract and systemic infections. The inci-dence of gram-negative infections has been increasing, due in part to higher numbers of hospital-acquired and resistant organisms (Shaikh, et al., 1982). In fact, one study reported that the four fatal infections in the population re-viewed (39 patients with myeloma) were hospital-acquired (Eperson et al., 1984).

A biphasic pattern of incidence has been documented for infection in mye-loma patients. Pneumonia, resulting from *S. pneumoniae* and *Haemophilus influenzae,* tends to occur within the first 8 months following diagnosis. Gram-negative organisms causing bacteremia predominate later, with advancing re-fractory disease (Savage, Lindenbaum, & Garrett, 1982). A fairly consistent finding was that infections developed in patients with normal neutrophil counts (Cohen & Rundles, 1975), indicating the important role of immunoglobulin impairment as a risk factor.

Efforts to increase immune protection against invasion by pathogenic or-ganisms include pneumococcal vaccination (Lazarus et al., 1980) and admin-istration of gamma globulin (Jacobson & Zolla-Paznur, 1986). The antibody response to vaccination was found to be highly variable among the 13 patients with myeloma studied, with overall response depressed. Based on these find-ings, the Health and Public Policy Committee of the American College of Phy-sicians has recommended that the vaccine be offered to patients with myeloma, at the same time cautioning them about the limitations of potential benefit (Health and Public Policy Committee, 1986).

Intramuscular injection of gamma globulin has shown no benefit in re-ducing the incidence of infection. Although a Phase I study of intravenous gamma globulin showed promise in decreasing risk, additional study is re-quired to determine its role in preventing infection in myeloma patients (Health and Public Policy Committee, 1986).

Skeletal Involvement

The most common symptoms associated with multiple myeloma are a con-sequence of bone destruction: intractable pain, hypercalcemia, pathologic frac-tures (particularly of the ribs and the clavicles) (Alexanian, 1985; Kintzer, Posenow, & Kyle, 1978), and vertebral collapse with spinal cord compression. Research reported by Mundy et al. (1974) revealed the presence of osteoclast-activating factors (OAF) in areas of the bone adjacent to myeloma cell deposits.

OAF is a cytokine associated with bone resorption, local destruction, and, in 20 per cent of patients with myeloma, secondary hypercalcemia (Mundy, 1987).

Patients typically present with bone pain exacerbated by movement. When pain is persistent during periods of inactivity, the presence of pathologic fracture must be considered.

Approximately 70 per cent of patients with myeloma will exhibit the characteristic "punched-out" lesions on x-ray films (Alexanian, 1985). The most common sites of skeletal involvement include the skull, ribs, pelvis, and long bones. Bone scans are generally not helpful in evaluating extent of disease, even in the presence of bone pain (Wahner, Kyle, & Beabout, 1980). Serum alkaline phosphatase, an indicator of osteoblastic rather than osteoclastic activity, is usually within normal limits unless pathologic fractures are present (Mundy and Bertolini, 1986).

A randomized double blind trial of sodium fluoride, 50 mg twice daily, and calcium carbonate, 1 gm four times daily, vs. placebo resulted in improved bone formation and volume in the treatment group (Kyle et al., 1975). No increased benefit was shown with the addition of vitamin D (Kyle & Jowsey, 1980).

Renal Failure

Hypercalcemia and excretion of Bence Jones protein are the primary causes of renal failure in patients with multiple myeloma (Alexanian, Barlogie, & Dixon, 1990a). Production of Bence Jones proteinuria places the patient at high risk for the development of "myeloma kidney," severe irreversible renal damage caused by precipitation of light chains in the renal tubules. Eventually, the protein deposits obstruct the distal and occasionally the proximal convoluted tubules of the kidney nephrons (Alexanian, 1985). Early evidence of renal tubule damage includes the inability of the kidney to acidify and concentrate the urine (Bergsagel & Rider, 1985). As renal damage progresses, the presence of casts, comprised of precipitated proteins, will be noted on routine urinalysis. Depending on the type of protein excreted, the urine may also test positive for the presence of albumin.

Any patient with an unexplained proteinuria should be evaluated for the presence of Bence Jones protein by urinary protein electrophoresis before other diagnostic procedures are initiated. Bence Jones proteinuria has been shown to increase significantly the risk of irreversible renal failure following intravenous pyelography (IVP) or the injection of other intravenous contrast material. The diagnosis of multiple myeloma must be excluded to prevent inadvertent precipitation of nephropathy (Osserman, Merlini, & Butler, 1987).

Other factors contributing to renal failure in patients with myeloma include hypercalcemia, urine acid nephropathy, dehydration, plasma cell infiltration of the kidneys, and the use of nephrotoxic antibiotics (Alexanian, 1985; Salmon & Cassady, 1989).

Blood and Bone Marrow Involvement

The major hematologic effects of multiple myeloma include anemia, hyperviscosity, and coagulation disorders. Infiltration and the replacement of bone marrow by plasma cells causes moderate to severe anemia in 25 per cent of patients with multiple myeloma (Alexanian, 1985). The anemia is compounded by other disease-related factors, including renal failure and gastrointestinal bleeding, and pancytopenia secondary to treatment (Ting et al., 1982). In some patients, elevated serum gamma globulins will result in an expansion of the plasma volume. The dilutional effect causes a further decrease in hematocrit (Alexanian, 1985). Excessive folate and vitamin B_{12} utilization by the plasma cell neoplasm may explain the increased incidence of pernicious anemia associated with myeloma (Salmon & Cassady, 1989).

Results of a pilot study indicate a possible role for erythropoietin in the treatment of myeloma-related anemia. Ludwig, Fritz, Kotzmann, Hocker, Gisslinger, & Barnas (1990) administered the agent to 13 patients with myeloma three times per week. The anemias resolved, with patients no longer requiring blood component therapy. The disease itself remained stable during the treatment. Moreover, the patients reported an increase in performance status and a subjective improvement in quality of life. Additional study is necessary to establish the efficacy of erythropoietin in this patient population.

Hyperviscosity syndrome is the result of the increased concentration of abnormal proteins in the blood and has been observed in approximately 5 per cent of patients with myeloma. The manifestations of hyperviscosity fall primarily into four subgroups:

1. Bleeding tendency, marked by bruising, epistaxis, purpura, and oozing from mucosal surfaces;
2. Dilation and segmentation of retinal and conjunctival veins, resulting in retinal hemorrhages and papilledema;
3. Neurologic symptoms, including weakness, fatigue, anorexia, headaches, visual disturbances, transient paresis, and coma; and
4. Distention of peripheral vessels, increased vascular resistance, and cardiac failure (Salmon & Cassady, 1989).

Hemorrhagic complications associated with myeloma result from altered platelet function and interaction of paraproteins with coagulation factors.

Neurologic Syndromes

Neurologic complications may result directly from the neoplasm via tumor growth and metastasis or indirectly as a paraneoplastic process, such as hypercalcemia.

Spinal cord compression due to the tumor encroachment or bony collapse was at one time reported in as many as one third of all patients treated for multiple myeloma (Silverstein & Doniger, 1963). However, with earlier diagnosis and improved treatment methods, the incidence has declined to 10 to 15 per cent. Patients at greatest risk, those with thoracic spine lesions, should be routinely assessed for back pain and sensorimotor impairment heralding the onset of cord compression (Dahlstrom, Jarpe, & Lindstrom, 1979).

Meningeal myelomatosis is a rare complication associated with accelerated growth during the late stages of the disease. Plasma cell infiltration of the meninges should be considered when other etiologies for neurologic symptoms have been ruled out (Spiers et al., 1980).

Four types of myeloma-related peripheral neuropathy have been described (Oken, 1984; Kelly et al., 1981). The first two, carpal-tunnel syndrome and diffuse sensorimotor polyneuropathy, are the result of amyloidosis. Amyloidosis is a comprehensive term used for a variety of conditions associated with tissue infiltrates comprised of insoluble proteins, protein–polysaccharide complexes, or both. Sites most commonly involved in patients with myeloma include tongue, heart, gastrointestinal tract, skeletal and smooth muscle, carpal ligaments, nerves, and skin (Osserman et al., 1987). With advancing disease, amyloid desposits may be found in the kidney, spleen, liver, and endocrine glands. Diagnosis is made on the basis of biopsy and special stains.

In addition to amyloid-induced impairment, progressive sensorimotor polyneuropathy occurs in less than 5 per cent of patients and does not respond well to treatment (Oken, 1984). Finally, osteosclerotic myeloma, accounting for less than 1 per cent of all cases of myeloma, frequently produces a predominantly motor neuropathy that improves following radiation of the osteosclerotic lesion or systemic chemotherapy.

TREATMENT

Multiple myeloma is an incurable, although sometimes treatable, disease. Approximately one third of all patients with myeloma will not respond to therapy, and some will succumb to aggressive disease within weeks of diagnosis (Kyle, Greipp, & Gertz, 1986; Sporn & McIntyre, 1986).

Evaluating the response to therapy has not always been easy. The nature of the disease does not readily lend itself to the identification of objective response criteria; however, criteria established by the Southwest Oncology Group (SWOG), listed in Table 9–2, have proved to be the most reliable.

Chemotherapy

Alkylating agents have historically shown activity in the treatment of multiple myeloma with cyclophosphamide or melphalan with or without prednisone the drugs of choice. Regimens combining alkylators, nitrosoureas, antitumor antibiotics, and mitotic inhibitors have not shown a consistent benefit

TABLE 9-2. Criteria for Determining Response to Therapy for Myeloma.

Definite improvement*
  Decrease serum M protein value to less than 25 per cent of pretreatment value
  Synthetic index of IgA, IgG M proteins equal to the serum value
  Decrease globulin concentration in 24-hour urine sample to less than 10 per cent of
    pretreatment value and less than 0.2 gm/24 hr on two occasions 4 weeks apart
  No increase in size or number of lytic skeletal lesions
  Recalcification lytic lesions
  Serum calcium within normal range
  Hematocrit greater than 27 per cent
Improved
  Decrease in serum M-protein synthesis to between 25 and 50 per cent of pretreatment
    value
Unresponsive
  Fail to meet the above criteria for responsive or improved patients.

*Must satisfy all listed criteria.
(Adapted from Plasma cell neoplasms by S.E. Salmon and J.R. Cassady, 1989. In V. Devita, S. Hellman,
and S. Rosenberg [Eds.], *Cancer: Principles and practice of oncology* [3rd ed.] [p. 1868]. Philadelphia: J.B.
Lippincott.)

for either response or survival. Cost for therapy and the risk of toxicity are important considerations prior to initiating multiple-agent treatment (Sporn & McIntyre, 1986).

There is evidence to suggest that patients with multiple myeloma are at an increased risk for development of nonlymphocytic leukemia, as the two diseases have been noted to occur simultaneously (Kyle, Pierre, & Bayard, 1970; Rosner & Grunwald, 1974). The use of alkylating agents in the treatment of myeloma adds an additional and substantial risk (Kyle, Pierre, & Bayard, 1975; Bergsagel et al., 1979). Intermittent, as opposed to continuous, administration of alkylators is less likely to result in leukemia development. It has been suggested that using an intravenous rather than an oral route may lessen the chance of leukemogenesis, although there is no documentation to provide support for this supposition (Sporn & McIntyre, 1986).

VAD-based regimens (vincristine, doxorubicin, and dexamethasone) have been recommended for patients with aggressive or advanced disease or who do not respond to meyshalan plus Preanisone (MP), (Alexanian, Barlogie, & Tucker, 1990b). Although these regimens produce rapid and dramatic tumor responses, they show no survival benefit as compared with MP (Kyle, 1990).

Corticosteroids

Prednisone is believed to have an effect on myeloma through steroid-induced hypercatabolism of proteins that produces a negative nitrogen balance and a nonspecific decrease in serum protein concentrations (Bergsagel & Rider, 1985). In addition, corticosteroids reverse hypercalcemia by blocking the action of OAF, thereby reducing bone resorption (Raisz et al., 1975).

Immunotherapy

Early research suggested responsiveness of myeloma to immunotherapy in a study of alternating courses of alkylating agents and bacille Calmette–Guérin (BCG) vaccine. Although remission and survival data did not indicate a significant improvement, a trend was evident in the direction predicted (Alexanian et al., 1981).

Phase II studies of recombinant interferon-α (rIFNa2, Intron A®) as a single agent for treatment of relapsing or refractory myeloma has demonstrated benefit for certain patients. As has been seen in other studies, heavily pretreated patients were less likely to achieve a response to therapy than those for whom treatment with a single alkylating agent had failed (Cooper & Welander, 1986).

More recently, in vitro studies have shown evidence of colony growth inhibition when standard regimens are given with recombinant interferon-α (Barlogie & Alexanian, 1989; Kyle, 1990). In a pilot investigation, Cooper and Welander (1986) examined the feasibility of combining varying doses of interferon-α with melphalan and prednisone. In this small series, an overall response of 75 per cent was noted; however, a large sample with long-term follow-up is indicated in order to determine what role, if any, immunotherapy has in the treatment of multiple myeloma.

A major factor limiting the use of chemotherapy is subsequent prolonged granulocytopenia, resulting in potentially fatal infections. Barlogie et al. (1990) attempted to induce granulocyte recovery following high-dose melphalan by administering granulocyte–macrophage colony-stimulating factor (GM-CSF). In patients with adequate marrow reserve (younger age, less prior chemotherapy) duration of neutropenia and thrombocytopenia was significantly reduced.

Autologous Bone Marrow Transplantation (ABMT)

Failure to achieve cure of myeloma has led researchers to investigate high-dose melphalan with or without total body irradiation followed by ABMT as a possible treatment strategy. However, relapse rates remain high, probably because of incomplete eradication of the disease and contamination of autologous marrow with myeloma cells or their precursors (Jagannath et al., 1990; Kyle, 1990). Further study of ABMT in patients with myeloma includes the use of monoclonal antibodies to purge myeloma cells from the marrow and more intensive chemotherapy prior to ABMT (Alexanian & Barlogie, 1990; Anderson et al., 1991).

Radiation Therapy

The role of radiation in multiple myeloma is limited to palliation, particularly in cases of skeletal destruction and lesions causing spinal cord or nerve root compression. Large osteolytic lesions in long bones may require surgical intervention for stabilization prior to radiation because of the high potential for pathologic fractures.

CASE STUDIES

Multiple myeloma may present as a slowly progressing disease, although some patients will have advanced disease at the time of diagnosis. The following case studies provide examples of the two different presentations for myeloma.

Case Study I

Mrs. B. is a 72-year-old black woman who has been treated by her family physician for left arm pain. Injections of nonsteroidal antiinflammatory agents were given for several months without improvement. When an x-ray film revealed a large lytic lesion in the left proximal humerus, she was referred to an orthopedic surgeon for evaluation and stabilization. Laboratory studies done on admission demonstrated pancytopenia. Bone marrow aspiration and a biopsy were performed, with results indicative of multiple myeloma. Normal hematopoietic contents were moderately decreased, with marked plasmacytosis. On the following day, Mrs. B. underwent biopsy of the lesion, with stabilization of the humerus. Pathologic studies were again consistent with the diagnosis of multiple myeloma.

Serum calcium, electrolytes, blood urea nitrogen, and creatinine were within normal limits. Her white-cell count was 2600, hemoglobin 10.7, and platelet count 84,000. Urine electrophoresis was normal, with Bence Jones protein absent. Serum immunoelectrophoresis demonstrated a monoclonal IgG, with both IgA and IgM decreased. Quantitative analysis revealed an IgG level of 4950 (normal, 530 to 1420), IgA 22 (normal, 70 to 290), and IgM 53 (normal, 50 to 375).

Mrs. B. was given pneumococcal vaccine polyvalent (Pneumovac®) prophylactically. Treatment was initiated with melphalan 10 mg and prednisone 100 mg (MP) orally daily for 4 days, followed by prednisone 20 mg orally every other day. Follow-up visits were scheduled every 2 weeks to reevaluate her hematologic and immunologic status. At the same time, radiation treatments were delivered to the involved area in the left humerus. Physical therapy two to three times weekly enabled Mrs. B. to recover use of her left arm.

Mrs. B. responded well to treatment over the next several months. Within 3 months, her IgG level had fallen to 1560 and she remained hematologically stable on MP. However, 5 months after diagnosis, Mrs. B. fell, slightly displacing the left humerus, but no new fractures were noted. Laboratory studies at that time included a white-cell count of 3000, hemoglobin 10.1, and 115,000 platelets, with IgG 1180. Electrolytes, blood urea nitrogen and creatinine remained within normal limits.

Mrs. B. is an example of stable disease, well controlled on oral chemotherapy. The primary nursing concern for her is safety, to minimize the risk of trauma to the left humerus. In addition, she is at risk of complications associated with the disease and treatment-induced alterations of immune function. A nursing plan of care specific for the needs of Mrs. B. would include patient care problems 1 (potential for systemic infection), 4 (potential for pulmonary dysfunction), 11 (potential for inadequate oxygenation), and 12 (potential for bleeding) as described in Chapter 15.

Case Study 2

Mr. P. is a 45-year-old white male with a history of chronic low back pain. When the pain began to increase in severity, he consulted a chiropractor. Over the next 3 months, his condition worsened until he was barely able to get out of bed. He presented to the emergency room, where x-ray films of the lumbosacral spine revealed multiple lytic lesions. A bone marrow biopsy confirmed the diagnosis of multiple myeloma. Other laboratory results included serum calcium 15.9, blood urea nitrogen 37, and creatinine 3.1. His urine tested positive for Bence Jones protein. Serum protein electrophoresis demonstrated the presence of a light-chain kappa protein. Mr. P.'s renal failure and hypercalcemia responded well to hydration and furosemide. He was fitted with an orthopedic back brace and started on a treatment regimen that included cyclophosphamide, vincristine, BCNU (carmustine), melphalan, and prednisone.

Six weeks later, Mr. P. was presented in the emergency room, complaining of severe back pain and an inability to walk for 2 days. Spine films revealed compression fractures at T4, T12, and L1. He was admitted for pain management and treatment of spinal cord compression. The nursing plan of care specific for the current needs of Mr. P. includes patient care problems 1 (potential for systemic infection), 4 (potential for pulmonary dysfunction), 10 (potential genitourinary infection), 11 (potential for inadequate oxygenation), and 12 (potential for bleeding) as described in Chapter 15.

SUMMARY

Patients with multiple myeloma experience immunosuppression as a result of both the disease pathology and the current methods of treatment. The type of immunosuppression related to the disease itself primarily involves defective antibody-mediated immune function with varied impairment of other specific leukocyte functions. Patients with multiple myeloma are at a greatly increased risk for a variety of infections, with gram-negative bacteria being the most common causative organism. Bacterial pneumonia and systemic infections are major causes of death in the patient with multiple myeloma. While many people experience such infections during cancer treatment as a result of neutropenia, patients with multiple myeloma experience these infections with near normal granulocyte/neutrophil counts. Thus, the standard complete blood count with differential white-cell count is not a reliable predictor of risk for infection among these patients. Generally, patients with multiple myeloma have some protection against viruses to which they were previously exposed; however, many patients are unable to generate antibodies against new viruses. This deficiency increases the patient's susceptibility to common viral infections such as colds, flu, and hepatitis A.

SELECTED BIBLIOGRAPHY

Alexander, L., & Benninghoff, D. (1965). Familial multiple myeloma. *Journal of the National Medical Association, 57,* 471.

Alexanian, R. (1985). Diagnosis and management of multiple myeloma. In P. Wiernik, et al. (Eds.), *Neoplastic diseases of the blood* (p. 529). New York: Churchill Livingstone.

Alexanian, R., & Barlogie, B. (1990). New treatment strategies for multiple myeloma. *American Journal of Hematology, 35*(3), 194.

Alexanian, R., Barlogie, B., & Dixon, D. (1990a). Renal failure in patients with multiple myeloma: Pathogenesis and prognostic implications. *Archives of Internal Medicine, 150*(8), 1693.

Alexanian, R., Barlogie, B., & Tucker, S. (1990b). VAD-based regimens as primary treatment for multiple myeloma. *American Journal of Hematology, 33*(2), 86.

Alexanian, R., Salmon, S., Gutterman, J., et al. (1981). Chemoimmunotherapy for multiple myeloma. *Cancer, 47,* 1923.

Anderson, K., Barut, B., Ritz, J., Freedman, A., Takvorian, T., Rabinowe, S., Soiffer, R., Heflin, L., Coral, F., & Dear, K. (1991). Monoclonal antibody purged autologous bone marrow transplantation therapy for multiple myeloma. *Blood, 77*(4), 712.

Barlogie, B., & Alexanian, R. (1989). Second international workshop on myeloma: Advances in biology and therapy of multiple myeloma. *Cancer Research, 49*(24, Part 1), 7172.

Barlogie, B., Jagannath, S., Dixon, D., Cheson, B., Smallwood, L., Hendrickson, A., Purvis, J., Bonnem, E., & Alexanian, R. (1990). High-dose melphalan and granulocyte-macrophage colony-stimulating factor for refractory multiple myeloma. *Blood, 76*(4), 677.

Bergsagel, D., Bailey, A., Langley, G., et al. (1979). Chemotherapy of plasma-cell myeloma and incidence of acute leukemia. *New England Journal of Medicine, 301,* 743.

Bergsagel, D., & Rider, W. (1985). Plasma cell neoplasms. In V. Devita, S. Hellman, & S. Rosenberg (Eds.), *Cancer: Principles and practice of oncology* (2nd ed.) (p. 1753). Philadelphia: J.B. Lippincott.

Blattner, W. (1980). Epidemiology of multiple myeloma and related plasma cell disorders: An analytical review. In M. Potter (Ed.), *Progress in myeloma* (p. 1). New York: Elsevier/North-Holland Press.

Broder, S., & Waldman, T. (1980). Characteristics of multiple myeloma as an immunodeficiency disease. In M. Potter (Ed.), *Progress in myeloma* (p. 151). New York: Elsevier/North-Holland Press.

Broder, S., & Waldman, T. (1985). Multiple myeloma and immunodeficiency. In P. Wiernik, et al. (Eds.), *Neoplastic diseases of the blood* (p. 483). New York: Churchill Livingstone.

Cohen, H., & Rundles, R. (1975). Managing the complications of plasma cell myeloma. *Archives of Internal Medicine, 135,* 177

Cooper, M., & Welander, C. (1986). Interferons in the treatment of multiple myeloma. *Seminars in Oncology, 13,* 334.

Cuzick, J. (1981). Radiation-induced myelomatosis. *New England Journal of Medicine, 304,* 204.

Dahlstrom, U., Jarpe, S., & Lindstrom, F. (1979). Paraplegia in myelomatosis: A study of 20 cases. *Acta Medico Scandinavica, 205,* 173.

Eperson, F., Birgens, H., Herta, J., et al. (1984). Current patterns of bacterial infection in myelomatosis. *Scandanavian Journal of Infectious Diseases, 16,* 169.

Gilbert, E., Petersen, G., & Buchanan, J. (1989). Mortality of workers at the Hanford site: 1945–1981. *Health Physics, 56*(1), 11.

Grufferman, S., Cohen, H., Delzell, E., Morrison, M., Schold, S., & Moore, J. (1989). Familial aggregation of multiple myeloma and central nervous system diseases. *Journal of the American Geriatrics Society, 37*(4), 303.

Health and Public Policy Committee of the American College of Physicians (1986). Position papers: Pneumococcal vaccine. *Annals of Internal Medicine, 104,* 118.

Ichimaru, M., Ishmaru, T., Mikami, M., & Matsunaga, M. (1979). Multiple myeloma among atomic bomb survivors, Hiroshima and Nagasaki, 1950–1976. Hiroshima, Japan: Radiation Effects Research Foundation.

Jacobson, D., & Zolla-Paznur, S. (1986). Immunosuppression and infection in multiple myeloma. *Seminars in Oncology, 13,* 282.

Jagannath, S., Barlogie, B., Dicke, K., Alexanian, R., Zagars, G., Cheson, B., Lemaistre, F., Smallwood, L., Pruitt, K., & Dixon, D. (1990). Autologous bone marrow transplantation in multiple myeloma: Identification of prognostic factors. *Blood, 76*(9), 1860.

Karle, H., Hansen, N., & Plesner, T. (1976). Neutrophil defect in multiple myeloma: Studies in intraneutrophilic lysozyme in multiple myeloma and malignant lymphoma. *Scandinavian Journal of Haematology, 17,* 62.

Kelly, J., Kyle, R., Miles, J., et al. (1981). The spectrum of peripheral neuropathy in multiple myeloma. *Neurology, 31,* 24.

Kennard, J., & Zolla-Paznur, S. (1980). Origin and function of suppressor macrophages in myeloma. *Journal of Immunology, 124,* 263.

Kintzer, J., Posenow, E., & Kyle, R. (1978). Thoracic and pulmonary abnormalities in multiple myeloma: A review of 958 cases. *Archives of Internal Medicine, 138,* 727.

Kyle, R. (1990). Newer approaches to the therapy of multiple myeloma. *Blood, 76*(9), 1678.

Kyle, R., Greipp, P., & Gertz, M. (1986). Treatment of refractory multiple myeloma in considerations for future therapy. *Seminars in Oncology, 13,* 326.

Kyle, R., Pierre, R., & Bayard, E. (1970). Multiple myeloma and acute myelomonocytic leukemia. *New England Journal of Medicine, 283,* 1121.

Kyle, R., Pierre, R., & Bayard, E. (1975). Multiple myeloma and acute leukemia associated with alkylating agents. *Archives of Internal Medicine, 135,* 185.

Kyle, R., & Jowsey, J. (1980). Effect of sodium fluoride, calcium carbonate and vitamin D on the skeleton in multiple myeloma. *Cancer, 45,* 1669.

Kyle, R., Jowsey, J., Kelly, P., et al. (1975). Multiple myeloma bone disease: The comparative effect of sodium fluoride and calcium carbonate or placebo. *New England Journal of Medicine, 293,* 1334.

Lazarus, H., Lederman, M., Lubin, A., et al. (1980). Pneumococcal vaccination: The response of patients with multiple myeloma. *American Journal of Medicine, 69,* 419.

Ludwig, H., Fritz, E., Kotzmann, H., Hocker, P., Gisslinger, H., & Barnas, U. (1990). Erythropoietin treatment of anemia associated with multiple myeloma. *New England Journal of Medicine, 322,* 1693.

Maldonado, J., & Kyle, R. (1974). Familial myeloma: Report of eight families and a study of serum proteins in their relatives. *American Journal of Medicine, 57,* 875.

Mundy, G. (1987). Bone resorption and turnover in health and disease. *Bone, 8,* Suppl. 9.

Mundy, G., & Bertolini, D. (1986). Bone destruction and hypercalcemia in plasma cell myeloma. *Seminars in Oncology, 13,* 291.

Mundy, G., Raisz, L., Cooper, R., et al. (1974). Evidence for the secretion of an osteoclast stimulating factor in myeloma. *New England Journal of Medicine, 291,* 1041.

Nishida, K., Taniwaki, M., Misawa, S., & Abe, T. (1989b). Nonrandom rearrangement of chromosome 14 at band q32.33 in human myeloid malignancies with mature B-cell phenotype. *Cancer Research, 49*(5), 1275.

Nishida, K., Yashige, H., Maekawa, T., Fujii, N., Taniwaki, M., Horiike, S., Misawa, S., Inazawa, J., & Abe, T. (1989a). Chromosome rearrangement, t(6:14)(p21.1;q32.3), in multiple myeloma. *British Journal of Haematology, 71*(2), 295.

Oken, M. (1984). Multiple myeloma. *Medical Clinics of North America, 68,* 757.

Oken, M., & Kay, N. (1981). T-cell sub-populations in multiple myeloma: Correlation with clinical disease status. *British Journal of Haematology, 49,* 629.

Osserman, E., Merlini, G., & Butler, V. (1987). Multiple myeloma and related plasma cell dyscrasias. *JAMA, 258,* 2930.

Penny, R., & Galton, D. (1966). Studies on neutrophil function. II. Pathological aspects. *British Journal of Haematology, 12,* 633.

Quesada, J., Alexanian, R., Hawkins, M., et al. (1986). Treatment of multiple myeloma with recombinant α-interferon. *Blood, 67,* 275.

Raisz, L., Luben, R., Mundy, G., et al. (1975). Effect of osteoclast activating factor from human leukocytes on bone metabolism. *Journal of Clinical Investigation, 56,* 408.

Rosner, F., & Grunwald, H. (1974). Multiple myeloma terminating in acute eukemia. *American Journal of Medicine, 57,* 927.

Salmon S., & Cassady, J. (1989). Plasma cell neoplasms. In V. Devita, S. Hellman, & S. Rosenberg (Eds.), *Cancer: Principles and practice of oncology* (3rd ed.) (p. 1853). Philadelphia: J.B. Lippincott.

Savage, D., Lindenbaum, J., & Garrett, T. (1982). Biphasic pattern of bacterial infection in multiple myeloma. *Annals of Internal Medicine, 96,* 47.

Shaikh, B., Lombard, R., Appelbaum, P., et al. (1982). Changing patterns of infections in patients with multiple myeloma. *Oncology, 39,* 78.

Silverberg, E., Boring, C., & Squires, T. (1990). 1990 cancer statistics. *CA—A Journal for Clinicians, 40*(1), 9.

Silverstein, A., & Doniger, D. (1963). Neurologic complications of myelomatosis. *Archives of Neurology, 9,* 534.

Spiers, A., Halpern, R., Ross, S., et al. (1980). Meningeal myelomatosis. *Archives of Internal Medicine, 140,* 256.

Spitler, L., Spath, P., Petz, L., et al. (1975). Phagocytes and C₄ in paraproteinaemia. *British Journal of Haematology, 29,* 279.

Sporn, J., & McIntyre, O. (1986). Chemotherapy of previously untreated multiple myeloma patients: An analysis of recent treatment results. *Seminars in Oncology, 13,* 318.

Tanake, H., Tanabe, O., Iwato, K., Asaoku, H., Ishikawa, H., Nobuyoshi, M., Kawano, M., & Kuramoto, A. (1989). Sensitive inhibitory effect of interferon-alpha on M-protein secretion of human myeloma cells. *Blood, 74*(5), 1718.

Ting, W., Cavill, C., Jacobs, A., et al. (1982). Anaemia in patients with myelomatosis. *British Journal of Cancer, 45,* 887.

Wahner, H., Kyle, R., & Beabout, J. (1980). Scintigraphic evaluation of the skeleton in multiple myeloma. *Mayo Clinic Proceedings, 55,* 739.

Waldman, T., & Strober, W. (1969). Metabolism of immunoglobulins. *Progress in Allergy, 13,* 1.

Ziegler, J., Hansen, P., & Penny, R. (1975). Leukocyte function in paraproteinaemia. *Australia New Zealand Journal of Medicine, 5,* 39.

Immunodeficiency Secondary to Medical Treatment

10

IMMUNOSUPPRESSION AS A RESULT OF CANCER TREATMENT

Cancer holds a unique position in its relationship with the immune system. First of all, immune system failure is thought to play a major part in the development and progression of malignancy. In addition, specific malignancies can cause alterations of the patient's immune response to the extent that some immunosuppression is evident. Finally, every form of cancer treatment alters the patient's immune function to some degree.

The diagnosis of cancer can and usually does fill a patient with fear. Along with the almost certain perception that all cancers are fatal are the patient's misgivings about cancer treatment. Most forms of cancer treatment have some temporary and some permanent unpleasant side effects.

CHEMOTHERAPY

Chemotherapy, the treatment of disease through the use of chemical agents, has assumed a major role in the treatment of oncology patients. Functions of chemotherapy as cancer treatment include:

1. assisting in providing for complete cure;
2. increasing mean survival time;
3. decreasing discomfort and the incidence of specific life-threatening complications.

Specific serious side effects associated with aggressive chemotherapy cause the patient distress. These side effects include alopecia, nausea and vomiting, the development of open sores on mucous membranes (mucositis), and various skin changes. Common side effects of chemotherapy on the hematopoietic system can be life threatening and are the most frequent dose-limiting factors in the use of chemical agents for cancer treatment. Chemotoxic effects on the blood-forming cells of the bone marrow also produce specific side effects that include anemia (decreased numbers of circulating red blood cells) and thrombocytopenia (decreased numbers of platelets). However, the possible and often inevitable suppression of immune function is the most life-threatening side effect for the patient and presents the nurse with a most serious challenge—to provide the patient with the understanding, environment, and support to withstand this potentially devastating complication.

Rationale for Use of Chemotherapy

A characteristic of cancer growth is the ability for cancer cells to separate from the original tumor, spread to new areas and establish new malignant cancers at distant sites (Oppenheimer, 1985). Documentation is clear that many, if not all, patients with disseminated or metastatic disease die of their cancers unless treatment focuses on the metastatic cancer cells as well as the original cancer cells (Fraser & Tucker, 1989). Chemotherapy is instrumental in the treatment of cancer because the effects of chemotherapy are exerted systemically and thus provide the opportunity to kill metastatic cancer cells that may have escaped local treatment.

Chemotherapy has joined surgery and radiation as an accepted major component in the medical management of cancer. The role for chemotherapy is clearly indicated in the treatment of some cancers but is less clear in the treatment of others. The following list indicates the general responsiveness of chemotherapy for specific malignancies (Guy, 1991).

Malignancies usually responsive to chemotherapy:
  Acute lymphocytic leukemia (ALL)
  Chronic lymphocytic leukemia (CLL)
  Lymphoma
  Choriocarcinoma
Malignancies often responsive to chemotherapy:
  Breast carcinoma
  Testicular carcinoma
  Prostatic carcinoma
  Head-and-neck carcinoma
  Acute myelogenous leukemia (AML)
  Chronic myelogenous leukemia (CML)
Malignancies occasionally responsive to chemotherapy:
  Colorectal carcinomas

Central nervous system tumors
Oat-cell carcinoma of the lung
Ovarian carcinoma
Uterine carcinoma
Malignancies usually nonresponsive to chemotherapy:
Renal-cell carcinoma
Pancreatic carcinoma
Bladder carcinoma
Liver carcinoma
Most carcinomas of the lung

Chemotherapy is a successful form of cancer treatment because it has some demonstrated selectivity for cancer cells over normal cells. The killing effect of chemotherapy on cancer cells appears to be related to two basic intracellular mechanisms. One mechanism is the inhibitory influence of chemotherapy on DNA synthesis. The second mechanism is the direct chemical interaction of chemotherapy with cellular DNA. The ultimate result of either of these mechanisms is cell death through interference with successful cell division. Because the mechanisms of killing by chemotherapy generally involve damaging the target-cell's DNA and interfering with cell division, the tumors most sensitive to chemotherapy are those that contain large numbers of individual cells in the active growth phase. Such cells are actively synthesizing DNA and undergoing cell division through the process of mitosis. Tumors that have large numbers of cells in this phase are said to have a *high mitotic index.*

Unfortunately, chemotherapeutic agents usually are administered systemically and exert their cytotoxic effects against normal cells as well as against malignant cells. Normal cells most profoundly affected by systemic chemotherapy are among the tissues that undergo frequent and rapid cell division. These tissues include skin, hair, epithelial lining of the gastrointestinal tract, spermatocytes, and hematopoietic cells (Tennenbaum, 1989).

Chemotherapy is a broad classification of drugs or chemical compounds that have demonstrated effectiveness in killing cancer cells. Agents used for chemotherapy are further classified both by the specific types of biologic action they exert in the cancer cell and by what specific period in the life of a cell the actions of chemotherapy are most likely to be successful in disrupting vital cell processes (Fig. 10–1). Most cancer treatment protocols are for *multiagent* or *combination chemotherapy* in that they involve the use of more than one specific antineoplastic drug. The purpose of multiagent therapy is to increase the killing of cancer cells in all phases of the cell cycle.

Antimetabolites

As a group, most antimetabolites exert their greatest cell killing or toxic effects on cells that are in S phase; therefore, most antimetabolites are both cell-cycle-specific and phase-specific. Antimetabolites are chemical substances

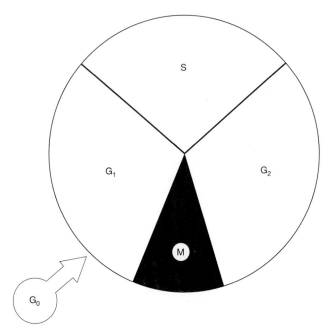

FIGURE 10-1. Cell phases during which chemotherapy may be effective. G_0—cell is in a reproductive "resting" state, in which the cell actively carries out its specific function but does not divide. G_1—cell is preparing for division, taking on extra nutrients and energy substrates. S—phase of doubling of the DNA content (DNA synthesis). G_2—synthesizes important protein components. M—nucleokinesis (division of the nucleus) followed by cytokinesis (division of the cell body).

that have molecular structures highly similar to normal metabolites that have essential roles in critical cell processes. Most enzymatic reactions require "cofactors" in order to begin or to continue the reaction. Many cofactors are vitamins. Antimetabolites resemble these cofactors and seem to work by one of several mechanisms:

competing with normal metabolites (cofactors)
replacing normal metabolites
antagonizing normal metabolites

In this way, the antimetabolite interferes with some critical cell process needed for successful cell division; therefore, cell division is either impaired or prevented. The vast majority of antimetabolites are structurally similar to vitamins, coenzymes, and actual neucleotides (purines and pyrimidines).

The following common chemotherapeutic agents are antimetabolites:

Methotrexate (amethopterin [old name], MTX; Mexate)
6-Mercaptopurine (Purinethol)

6-Thioguanine (6-TG; Tabloid)
5-Fluorouracil (5-FU; Adrucil, Efudex, Fluoroplex)
FUDR (Floxuridine)
Cytarabine (cytosine arabinoside [old name], Ara-C; Cytobar)

Antibiotics

This class of antineoplastic drugs was initially developed to combat standard bacterial infections. Many of these drugs can still be used for their bacteriocidal capacities. However, these drugs usually inflicted significant damage on the DNA of the bacteria. Because this DNA damage was not limited to bacterial DNA but also to host DNA, their general use as antibacterial agents was somewhat limited. Most of these antitumor antibiotics were developed as fermentation byproducts of other microorganisms (usually nonpathogenic bacteria or fungus). The mechanism of action for most of the antitumor antibiotics is to damage the tumor cell by interrupting either DNA or RNA synthesis (and sometimes both) although exactly how these tasks are accomplished varies with the individual antibiotic.

The following common chemotherapeutic agents are antitumor antibiotics:

Bleomycin (Blenoxane)
Dactinomycin (Actinomycin D; Cosmegen)
Doxorubicin (Adriamycin)
Daunorubicin (Cerubidine)
Mithromycin (Mithracin, Plicamycin)
Mitomycin-C (Mutamycin)
Mitoxantrone

Alkylating Agents

Alkylating agents all cause cross linking of DNA by various means. They may form electrophilic bonds, covalent bonds, dimethylation between side groups, or all three. Whatever the mechanism, the result is that the double strands of DNA are more tightly bound together (usually in intermittent areas rather than continuously down the whole stand). This tight binding will cause some areas of the DNA either to be misread or not read at all during DNA and RNA synthesis, resulting in the cell not being able to divide properly (if at all). These agents can bind to the DNA any time, even when the cells are taking a breather during the G_0 phase, so these agents are (as a group) cell-cycle-nonspecific.

The following common chemotherapeutic drugs are alkylating agents:

Cyclophosphamide (Cytoxan, Endoxan)
Cisplatin (Platinol)
Mechlorethamine (Nitrogen mustard; Mustargen)

Busulfan (Myleran)
Chlorambucil (Leukeran)
Melphalan (Alkeran)
Carmustine (BCNU)
Lomustine (CCNU)
Triethylenethiophosphoramide (Thiotepa)
Streptozocin (Zanosar)

Plant Alkaloids

Plant alkaloids (some of them vinca alkaloids) are derived from specific plants. The vinca alkaloids are derived from the periwinkle plant. The primary mechanism of action is interfering with the proper formation of microtubules. Some of the plant alkaloids destroy completed microtubules or inhibit microtubular assembly. Either way, there are no microtubules present to form the spindles necessary for pulling apart the double chromosomes. Other alkaloids appear to promote improper microtubule formation. As a result of any of these actions, the cell either does not divide at all or it divides only once, resulting in two daughter cells that have unequal (and nonproductive) amounts of DNA in them so that they cannot divide.

The following chemotherapeutic drugs are plant alkaloids:

Vincristine (leurocristine, VCR; Oncovin)
Vinblastine (VLB; Velban, Velbe)
Vindesine (DAVA; Eldisine)
Etoposide (VP16; Vepesid)
Taxol

Hormonal Manipulation

Hormone Therapy

Hormones are naturally occurring chemicals secreted by endocrine glands (ductless) and picked up by capillaries. Once in the bloodstream the hormones are distributed to all body areas but exert their effects only on specific target tissues (different for each hormone). Hormones can be used therapeutically against some cancer cells. The endocrine system usually keeps all of the hormones within narrow ranges, and a balance is maintained. When a large amount of one hormone is administered, it upsets the balance and disturbs the uptake of some other hormones. If a tumor depends on hormone A for growth, and lots of hormone B (structurally but not functionally related to A) is given to the person, hormone B will interfere with the tumor's uptake of hormone A or will limit the amount of hormone A produced (through competition or feedback inhibition) so that tumor growth is slowed (but not usually stopped or killed). Thus, hormonal therapy may increase survival time, often with decreasing tumor side effects.

The following drugs are used in hormonal manipulation for cancer therapy:

Estrogens (estradiol, diethylstilbestrol [DES], chlorotrianisene; Estrace, Premarin)
Androgens (fluoxymesterone; halotestin)
Progestins (progesterones; Megace, Provera, Depo-provera, Amen)
Adrenal corticosteroids

Antihormone Therapy

The antihormone drugs are receptor antagonists and are actually competitors for the hormones at the receptor sites. Often they are monoclonal antibodies specific for the receptor. When administered, antihormones will bind to the specific hormone receptor of the tumor cell and largely prevent the actual hormone from binding to the receptor. Therefore, if a tumor requires the presence of a certain hormone to grow, and the hormone can only enter the cell through a receptor, the use of an antireceptor antibody can effectively slow the growth of the tumor (and may even cause its death).

The following drugs are specific antihormone drugs used as chemotherapy for cancer:

Antiestrogen receptor (tamoxifen)
Antiandrogen receptor (flutamide)
Antiadrenal receptor (Lysodrene [mitotane])

Miscellaneous Chemotherapeutic Agents

The action of these specific drugs does not fit any of the broad categories of chemotherapeutic agents. Because the actual number of these agents is relatively small, they are described here individually.

Procarbazine

Procarbazine (Matulane, Natulanar) is a monoamine oxidase inhibitor; it appears to have several effects on DNA. In some not-well-understood way it inhibits both DNA and RNA synthesis and it also causes the direct depolymerization of DNA, possibly through the formation of a DNA-specific type of peroxide. This drug is non-phase-specific.

Dacarbazine

Although the exact mechanism of action of dacarbazine (DTIC-Dome) is not known, this drug does exert some cross linking or alkylating of nucleotide effects on DNA and to a more limited extent on RNA (so sometimes it is classified as an alkylating agent although it does do more than that). It is non-phase-specific.

Hydroxyurea

Hydroxyurea (Hydrea) interferes with DNA synthesis in much the same way that certain antimetabolites do, although it is not really similar to any known metabolite. Its actions are specific to the S phase of the cell cycle.

Asparaginase

Asparaginase (Elspar) is an enzyme that degrades the amino acid asparagine. Some tumor cells require this amino acid in order to survive and divide as do most normal cells. However, normal cells have an additional "survival pathway" that can convert other asparagine precursors into asparagine in the cell whereas some tumor cells are not able to do this. This drug is non-phase-specific.

Immunologic Consequences of Chemotherapy

Pretreatment Considerations

It is important to understand that the chemotherapy recipient may present as an already immunocompromised host as a result of a variety of factors influencing immune function. The malignant process itself has been found to directly and indirectly suppress the activity of some immune system cells. Patients with widespread malignant disease may have suppression of the bone marrow and lymphoreticular system before treatment is even started (Hancock & Bradshaw, 1986). Adding chemotherapy may worsen the situation. The following specific factors place the patient with cancer at additional risk for immunosuppression prior to receiving chemotherapy.

OVERALL HEALTH OF THE PATIENT. The patient who is already severely debilitated because of the malignancy or any other chronic health problem will be less tolerant of the side effects of chemotherapy.

AGE. The magnitude of chemotherapy's impact on the peripheral blood cell counts depends on the degree of bone marrow cellularity. With aging there is atrophy and hypoplasia of the bone marrow, with a subsequent decrease in the number of leukocytes produced. This phenomenon is associated with functional marrow being replaced with fat and fibrous tissue (Diekmann, 1988). The elderly patient has a diminished capacity for antibody-mediated and cell-mediated immune responses (see Chapter 13).

UNDERLYING CANCER. Patients with metastatic disease may already have bone marrow suppression with consequent decreases in phagocytic and cytotoxic cell reserves. These changes can occur as a result of direct bone marrow invasion or as a result of proteins produced by more remote tumors (Pitot, 1987). Invasion of the bone marrow by cancer cells makes the bone marrow far less able to carry on its normal function. Therefore, the number of cells that can be involved in an immune response is decreased, generally resulting in both lymphopenia and neutropenia. Some tumors release factors that selectively enhance the activity and number of T suppressor cells so that the T suppressors constitute a larger percentage of circulating leukocytes. These T suppressors function in at least two ways that cause an overall immunosuppression and favor tumor growth: they suppress the proliferative response of other T cells and they suppress immunoglobulin production.

CRITICAL ORGAN DYSFUNCTION. Most chemotherapeutic agents are metabolized for activation or degradation (or both) by the liver and kidneys. Functional impairment of either organ can lead to a prolonged circulation time for chemotherapeutic agents, increasing the intensity and duration of side effects.

PREVIOUS CANCER TREATMENT. Patients who already have had radiation or chemotherapy tend to be more sensitive to all the side effects of chemotherapy. In addition, previous cancer treatments may have permanently altered (decreased) cell-mediated immune response to the extent that a new course of treatment results in an additive or even a synergistic immunosuppression.

HOSPITALIZATION. Residing in an acute care setting increases the susceptible host's exposure to pathogens and increases the risk for nosocomial infections.

INVASIVE DIAGNOSTIC PROCEDURES. The more seriously ill the patient is, the more likely he or she is to have to undergo invasive diagnostic or therapeutic procedures. These procedures increase the risk for infection by potentially introducing pathogens.

Short-Term Immunologic Consequences

The immediate effect of combination chemotherapy (use of several different agents during a specified treatment regimen) on immune function is a decreased total leukocyte count. Especially affected are leukocytes that normally have a rapid turnover and a relatively short lifespan (12 to 36 hours), such as granulocytes (DiJulio, 1991). Leukocytes with longer lifespans (months to years), such as the T and B memory cells, and the actual products that some leukocytes synthesize and release into the blood (antibodies and cytokines) appear to be affected to a lesser degree.

While most antineoplastic drugs (chemotherapeutic agents) do suppress bone marrow activity and immune function to some degree, some agents affect this function more profoundly than do others. The following agents are examples of drugs considered profoundly immunosuppressive or myelosuppressive: busulfan, cyclophosphamide, etoposide, dactinomycin, doxorubicin, and mechlorethamine. The following agents are examples of drugs considered mildly immunosuppressive or myelosuppressive: cisplatin, streptozocin, mithramycin, and vincristine. In addition to variation in the degree to which chemotherapeutic agents suppress immune function there is also variation in the timing of this drug-induced immunosuppression. The time when bone marrow activity and peripheral white-cell counts are at their lowest levels following chemotherapy is referred to as the *nadir*. The nadir occurs at different times for different chemotherapeutic agents. For instance the expected nadir following cytosine arabinoside is 5 to 7 days, the nadir following methotrexate administration is 10 to 14 days, and the nadir following mitomycin C is about 4 weeks. When planning combination chemotherapy, care should be taken to avoid prescribing drugs that all have their nadir at or near the same time in order to minimize immunosuppression.

The clinical problems associated with the immediate effects of cancer treatment on immune function are related primarily to a transient loss or impairment of inflammatory responses to tissue injury or invasion by microorganisms. The severity and duration of the impairment are related directly to the dosage of specific chemotherapeutic agents. Although this impairment is usually temporary, with good recovery of inflammatory responses evident within weeks or months of the completion of therapy, the seriousness of the potential infectious complications makes this a major treatment concern. The infectious processes most commonly observed during this period include those of fungal origin, yeast, some residual viral breakthrough, and a wide variety of bacteria. After treatment, as the inflammatory responses recover, the risk of infection decreases inversely to the increase in the number of mature granulocytes. Although antibody-mediated and cell-mediated immune function are also depressed to some degree during and immediately after a typical chemotherapy regimen, any associated problems are usually overshadowed or even masked by the complications that arise as a result of depressed inflammatory responses.

An innovation showing great promise in reducing the intensity or duration (or both) of neutropenia among patients receiving chemotherapy is the addition of stimulating factors to the treatment regimen. Currently, both granulocyte–macrophage colony-stimulating factor (GM-CSF) and granulocyte colony-stimulating factor (G-CSF) are approved for use in patients with neutropenia. The administration of these factors, while probably not antitumor in their own right, dramatically increases the rate at which patients' leukocytes, especially neutrophils, rebound after bone marrow suppressive action resulting from chemotherapy (Rostad, 1991). This prevention or amelioration of drug-induced neutropenia not only reduces patients' risks for infection but also permits greater or more frequent doses of chemotherapy to be administered. By this action, the colony-stimulating factors may assist the killing of tumor cells and improving overall long-term survival of individuals with cancer. It is anticipated that the role of these stimulating factors will expand to include other disorders that cause the host to be immunocompromised, such as myelodysplastic syndromes, bone marrow transplantation, and the acquired immunodeficiency syndrome (AIDS) (Haeuber, 1991).

Long-Term Immunologic Consequences

As techniques for distinguishing various subpopulations of leukocytes and for determining leukocyte responsiveness have became more readily available, studies examining immune function after cancer treatment are beginning to indicate interesting patterns of functional impairment. Many of these studies also examine the functional capacity of bone marrow cells rather than relying solely on evaluation of circulating peripheral leukocytes. The majority of studies noting long-term immune system effects after cancer treatment examined patients with acute lymphocytic leukemia and Hodgkin's lymphoma (Borella, Green, & Webster, 1972; Simone, Aur, Hustu, Verzosa, & Pinkel, 1978). These studies noted that lymphocyte counts were slower to return to normal than neutrophils. An interesting finding was that frequently the total number of lymphocytes "rebounded" to above normal levels within 1 year of treatment, but when the proliferative responsiveness or the actual activity of these lymphocytes was examined, the T lymphocytes (cell-mediated immunity) were found to be impaired.

Chemotherapy, especially regimens including relatively high or long-term doses of alkylating agents, does induce immunologic impairment in children and adults treated for cancer. Some of these impairments persist for up to 10 years after treatment cessation. These immunologic impairments are expressed more as abnormalities in specific leukocyte function rather than just as abnormalities in leukocyte numbers. The division of immunity that consistently shows the most persistent abnormalities is cell-mediated immunity. Abnormalities include depressed activity of T-lymphocyte helper cells and cytotoxic/cytolytic T-lymphocyte cells along with increased T-lymphocyte suppressor cell activity. It is thought that this specific impairment may put the treated person at higher risk for having a recurrence of the original malignancy or may predispose these individuals to the development of new malignancies (Fraser & Tucker, 1989; Penn, 1982). The long-term impairments of immune function resulting from chemotherapy are dose dependent and intensified when chemotherapy is coupled with radiation therapy (Workman, 1989).

RADIATION THERAPY

The ultimate purpose of all types of radiation therapy for cancer is to destroy malignant cells with minimal exposure of the normal cells to the cell-damaging activities of radiation. Most of the radiation used for treatment of malignancy is *ionizing radiation*. During cellular or tissue absorption, this type of radiation causes the "kicking out" of an orbital electron from the atom of elements, resulting in ionization and release of energy. Cellular damage by radiation appears to occur by the following two mechanisms:

1. Formation of oxygen free radicals that can be combined with water through the action of superoxide dismutase to form intracellular hydrogen peroxide;

2. Ionization of the DNA, directly causing alkylation of the double strands of DNA.

Radiation damage is not really cell cycle phase-specific, although some phases are more sensitive than others. The cell cycle sensitivity to radiation in descending order is M, G_2, G_1, and S.

There are two major categories of ionizing radiation: particulate radiation and electromagnetic radiation. The type of radiation primarily used as cancer therapy is electromagnetic radiation and there are two basic types: gamma radiation and roentgen radiation.

Gamma Radiation

Gamma radiation is produced intranuclearly, by the decay of radioisotopes, which are unstable compounds because they contain an imbalance of nuclear particles (usually electrons), so that they actually carry an overall charge. As they decay, they give up these particles, release energy, and become stable. Three different types of energy or rays are produced as a result of gamma radiation: gamma rays, beta rays, and alpha rays (Hilderley & Dow, 1991).

Gamma Rays

Gamma rays are very light, with a low energy-transfer potential. They travel very rapidly (speed of light), allowing them to be concentrated and to penetrate deeply.

Beta Rays

Beta rays are heavier, with moderate to high speed. They have a high linear-energy-transfer potential and do not penetrate tissues or other substances well. Most gamma emitters also emit beta rays as a side product.

Alpha Rays

Alpha rays are very heavy and slow. They easily transfer energy to surroundings and quickly lose their ability to penetrate tissues (0.04 mm into tissue).

Roentgen Radiation

Roentgen radiation differs from gamma radiation only in how it is produced—extranuclearly, not by decay of unbalanced isotopes, but by linear acceleration with electrical machines. This type of radiation still causes ionization in absorbing atoms.

The intensity of the radiation emitted with either type (roentgen or gamma radiation) decreases with the inverse square of the distance from the radiation source. In practice, this means that the dose of radiation received at a distance of 2 in. from the radiation source is only 25 per cent of the dose received at a distance of 1 in. and that the dose of radiation received at 3 in. from the source is only 1/9 of the dose received at a distance of 1 in. (Hassey, 1987).

The amount of radiation delivered to a recipient cell or tissue is called *exposure;* how much of this exposure is absorbed by the recipient cell or tissue is called the *dose.* Therefore, the dose is always some fraction or percentage of the exposure and will depend on the energy level, absorption type, intensity, proximity, and duration of exposure. The following terms are used to described absorbed doses of radiation (Iwamoto, 1991):

rad = radiation absorbed dose
Gray (Gy) = 100 rad (calculated as joules per kilogram)
rem = roentgen equivalents in man
R (roentgen) = unit of radiation that can ionize a certain amount of air.
  (1R = a dose less than 1 rad or less than 0.01 Gy.)

Killing Effects of Radiation

If the absorbed dose of radiation is high enough, all cells will be killed immediately, but this is not what usually happens with therapeutic radiation. Instead, radiation damage to the DNA is usually not apparent until the cells attempt to divide (Strohl, 1990). In a population of tumor cells blasted with a single exposure of radiation, all cells within the tumor would absorb the radiation slightly differently, and thus their overall response to the radiation would be slightly different. The following list outlines various possible fates of tumor cells after a single exposure of radiation.

1. A small percentage of tumor cells will die immediately on absorption of the radiation.

2. More cells will die a little later (when they attempt to divide).

3. Other cells will produce abnormal forms as they try unsuccessfully to divide.

4. Still other cells may remain functional but are sterile and completely unable to divide.

5. Some cells are able to divide successfully for several generations before all progeny are rendered sterile.

6. A certain percentage of radiated tumor cells (after a single dose of radiation) will repair, recover, and go on for many cell generations with no apparent problem. This possible outcome of radiation therapy forms the basis for the traditional daily small doses of radiation.

In all tissues, some of the effects of radiation are cumulative, and whether or not they prove lethal depends to a large extent on the cell's ability to perform error-free DNA repairs. This repair ability varies with tissue type, developmental stage, and inherent and acquired individual characteristics.

In general, two types of radiation delivery are used most commonly for cancer therapy: teletherapy and brachytherapy. The type to be used depends on:

1. site of the tumor;

2. stage of the tumor (including size and depth of lesion);

3. radiosensitivity of the tumor;

4. general condition and state of health of the patient. (Remember, sometimes surgery would be the treatment of choice for the disease but the patient's condition is such that surgery would not be well tolerated.)

Regardless of how radiotherapy is administered, the optimal dose of radiation is one that cures or produces the desired physiologic effect on the cancer cells with an acceptable level of morbidity on normal tissues. (We don't want the cure to be worse than the disease.)

Teletherapy

The term *teletherapy* is derived from the Greek prefix "tele," meaning far or distant. With teletherapy the actual radiation source is external from the patient and remote from the tumor site. Because the source is external, the patient is never radioactive and poses no radiation hazard to anyone else. This type of therapy may also be referred to as *beam radiation.* Some of the sources for this type of radiation are high-energy photons (usually provided by linear accelerators), electrons, cobalt 60 megavolt radiation, and more recently, fast neutrons generated by cyclotrons.

With all types of teletherapy, the actual beam of radiation does not deliver the radiation to the target tissue uniformly. The center of the beam has the greatest intensity of radiation; therefore, calculations that include the angle of the beam, number of treatments, and wedging are critical for delivery of the optimal dose to all areas of a deep and irregularly shaped tumor. Often the beam will be delivered from more than one angle; this increases the amount of normal tissues exposed, while decreasing the amount of radiation any one normal tissue area receives (without decreasing the dose to the tumor). Wedging is accomplished using wedge-shaped pieces of different types of metal that all absorb radiation differently (lead, tin, cadmium, alloys). By using wedges, radiation beams can be more accurately directed to the target site. The total dose of radiation prescribed for a given tumor varies with the type, size, location, and degree of radiation sensitivity of the tumor and the radiation sensitivity of the surrounding normal tissues. For example, a total dose of 1200 rad may be prescribed for a primary liver tumor, whereas a 5000- to 6000-rad total dose may be prescribed for a breast carcinoma.

In order to increase the accuracy of radiation delivery to the cancer cells, before teletherapy is administered the exact location of the tumor must be determined. Techniques used for localization include computed tomographic (CT) scans, nuclear magnetic resonance imaging (MRI), ultrasonography, and standard diagnostic x-ray scans. After the dosage and approach have been individually calculated for each patient by the team consisting of radiation oncologist, radiologic physicists, and dosimetrist, a "dry-run" or *simulation* is done to define and refine positions, exposures, and intensities (Iwamoto, 1991). The simulator mimics the beam distribution of the actual machines used for therapy, but it produces only weak superficial radiation. This superficial radiation can be easily picked up on radiosensitive film, and the picture is intensified or enhanced to produce an image that will clearly show radiation beam patterns. Once the pattern of radiation delivery has been confirmed, the patient must always be in the same exact position for all treatments (making certain that the patient can get into and maintain this position with relative ease). Position-fixing devices and markings (either on the patient's body or on the position-fixing devices) are used to ensure that exactly the proper position can be assumed each day of the treatment.

Because the efficacy of radiation has been demonstrated to increase if many smaller doses of radiation are given rather than a single high dose, most teletherapy is fractionated. Standard radiotherapy is usually fractionated between 180 and 250 rad per day times as many days as necessary to achieve the optimal prescribed dose with the least amount of short- and long-term effects to normal tissues. Some newer techniques being tested experimentally further fractionate the normal daily dose so that two to four smaller doses are given each day. This technique is called *hyperfractionation,* where smaller-sized doses are administered more than once each day, usually separated by at least 6 hours (Strohl, 1990).

Depending on the total prescribed dose, sometimes teletherapy will be given as a "split course." This regimen requires that half the dose be delivered on a specific daily schedule followed by a rest period of 2 to 3 weeks before the other half is administered. The split course technique is much better tolerated by patient, with much quicker recovery of normal tissues. However, it appears that tumor tissues also recover better and faster with this technique; thus it is not as effective as straight-course radiation administration unless the later dose is greater than the first dose.

Most of the side effects for all types of teletherapy radiation are limited to the local tissues subjected to the actual radiation, so these side effects vary with the site. Skin changes and alopecia are local but are more likely to be permanent (depending on total absorbed dose) than those resulting from chemotherapy (Hilderley & Dow, 1991). Two systemic side effects commonly seen with external beam radiation (depending on dose) regardless of the site of radiation are altered taste sensations and fatigue. The basis for the changes in taste sensation or appreciation has been attributed to the metabolic byproducts that are rapidly released and absorbed systemically from dead and dying cells (both tumor cells and normal cells). In particular, many people acquire an aversion to the taste of red meats and other protein food sources. The symptom of fatigue is thought to be related to the hypermetabolism and increased energy demands of the radiation-damaged cells (normal and malignant) required to attempt cell repair continuously (Hilderley & Dow, 1991).

Brachytherapy

The term *brachytherapy* is derived from the Greek word "brach," meaning short. Essentially, brachytherapy requires the radiation source to come into direct continuous contact with the tumor target tissues for a specific period of time. The rationale for this treatment plan is to provide a high absorbed dose of radiation in the tumor tissues and a very limited absorbed low dose in surrounding normal tissues (Strohl, 1990). There are several ways brachytherapy can be delivered to the tumor tissues. With all types of brachytherapy, the radiation source is within the patient, and thus, for a time the patient can pose a radiation hazard to others (directly or indirectly). Brachytherapy involves the use of radioactive isotopes, and these isotopes can be either in solid form or may be soluble in body fluids. Brachytherapy is used to deliver radiation to the body surface, interstitial tissues, and body cavities.

Soluble isotopes are unsealed radioactive sources and are usually administered orally, intravenously, or as an intracavitary instillation. Because they are unsealed, soluble isotopes are not completely confined to any one area of the body (although they may concentrate more in some specific body tissues than in others). These soluble isotopes are not deliberately recovered from the individual but may enter other body fluids and eventually be eliminated from the body in various excretions. These excretions are radioactive and can be harmful to other individuals. An example of this type of therapy is the ingestion or injection of the radionuclide iodine-131 (iodine base with a half-life of 8.05 days) for the treatment of hyperthyroidism and certain thyroid malignancies. Although the radioactive iodine does initially circulate to all areas of the body, most of it becomes sequestered in the thyroid gland (remember, the hormones the thyroid produces require large amounts of iodine for activity). The radioactivity of the iodine-131 will destroy some of the thyroid cells. Most of this isotope will be eliminated from the body within 48 hours. Once the isotope is eliminated, neither the patients nor their excretions are radioactive. Another commonly used soluble isotope is phosphorus-32. In general, the soluble isotopes are used more for diagnosis and treatment of nonmalignant conditions rather than for radiation therapy of malignancies.

The solid forms of brachytherapy involve the use of sealed radiation sources implanted either within or very close to the tumor target tissues. These implants may be temporary or permanent. Most emit lower-energy radiation continuously to the tumor tissues. Some devices, such as seeds or needles, can be placed into the tissues and will stay in place alone. Other solid isotope devices must be held in place within the tissue or cavity by other pieces of equipment. The needles and seeds are radioactive at the time of insertion or implantation; they have been preloaded with the radioactive isotope. This type of procedure is called *hot implantation.* Some of these devices are so small and the half-life of the isotope so short that the device is left in place permanently (most commonly for prostate cancer). Others are removed from the patient and reused in other patients.

Afterloading is a technique (generally used when radiation is to be delivered within an organ or cavity) in which the implant, without the radioactive isotope, is placed within the cavity and special devices (applicators) hold it in position. When placement has been ascertained and the patient is in the proper environment, the implants are loaded with the radioisotope. After the prescribed dose has been delivered, the implant, isotopes, and position-holding devices are removed. With solid implants, the patient is radioactive while the implant is in place but the excretions are not radioactive.

Dose delivery by brachytherapy has some of the same limitations as doses delivered by external radiation sources. Implants are not symmetrical with regard to their geometric placement of the radioactive isotope content. Because of this asymmetry, there is some degree of nonhomogeneity in the dose delivery from area to area on any single implant (not to mention the variance that can be seen from one implant to another). Also, depending on the isotope used, the radioactive decay does not occur uniformly within one implant (this is much more of a problem for isotopes with a very short half-life as compared with those with extremely long half-lives). The dosage most commonly prescribed for delivery by brachytherapy is between 30 and 100 rad per hour times the number of hours it takes to receive the calculated total dose.

Radiation delivered by brachytherapy is ionizing radiation and has the same tissue effects and limitations as ionizing radiation delivered by external sources. Most commonly, brachytherapy is used in conjunction with teletherapy for maximum tumor kill with better cosmetic and functional results than delivery solely by external sources (Strohl, 1990).

Immunologic Consequences of Radiation Therapy for Cancer

Short-Term Consequences

Short-term consequences resulting from radiation therapy for cancer are those that manifest during and up to 6 months after the initiation of radiation therapy (Hilderley & Dow, 1991). Whether or not immune function impairment occurs after radiation therapy is dependent on the location and the dose of radiation received. Therefore, in order for radiation therapy to influence bone marrow activity and immune function significantly, active marrow sites must be within the radiation field. (In children, bone marrow throughout most of the body is active in the synthesis of red and white blood cells. In adults, the vast majority of this activity is limited to the iliac crests and the sternum.) When active sites lie within the radiation field total white-cell counts are greatly diminished, with neutrophils most profoundly affected. As a result, the patient is at risk for infection, especially bacterial, fungal, and viral infections to which they have not been previously exposed. The neutropenia appears to resolve completely within 6 months after radiation therapy is completed (Hilderley & Dow, 1991).

Long-Term Consequences

Long-term consequences or effects of radiation therapy for cancer are those that manifest 6 months or later after initiation of radiation therapy (Hilderley & Dow, 1991). Studies of long-term survivors of Hodgkin's lymphoma, breast cancer, and cervical carcinoma treated with radiation have shown immune function impairment along with other tissue specific problems (Job, Pfreund-schuh, Bauer, Zum Winkel, & Hunstein, 1984). Most of these studies indicated that extensive radiation was associated with prolonged T-lymphocyte impairment while B-lymphocyte function returned to or remained normal (Wasserman, Petrini, & Blomgren, 1982; Rotstein, Blomgren, Petrini, Wasserman, & Baral, 1985; Rotstein, Blomgren, Petrini, Wasserman, & Baral, 1986). One postulated mechanism for this finding was that since T-lymphocyte activity was thymus-dependent, radiation to the thymus was more likely to result in T-lymphocyte impairment. Other studies suggested an age-dependent relationship between thymic radiation and T-lymphocyte impairment. An apparent dose–response relationship was seen with radiation-induced immune impairment (Parmentier, Morardet, & Tubiana, 1983; Thierry, Jullien, Rigaud, Hardy, Vicoq, & Magdelenat, 1985), larger doses, and larger volumes of exposed areas correlated with greater immune impairment. Although few children were included in these studies, Sacks et al. (1978) reported a clear age-dependent relationship in the ability of bone marrow to regenerate after extensive radiation therapy. Regeneration occurred more quickly and to a greater extent among patients under age 20 regardless of the absorbed dose. More T-lymphocyte function abnormalities were noted when the upper body was heavily irradiated as compared with lower irradiation levels. Immune function impairment appeared more frequently and more profoundly among patients who had received a combination of radiation therapy and multiagent chemotherapy as treatment for their malignant conditions.

The overall effects of this immune function impairment secondary to radiation therapy are not known. Because these impairments are long-term and possibly permanent, it is postulated that the major outcome will be an increase in the incidence of second malignancies among individuals receiving extensive or high-dose radiation therapy for cancer.

CASE PRESENTATION

Mr. Rock is a 29-year-old white male chemical engineer employed by a large pharmaceutical company. He has no history of any serious illness and was hospitalized only once at age 7 for a closed reduction of a broken arm. He is married to a high school math teacher.

Mr. Rock sustained a severely sprained right ankle during a softball game at the annual company picnic. Bruising and edema were extensive. The company physician examined the ankle and took x-ray films, ruling out a bone fracture and recommending ice applications, elevation, and no weight-bearing activity for at least 2 weeks.

One week after the sprain Mr. Rock noticed a painless, "rubbery" lump about the size of a grape in his right groin area. He called the company physician, who told him that the lump was probably an enlarged lymph node related to the massive inflammatory reaction occurring at the site of the ankle injury and that it would probably stay enlarged for several weeks.

Six weeks after the injury Mr. Rock found another lump slightly higher up from the first one. Later that same morning his wife pointed out a similar swelling just above Mr. Rock's collar bone on the left side. Mr. Rock reported to the employee health department that morning, where the lumps were examined by an adult nurse practitioner. Later in the day Mr. Rock was seen by the company physician who referred Mr. Rock to a surgeon. The surgeon scheduled Mr. Rock for a biopsy of the enlarged lymph node above the left clavicle.

The pathology report of the lymph node revealed the presence of Reed–Sternberg cells with nodular sclerosis. On the basis of these findings, Mr. Rock was diagnosed with Hodgkin's lymphoma (Cotran, Kumar, & Robbins, 1989) and referred to a hematologist/oncologist. Biopsy of the groin nodes was also positive. Lymphangiography revealed probable involvement of other nodes above and below the diaphragm. Based on these findings, along with the fact that Mr. Rock was essentially asymptomatic (had no fever, night sweats, or significant weight loss), his disease was considered Stage IIIa. The treatment plan included total nodal irradiation followed by chemotherapy.

Before treatment was started, Mr. and Mrs. Rock were informed of the probable and potential side effects of both the radiation therapy and the chemotherapy. Because of the probability of infertility/sterility and the possibility of impotence, Mr. Rock had seven semen specimens banked in liquid nitrogen before the treatment regimen was started for possible later use.

Mr. Rock received 4500 rad total nodal irradiation (TNI) over a 5-week period. The areas irradiated are those shown as "extended field" radiation in Figure 10–2.

Because the chemotherapeutic regimen selected involved the use of drugs known to cause venous fibrosis and scarring and was planned to be delivered for about 1 year, Mr. Rock was hospitalized for 1 day for the surgical placement of an implanted venous access device (IVAD). He tolerated the procedure well and began his chemotherapy on an outpatient basis. Mr. Rock's chemotherapeutic regimen was the MOPP alternated with the ABVD regimen. The following schedule of drugs was initiated (Carson & Callaghan, 1991):

MOPP

M = mechlorethamine (nitrogen mustard)
   6 mg per square meter of body = surface area intravenously on
   Days 1 and 8
O = Oncovin (vincristine)
   2.0 mg per square meter intravenously on Days 1 and 8

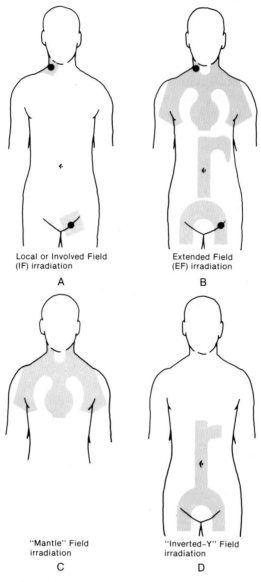

FIGURE 10-2. Typical radiation fields used in the treatment of Hodgkin's lymphoma. (From Hodgkin's disease by C. Haskell and R. Parker, 1990. In C. Haskell [Ed.], *Cancer treatment* [3rd ed.] [p. 669]. Philadelphia: W.B. Saunders.

P = procarbazine (Matulane)
    100 mg per square meter orally continuously on Days 1 through 14
P = prednisone
    40 mg per square meter orally continuously on Days 1 through 14
    (only during cycles 1 and 4)

These drugs were given together as a "cycle." The cycle was administered for the first 2 weeks followed by a resting or recovery period of 2 weeks. After the recovery period, the ABVD regimen was administered (on 1 day) followed by a 2-week recovery period.

ABVD

A = Adriamycin (doxorubicin)
    25 mg per square meter of body = surface area intravenously
B = bleomycin (Blenoxane)
    10 units per square meter intravenously
V = vinblastine (Velban)
    6 mg per square meter intravenously
D = dacarbazine (DTIC)
    375 mg per square meter intravenously

He tolerated the chemotherapeutic regimen very well, with a chief complaint of mouth soreness after four treatments. Mr. Rock's red blood counts remained relatively stable. His white-cell counts were too low at the time for his second ABVD cycle, and treatment was delayed for an additional 2 weeks (prolonged nadir). He was not hospitalized during the treatment and missed few work days. Nausea and vomiting were controlled with a combination of antiemetics, lorazepam (Ativan) and intravenous dexamethasone (Decadron). Mr. Rock received his chemotherapy on Friday afternoons, which gave him 2 days to recover from the acute side effects before going back to work. Mr. Rock suffered total scalp and body alopecia. He elected to wear a baseball cap rather than a wig.

After 10 months of chemotherapy (12 alternating MOPP and ABVD cycles) Mr. Rock's treatment was complete. He had no evidence of disease at that time and has remained disease-free for 4 years since therapy was complete. Mr. Rock has some numbness of the fingers and toes. His sperm count is less than 50,000 per ejaculate. Two years after his therapy was complete, Mr. Rock's wife was impregnated twice with his frozen semen. The couple have a healthy 16-month-old daughter.

SELECTED BIBLIOGRAPHY

Abbas, A., Lichtman, A., & Pober, J. (1991). *Cellular and molecular immunology.* Philadelphia: W.B. Saunders.
Borella, L., Green, A., & Webster, R. (1972). Immunologic rebound after cessation of long-term chemotherapy in acute leukemia. *Blood, 40*(1), 42.

Braun, D., & Harris, J. (1986). Effect of chemotherapy on NK function in the peripheral blood of cancer patients. *Cancer Immunology and Immunotherapy, 21,* 240.

Carson, C., & Callaghan, M. (1991). Hematopoietic and immunologic cancers. In S. Baird, R. McCorkle, & M. Grant (Eds.), *Cancer nursing: A comprehensive textbook* (p. 536). Philadelphia: W.B. Saunders.

Cotran, R., Kumar, V., & Robbins, S. (1989). *Robbins pathologic basis of disease* (4th ed.). Philadelphia: W.B. Saunders.

Diekmann, J. (1988). Cancer in the elderly: Systems overview. *Seminars in Oncology Nursing, 4*(3), 169.

DiJulio, J. (1991). Hematopoiesis: An overview. *Oncology Nursing Forum, 18*(2 Suppl), 3.

Fraser, M., & Tucker, M. (1989). Second malignancies following cancer therapy. *Seminars in Oncology Nursing, 5*(1), 43.

Fried, W., & Barone, J. (1980). Residual marrow damage following therapy with cyclophosphamide. *Experimental Hematology, 8,* 610.

Goodman, M. (1991). Delivery of cancer chemotherapy. In S. Baird, R. McCorkle, & M. Grant (Eds.), *Cancer nursing: A comprehensive textbook* (p. 291). Philadelphia: W.B. Saunders.

Guy, J. (1991). Medical oncology—The agents. In S. Baird, R. McCorkle, & M. Grant (Eds.), *Cancer nursing: A Comprehensive textbook* (p. 266). Philadelphia: W.B. Saunders.

Haeuber, D. (1991). Future strategies in the control of myelosuppression: The use of colony-stimulating factors. *Oncology Nursing Forum, 18*(2 Suppl), 16.

Hancock, B., & Bradshaw, J. (1986). *Lecture notes on clinical oncology* (2nd ed.). London: Blackwell Scientific.

Hassey, K. (1987). Principles of radiation safety and protection. *Seminars in Oncology Nursing, 3,* 23.

Hilderley, L., & Dow, K. (1991). Radiation oncology. In S. Baird, R. McCorkle, & M. Grant (Eds.), *Cancer nursing: A comprehensive textbook* (p. 246). Philadelphia: W.B. Saunders.

Iwamoto, R. (1991). Radiation therapy. In S. Baird, M. Donehower, V. Stalsbroten, & T. Ades (Eds.), *A cancer source book for nurses.* (p. 63). Atlanta: American Cancer Society.

Job, G., Pfreundschuh, M., Bauer, M., Zum Winkel, K., & Hunstein, W. (1984). The influence of radiation therapy on T-lymphocyte subpopulations defined by monoclonal antibodies. *International Journal of Radiation Oncology and Biological Physics, 10,* 2077.

Katz, J., Walter, B., Bennets, G., & Cairo, M. (1987). Abnormal cellular and humoral immunity in childhood acute lymphoblastic leukemia in long-term remission. *Western Journal of Medicine, 146,* 179.

McGeorge, M., Russell, E., & Mohanakumar, T. (1982). Immunologic evaluation of long-term effects of childhood ALL chemotherapy: Analysis of in vitro NK and K cell activities of peripheral blood lymphocytes. *American Journal of Hematology, 12,* 19.

Oppenheimer, S. (1985). *Cancer: A biologic and clinical introduction* (2nd ed.). Boston: Jones & Bartlett.

Parmentier, C., Morardet, N., & Tubiana, M. (1983). Late effects on human bone marrow after extended field radiotherapy. *International Journal of Radiation Oncology and Biological Physics, 9,* 1303.

Penn, I. (1982). Second neoplasma following radiation or chemotherapy for cancer. *American Journal of Clinical Oncology, 5,* 83.

Phillips, T., & Fu, K. (1976). Quantification of combined radiation therapy and chemotherapy on critical normal tissues. *Cancer, 37,* 1186.

Pitot, H. (1987). *Fundamentals of oncology* (3rd ed.). New York: Marcel Dekker.

Rostad, M. (1991). Current strategies for managing myelosuppression in patients with cancer. *Oncology Nursing Forum, 18*(2 Suppl), 7.

Rotstein, S., Blomgren, H., Petrini, B., Wasserman, J., & Baral, E. (1985). Long term effects on the immune system following local radiation therapy for breast cancer. I. Cellular composition of the peripheral blood lymphocyte population. *International Journal of Radiation Oncology and Biological Physics, 11,* 921.

Rotstein, S., Blomgren, H., Petrini, B., Wasserman, J., & Baral, E. (1986). Long term effects on the immune system following local radiation therapy for breast cancer. 4. Proliferative responses and induction of suppressor activity of the blood lymphocyte population. *Radiotherapy and Oncology, 6,* 223.

Sacks, E., Goris, M., Glatstein, T., Gilbert, E., & Kaplan, H. (1978). Bone marrow regeneration following large field radiation. *Cancer, 42,* 1057.

Simone, J., Aur, R., Hustu, O., Verzosa, M., & Pinkel, D. (1978). Three to ten years after cessation of therapy in children with leukemia. *Cancer, 42*(2), 839.

Strohl, R. (1990). Radiation therapy: Recent advances and nursing implications. *Nursing Clinics of North America, 25*(2), 309.

Tennenbaum, L. (1989). *Cancer chemotherapy.* Philadelphia: W.B. Saunders.

Thierry, D., Jullien, D., Rigaud, O., Hardy, M., Vilcoq, J., & Magdelenat, H. (1985). Human blood granulocyte progenitors (GM-CFU) during extended field radiation. *Acta Radiologica Oncologica, 24*, 521.

Wasserman, J., Petrini, B., & Blomgren, H. (1982). Radiosensitivity of T-lymphocyte subpopulations. *Clinical Laboratory Immunology, 7*, 139.

Workman, M. (1989). Immunologic late effects in children and adults. *Seminars in Oncology Nursing, 5*(1), 36.

SOLID ORGAN TRANSPLANTATION

Some organs perform specific and vital life processes (brain, heart, liver, lung, kidney). If these organs fail, no other organ is capable of performing the vital functions to the degree necessary to maintain life. Therefore, failure of these organs, without intervention, leads to death of the individual. A curative intervention for failure of a vital organ is the acquisition of a healthy organ through transplantation from another person or animal. The concept of solid organ transplantation is very old; its acceptance and success as a relatively common procedure is quite new.

The actual surgical technique required for the physical transplantation of a solid organ from one individual to another was available during the 19th century, although supportive therapies for associated complications and side effects were not available until the mid 20th century. Thus, solid organ transplantation in the 19th century was held back by a lack of asepsis, anesthesia, antibiotic therapy, fluid and electrolyte replacement therapy, and blood component therapy.

During the 20th century supportive therapy became available, and solid organ transplantation was attempted in the second half of the century. Technical success was possible immediately. Organ recipients survived the trauma associated with surgery. Healthy organs transplanted from one individual to another were capable of normal function for short periods in the recipient. However, the transplanted organs could not be maintained. The immune system of the recipient attacked and destroyed the transplanted organ, making the technical success a clinical failure.

During the 1960s interest in solid organ, particularly kidney, transplantation resurfaced. Great technical and clinical successes were seen when the

168

organ donor and recipient were identical twins. However, such resources were available only on an extremely limited basis. Increased clinical success was seen with the advent of histocompatibility testing and of increased availability of pharmacologic agents with the capacity to artificially suppress the immune response. Immunosuppressive techniques and agents were the key to moving solid organ transplantation from the realm of "experimental" to that of accepted standard therapy for many specific pathologic conditions. However, these same techniques/agents were and continue to be detrimental to other aspects of the recipient's general health resulting in an immunocompromised condition.

OVERVIEW

The number of solid organ transplantations performed in the United States in the year 1990 totalled 14,617 (United Network for Organ Sharing). The transplantations, categorized by organ were: heart, 1988; lung, 185; liver, 2524; pancreas, 528; heart and lung, 52; and kidney, 9340 (living, related donors, 1927; cadaveric donors, 7413).

Many more individuals need a solid organ transplant than receive one. The availability of organs for transplantation is limited by a variety of factors, and many patients die while waiting.

While the actual number of transplantations performed during any one year does not comprise a large percentage of this nation's citizens, it is important to remember that many of these individuals will live 20 years or longer. Though they may be cured of the specific condition or disorder that initially necessitated the transplant and lead very active and useful lives, these individuals continue to be followed within the health care system. Some of the agents used for immunosuppression increase the patients' risks for other health problems. In addition, these individuals are just as susceptible to traumatic and age-related health problems as anyone else. Therefore, nurses can expect to be caring for these individuals in nearly any clinical setting for almost any type of health problem. Because these individuals must remain on their immunosuppressive regimens for the rest of their lives, it is essential that all nurses have a strong, basic understanding of the physiologic and immunologic consequences of solid organ transplantation.

TRANSPLANTATION IMMUNOLOGY

The patient receiving a donated organ is called a *recipient* or *host,* because the donated organ resides as a guest within the patient's body. In actuality, the donated organ is grafted directly onto (into) the host's body and, therefore, is a *graft.* In order for this graft to be functional it must be accepted by the host's body. The process of being accepted by the host's body is termed a *take* or *engraftment.*

As described in Chapter 1, each individual has a unique set of identification proteins on the surfaces of all nucleated cells. These proteins are termed *human leukocyte antigens (HLAs)* and enable the cells of the immune system to distinguish between self and nonself cells, tissues, and proteins. Because these proteins are inherited from an individual's parents, usually a person will share some (and very occasionally all) of these proteins with a parent or full sibling. Figure 11–1 depicts some possible combinations of HLA inheritance within one family group. Engraftment and acceptance occur best when the transplanted organ is a perfect match for all the major and minor HLAs of the recipient.

Syngeneic Transplantation

When the donor of the solid organ for transplantation is a person who is genetically identical to the recipient, a perfect HLA match for all major and minor antigens (see Chapter 1), the graft is described as *syngeneic.* Most commonly the donor for this type of graft is an identical twin sibling. The best rate of successful graft "take" accompanied by the fewest posttransplantation complications is achieved with this type of transplant. Because this type of transplantation results in the recipient receiving an organ with all the surface proteins identical to his or her own, the host's body does not recognize the transplanted organ as foreign tissue and mounts no immunologic actions against it. Therefore, the host requires no immunosuppressive therapy for graft take. Because total heart, lung, or pancreas transplantations from the donor would result in the death of the donor, only kidney transplantations are being performed between identical twins, although partial liver transplantation and

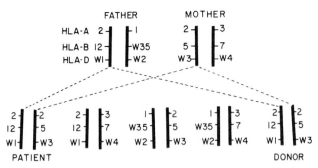

FIGURE II–I. Examples of possible combinations of human leukocyte antigens (HLAs) within one family. (From Bone marrow transplantation by R. Ford, 1991. In S. Baird, R. McCorkle, and M. Grant [Eds.], *Cancer nursing: A comprehensive textbook* [p. 387]. Philadelphia: W.B. Saunders.)

segmental pancreatic transplantation have been successful (Garovoy, Melzer, Gibbs, & Bozdech, 1987).

Allogeneic Transplantation

Allogeneic transplantation is the type in which the donor organ comes from another human being who is not genetically identical to the recipient. Some attempts are made to have the donor and recipient match HLA-A, HLA-B, and HLA-C types as closely as possible (Chapter 1), along with a blood-type match (ABO). The most successful transplants, requiring less recipient immuno-suppression, are those from donors who perfectly match at least three of the four major HLAs. The probability of finding a good match among full siblings ranges between 25 and 35 per cent (Ford, 1991). The most common donors for this type of transplantation are siblings or parents of the recipient; however, like syngeneic transplants, only kidney transplantation or partial liver and segmental pancreatic transplants are possible from a living, related donor.

Most solid organ transplantations are performed using allogeneic organs from unrelated, brain-dead donors. Finding good matches between a potential donor and the person who needs the organ is much more difficult with unre-lated people. Fewer than 1 person in 100 would share three of four major HLAs with any given individual (Abbas, Lichtman, & Pober, 1991). Fortunately, through various organ procurement agencies, computerized lists of future re-cipient tissue types and potential donor tissue types are analyzed for the closest match. This way, as soon as an organ becomes available, the potential recipient with the closest HLA and blood-type match has the greatest chance to receive the organ.

Histocompatibility matching between donor and recipient is determined through two tests, actual HLA typing and response to mixed lymphocyte cul-ture (MLC), also called a "lymphocyte crossmatch." The principle here is to find a donor who most closely matches the patient. The more closely the two match; the better the odds for a successful transplant and the less immuno-suppressive agents are needed by the recipient (Jackson, 1991).

Actual HLA typing involves using antibodies against specific HLA-A, HLA-B, and HLA-C types. HLA-D compatibility is determined by mixed lymphocyte culture. This test is more complicated and involves obtaining live lymphocytes from both the prospective donor and the patient and allowing these lympho-cytes to mix or incubate together in a culture. If they are incompatible, the lymphocytes will react with each other, stimulating cell division (mitosis). A positive reaction to MLC is determined by an assay that measures the amount of new DNA being synthesized during mitosis. Greater mitotic activity indi-cates less HLA-D compatibility between donor and recipient cells. Total com-patibility is shown if no reaction (no cell division) occurs. Usually this test is performed only when considering a transplant between living, related poten-tial donors and recipients (Smith, 1990).

TRANSPLANTATION

Transplantation involves removing all or part of an organ from one individual and placing it in the body of another. Except for syngeneic transplantation, success is not ensured and some immunologic modulation of the host is necessary. This modulation must be continuous throughout the life of the transplanted organ.

For some organs, the nonfunctional recipient organ is not completely removed unless it is infected (kidney and heart). Usually a kidney is not placed in the normal anatomical position for a kidney in the host. Instead, it is placed in a position easily accessible for monitoring and that has a good blood supply. Most kidneys are transplanted to the anterior abdominal region in the iliac fossa, where it can easily be palpated through the abdominal wall. The heart, on the other hand, cannot be placed anywhere else but the normal anatomical cardiac position in order to carry out proper cardiac function. Lungs and livers must also be transplanted to their normal anatomical locations.

Criteria

Solid organ transplantation is a major surgical procedure for both the donor and the recipient. Because of the potential for complications from the surgery, anesthesia and postoperative sequelae is significant, rigid criteria for donor and recipient selection are maintained.

Donor

The donor (whether living, related or unrelated, brain-dead) must be in reasonably good health. The donor must be free from malignancies and infectious diseases, especially those with a viral origin. For kidney transplantation, when the donor is living and may be related to the recipient, it is necessary to make certain that the donor can live well with only one kidney.

For transplantation of heart, lungs, or both, the donor and recipient must be of a similar size (not really a factor in adult kidney transplants). Most of the cadaveric or unrelated potential organ donors have sustained severe traumatic injuries leading to brain death as a result of cerebral vascular accidents and head trauma.

Age alone is not a qualifying factor for organ donation, especially among cadaveric donors. However, the donated organ must be anatomically normal and functionally acceptable. Older individuals may have at least one of a myriad of health problems that result in some functional impairment of the heart, lungs, liver, or kidneys.

When an otherwise healthy individual has suffered irreversible and total brain damage to the extent that recovery of the brain is not possible, brain death is diagnosed. For a period of time, the vital organs can be supported through aggressive life-support mechanisms while consideration is given to the possibility of organ transplant.

Once brain death is diagnosed, permission to use the organs for transplantation is usually sought from the closest surviving relative. When permission is obtained, and disease and organ status of the potential donor meet the criteria, the search for compatible recipients is made. Until the organs are recovered for transplantation, the organ donor is maintained and steps are taken to ensure adequate perfusion of all transplantable organs. Usually, the last of the vital organs to be recovered from the donor are the heart and lungs.

Recipient

Because transplantable organs, as resources, are in limited supply, a variety of recipient criteria help to determine which of the needy potential recipients will receive a specific donated organ. One criteria is a close histocompatibility match with the donor. When more than one person is a good or equal match, severity of the patient's current conditions is taken into consideration. Age can be a limitation, although this is not uniform in all states. Usually, individuals over age 60 are not given first priority for transplantation. The nature of the underlying disease process is also a factor in recipient selection. Individuals with significant pathologies of multiple organ systems are not viewed as favorably as transplantation candidates as are people who have major pathology of only one organ. Potential recipients also undergo some psychologic testing to determine whether the process is acceptable to them.

ORGAN REJECTION (GRAFT-VERSUS-HOST DISEASE)

Because the solid organ transplanted into the host seldom is an identical match of universal product codes (HLAs) between the donated organ and the recipient host, the patient's immune system cells will recognize any newly transplanted organ as nonself. Unfortunately, even though the transplanted organ is quite beneficial to the host patient, without intervention the host's immune system will initiate standard inflammatory and immunologic actions to destroy, eliminate, or neutralize these nonself cells. This activity is responsible for rejection of the transplanted organ. Graft rejection is actually a complex series of responses that change over time and involve different components of the immune system. Graft rejection is categorized into three different types: hyperacute, acute, and chronic. Organ function, management, and outcome vary significantly among the types.

Hyperacute Rejection

Description

Hyperacute graft rejection begins immediately upon transplantation and is an antibody-mediated response (Abbas et al., 1991). The underlying mechanism of action is the formation of antigen–antibody complexes within the blood vessels of the transplanted organ. The host's blood has preexisting antibodies to one or more of the antigens (including blood-group antigens) present in the donated organ. The antigen–antibody complexes adhere to the endothelial lining of blood vessels and stimulate complement activation (see Chapter 1). The activated/fixated complement on and in the blood vessel linings initiates the blood clotting cascade with microcoagulation occurring throughout the organ vasculature. Widespread coagulation and occlusion lead to ischemic necrosis and inflammation, with degranulization of phagocytes releasing hydrolytic enzymes into the tissue of the organ (Smith, 1990). These enzymes contribute to massive cellular destruction and graft loss.

Hyperacute rejection occurs primarily in transplanted kidneys. Individuals at greatest risk for hyperacute rejection are those who have received donated organs of an ABO blood type different from their own, those who have received multiple blood transfusions at any time prior to transplantation, those who have a history of multiple pregnancies, and those who have received a previous transplant (Smith, 1990).

Management

The manifestations of hyperacute rejection are apparent within minutes to hours of attaching the donated organ to the host's blood supply. The process cannot be stopped once it is initiated, and the rejected organ may be removed when hyperacute rejection is diagnosed.

Because the underlying mechanism for this type of rejection is known and the factors can be avoided, the best management is prevention. When the donated organ is of the same ABO type, MLC is negative, and IgG antibodies present in the host's serum do not react with the donor's cells, hyperacute rejection reactions do not occur (Abbas et al., 1991).

Acute Rejection

Description

Acute graft rejection occurs sporadically following transplantation and can occur within days after transplant. Two different mechanisms have been identified as responsible for this type of transplant rejection. The first mechanism is antibody-mediated and results in a vasculitis within the transplanted organ. This reaction differs from that of hyperacute rejection in that blood vessel necrosis rather than thrombotic occlusion leads to the organ destruction (Abbas et al., 1991). The second mechanism for acute graft rejection is cellular. Host cytotoxic/cytolytic T cells and natural killer cells enter the transplanted organ through the blood and other extracellular fluid, infiltrate the organ parenchymal cells (rather than the blood vessel cells), and initiate both direct and macrophage-mediated lysis of the graft cells.

Management

Acute rejection is diagnosed by laboratory tests indicating impaired function of the specific organ, along with biopsy of the grafted organ. Manifestations of this type of rejection vary with the individual patient and with the specific organ transplanted. For example when this type of rejection occurs in transplanted kidneys, the host usually experiences some tenderness in the kidney area and may manifest other general symptoms of inflammation.

An episode of acute rejection after solid organ transplantation does not usually mean the host will lose this transplant. Pharmacologic manipulation of host immune responses at this time can limit the damage to the organ and allow maintenance of the graft. Several different courses of action can be successful as an intervention for this problem, depending on which organ is affected and the severity of the rejection episode.

Specific actions of individual pharmacologic agents used for temporary and long-term immunosuppression after solid organ transplantation are described more completely in the section on immunosuppressive agents below. High-dose corticosteroids have been successful in halting acute graft rejection (Garovoy et al., 1987). If the rejection episode is only partially ameliorated or remains unaffected by high-dose corticosteroid therapy, administration of antilymphocyte globulin (ALG) may be successful in suppressing the rejection reaction. However, most of these antibodies are raised in animals and can provoke a progressively increased immune reaction in the host receiving it. Therefore, the number of times this agent can be administered is limited by the severity of the host's immunologic reactions to it. Thus, this agent is more effective at controlling an episode of acute rejection the first time it is administered than it is during subsequent episodes (Hooks, 1990). A more specific agent designed to suppress acute rejection activity is a monoclonal antibody to the CD3 antigen present on all T cells (Vaska, 1991). These agents alone or in combination are usually able to control episodes of acute rejection and assist the host in maintaining the graft from months to years.

Chronic Rejection

Description

The actual pathogenesis of chronic rejection is not clear but resembles the aftermath of chronic inflammation and scarring. Functional tissue of the transplanted organ is replaced with fibrotic, scarlike tissue. Because this fibrotic tissues does not resemble the organ tissue in either structure or function, the ability of the transplanted organ to perform differentiated tasks diminishes in proportion to the percentage of normal tissue replaced by fibrotic tissue. It has been postulated that this type of reaction is longstanding and occurs continuously as a response to chronic ischemia caused by blood vessel injury (Abbas et al., 1991). In addition, the process of chronic rejection differs among organ types.

Management

It is thought that good control over host immune function can delay the manifestations of this type of rejection but that the process probably occurs to some degree in all allogeneic transplants. The fibrotic changes are permanent, thus chronic graft rejection has no cure. When the fibrosis increases to the extent that there is significant interference with the functional capacity of the transplanted organ, the only recourse is retransplantation.

IMMUNOSUPPRESSIVE AGENTS

Rejection of transplanted solid organs involves all three components of immunity, although cell-mediated immune responses are most significant in the rejection process. Early in the history of successful transplantation recipients were on a pharmacologic regimen that profoundly suppressed general immune function. The hazards associated with this therapy, primarily increased susceptibility to infection and malignancy, led clinicians and researchers to search for alternative agents for immunologic manipulation.

Maintenance Therapy

The following group of pharmacologic agents generally are used as routine immunosuppressive therapy after solid organ transplantation. The doses of the drugs are adjusted for the immune responses of the individual patient. A regimen of these agents increases the patient's risk for bacterial, fungal, viral, and protozoal infections.

Corticosteroids

Corticosteroids decrease the numbers of circulating monocytes, lymphocytes, and basophils. They most profoundly diminish inflammatory responses but, because they inhibit the activation of T cells and suppress the release of interleukin-1, interleukin-2, and interferon, cell-mediated immune function also is diminished (Garovoy et al., 1987; Hooks, 1990).

Azathioprine

When metabolized, azathioprine is converted to the antimetabolite 6-mercaptopurine (Hooks, 1990). This agent is incorporated as a purine into the growing DNA strand during DNA synthesis, which must take place during cell division. Because 6-mercaptopurine is not a proper purine, its incorporation into the DNA strand halts further DNA synthesis and inhibits RNA synthesis. Therefore, dividing cells cannot divide and proliferate. This drug slows the proliferation of all dividing cells, including bone marrow cells. Pancytopenia (anemia, thrombocytopenia, and leukopenia) is a common side effect of this therapy.

Cyclosporine

The biologic activity of cyclosporine results in selective immunosuppression of T lymphocytes. B lymphocytes and the granulocyte–macrophages are affected only indirectly by this agent's effects on T-cell release of various lymphokines (see Chapter 4). The primary mechanism of action for cyclosporine is not known; however, in the presence of cyclosporine, T cells do not produce interleukin-2 receptors. Because the most damaging immunologic attacks on transplanted organs are mediated through T-lymphocyte actions, cyclosporine therapy has significantly reduced the number and severity of acute graft rejections. In addition, the use of cyclosporine has enabled transplant recipients to decrease, and in some instances, completely eliminate the use of corticosteroids or azathioprine after transplantation (Hooks, 1990). However, even though graft survival is increased, cyclosporine induces many serious changes in the host, particularly in the vasculature, increasing the risk for the development of serious side effects and other pathologies. These problems include nephrotoxicity, hepatotoxicity, increased rate of atherosclerosis, gingival hyperplasia, hirsutism, hypercholesterolemia, tremors, muscle weakness, paresthesia, and seizure activity (Hooks, 1990).

Rescue Therapy

The following group of agents are not used to maintain the graft within the host but are used to reduce the host's immunologic responses during rejection episodes, especially acute rejection. These agents may be used in addition to or in place of any of the maintenance drugs in the host's regimen. In addition, some transplant centers use these agents as initial therapy to prevent rejection in the early post transplant period.

Antilymphocyte Globulin

Antilymphocyte globulin (ALG) is an antibody (or antibodies) generated in an animal after exposure to human lymphocytes. The globulin can be made more specific by exposing the animal to human T lymphocytes instead of mixed lymphocytes. When these antihuman lymphocyte antibodies are administered to humans, the antibodies selectively attack and clear lymphocytes from the blood, extracellular fluids, and the tissues to which they have infiltrated (such as the transplanted organ). This agent is given only for a short time to combat the acute rejection episode (Garovoy et al., 1987).

Most individuals receiving ALG have some associated immunologic response, ranging from low-grade fever and malaise to serum sickness and anaphylaxis. Usually the responses increase with intensity on repeated exposure to ALG.

OKT3

OKT3 is another antibody. It differs from ALG in a variety of ways. First, it is a monoclonal rather than a polyclonal antibody, so it is very specific to the human T-cell surface antigen CD3. In addition, OKT3 is generated with a murine (mouse) model rather than a horse or rabbit model. This agent acts as a lytic antibody and an activator of complement to eliminate T cells, especially cytotoxic/cytolytic T lymphocytes (Abbas et al., 1991; Vaska, 1991).

Because the agent is generated in mice, antimouse antibodies rapidly develop in humans receiving it. These antimouse antibodies attack the OKT3 and prevent its anti-T-cell activities. Thus, OKT3 has the best action against rejection during the first episode for which it is used. Its utility in combating graft rejection may decrease with each subsequent use.

Corneal Transplantation

Corneal transplantation, although technically a solid tissue transplant, has some basic immunologic differences that have an impact on patient care as compared with organ transplant. These differences, on the whole, are responsible for making corneal transplantation a more successful and widespread therapy than is solid organ transplantation.

Keratoplasty, or corneal transplant, is the surgical removal of the patient's diseased corneal tissue, and replacement with tissue from a human donor cornea. It is performed to restore vision by removing corneal opacities or scars created by injury or infection, or to correct a corneal dystrophy. There are two approaches to performing a keratoplasty. In *lamellar (partial-thickness) keratoplasty,* the superficial cornea is removed and replaced with donor tissue. *Penetrating keratoplasty* involves removing the full thickness of the patient's cornea and replacing it with donor tissue. Penetrating keratoplasty is the most frequently used procedure since it produces clearer vision. The donor corneal button, also called the *graft,* is positioned on the recipient's eye and sutured in place.

Immunologically, corneal transplantation is very different from solid organ transplants. The cornea of the eye does not have a separate, direct blood supply and, therefore, has very little contact with any type of leukocytes, including cytotoxic/cytolytic T cells. Consequently, the cornea is considered an "immunoprivileged site." Even though corneal cells do have HLAs on their surfaces, transplanted unmatched HLA corneas do not usually stimulate rejection responses in the host. The success rate in corneal transplantation between unmatched donors and recipients is about 90 per cent (Heberlein & Walsh, 1990). In addition, corneal transplant recipients do not require systemic immunosuppression.

Tissue for a keratoplasty is obtained from a local eye or tissue bank. The eye bank obtains its supply of corneal tissue from volunteer donors at the time of their deaths. These volunteer donors must be free of infectious disease at the time of their death, and must meet the requirements set forth by the local chapter of the Eye Bank Association of America (Ignatavicius & Bayne, 1991). All donors are checked for the presence of human immunodeficiency virus and other infectious diseases. Unlike other transplant donors, age is not a factor in corneal transplantation. The major criteria is that the donor cornea is healthy and completely clear.

Although the cornea has no direct blood supply and presumably is somewhat protected from T-cell invasion, graft rejection is still possible and does occur in a small percentage of corneal transplants. The inflammatory process of rejection starts in the donated cornea near the graft margin and moves toward the center. Vision is reduced significantly. The cornea becomes slightly cloudy. Treatment consists of the frequent topical use of corticosteroids administered to the conjunctiva (Newell, 1986). If the rejection process continues, the cornea becomes opaque and blood vessels may begin to branch into the opaque tissue. The patient may lose this graft and require a new transplant. For patients who have had graft rejection unrelated to the presence of infection, a new corneal transplantation from an HLA-matched donor increases the chance of engraftment (Heberlein & Walsh, 1990).

CASE PRESENTATION

Jean was a 38-year-old registered nurse and mother of three children with no previous history of renal disease or other significant health problems. She had been hospitalized only for the deliveries of her three children, each by cesarean section, and had never received a blood transfusion.

Jean notice a gradual change in her voiding patterns (diminished as compared with intake) and a corresponding increase in weight. Jean sought advice from her internist. On examination, Jean was found to have elevated blood pressure, generalized edema, and a bounding pulse. Blood studies showed an increased blood urea nitrogen, serum creatinine, and electrolytes (sodium, potassium, and chloride). A tentative diagnosis of renal insufficiency was made, and Jean was sent to a nephrologist.

After an intravenous pyelogram and kidney biopsy Jean was discovered to have end-stage renal disease. The probable cause was long-term sequelae of a previous streptococcal infection; both kidneys were affected. Jean was started on biweekly hemodialysis while she explored other treatment options.

After 6 months of hemodialysis, Jean decided to attempt a kidney transplant and approached her only sibling, 42-year-old Ann, with the possibility of being a donor. Ann, a mother of two, had no signficant health problems except for von Willebrand's disease, a clotting disorder that would not affect kidney function. Ann had previously had major surgeries (a cholecystectomy and a hysterectomy). The anesthesia and postoperative recovery period for Ann with these surgeries had been uneventful.

Ann underwent tissue typing and was found to be histocompatible with Jean for 3 of the 4 HLAs. In addition, both she and Jean had O + blood types. Ann agreed to donate her kidney to her sister, and the surgery was planned to take place in 3 weeks, pending the outcome of psychologic and physiologic testing.

Ann and Jean were admitted to the hospital on the same day. Jean underwent one last round of hemodialysis and then received one unit of Ann's blood on the evening before the transplant.

On the day of the transplant, Ann was anesthetized and a flank incision made to remove the right kidney. The procedure took a little over 3 hours, with no untoward occurrences.

Because Jean's chronic renal failure may have been caused by an infectious organism and the diseased kidneys might serve as reservoirs for the organism, the decision was made to remove both of Jean's kidneys immediately prior to receiving the donated kidney. Ann's kidney was anastomosed to Jean's right hypogastric artery and Jean's right ureter. The kidney was nested in Jean's right iliac fossa. The entire procedure lasted 7 hours. The transplanted kidney began excreting pink-tinged urine within the first 10 minutes after anastomosis. By the time Jean was taken to the recovery room more than 300 ml of urine was produced.

After coming back to the medical–surgical floor from the recovery room, Ann's postoperative course was uneventful. She was discharged to home on the 4th postoperative day and planned to be back at work by the 21st postoperative day. Over the next 3 months Ann had some problem with fluid retention and mild hypernatremia. She limited her sodium intake to 3 g per day during this time. These manifestations gradually diminished and have not been a problem since 6 months after nephrectomy.

Jean went to the surgical intensive care unit within the transplant unit on discharge from the recovery room. Her immunosuppressive regimen included prednisone 50 mg/day, cyclosporine 10 mg/kg/day, and azathioprine 3 mg/kg/day. The kidney continued to function well and her blood urea nitrogen, serum creatinine, and serum electrolytes were maintained within normal levels.

On the sixth postoperative day Jean spiked a temperature of 102.4°F. A reddened and open area of her incision was found on culture to be positive for *Staphylococcus aureus,* and she was started on ampicillin IVPB (administered by intravenous piggy-back infusion). Delayed wound healing resulted from the corticosteroid therapy. The rest of the postoperative period was uneventful, and Jean was discharged to home on the 23rd postoperative day.

Jean was followed at the transplant clinic every 2 weeks for the first 2 months after discharge. At 7 weeks after transplantation, Jean experienced general malaise, a low-grade fever, pain over the kidney site, and a 3-lb weight gain in a 24-hour period. She called her transplant team coordinator and was seen in the emergency room.

Her laboratory work revealed elevations of potassium, blood urea nitrogen, and serum creatinine. A kidney biopsy revealed histologic evidence of acute rejection. Jean was hospitalized and treated with antilymphocyte globulin. Within 3 days the acute rejection episode appeared under control. On Day 7 Jean was discharged to home.

For the next 2 years the kidney worked well. The only complication was a fungal infection (candida), which responded well to ketoconazole. Jean remains in good health and is currently working full-time.

SELECTED BIBLIOGRAPHY

Abbas, A., Lichtman, A., & Pober, J. (1991). *Cellular and molecular immunology*. Philadelphia: W.B. Saunders.

Bartell, B., & Ferguson, R. (1984). Infectious complications and lymphomas in cyclosporine patients. In B. Kahan (Ed.), *Cyclosporine: Nursing and paraprofessional aspects* (p. 68). New York: Grune & Stratton.

Cotran, R., Kuman, V., & Robbins, S. (1989). *Robbins pathologic basis of disease* (4th ed.). Philadelphia: W.B. Saunders.

Ford, R. (1991). Bone marrow transplantation. In S. Baird, R. McCorkle, & M. Grant (Eds.), *Cancer nursing: A comprehensive textbook.* (p. 385). Philadelphia: W.B. Saunders.

Futterman, L. (1988). Cardiac transplantation: A comprehensive nursing perspective. Part 1. *Heart and Lung, 17*(5), 500.

Futterman, L. (1988). Cardiac transplantation: A comprehensive nursing perspective. Part 2. *Heart and Lung, 17*(6), 631.

Garovoy, M., Melzer, J., Gibbs, V., & Bozdech, M. (1987). Clinical transplantation. In D. Stites, J. Stobo, & J. Wells (Eds.), *Basic and clinical immunology* (6th ed.) (p. 420). Norwalk CT: Appleton & Lange.

Guyton, A. (1991). *Textbook of medical physiology* (8th ed.). Philadelphia: W.B. Saunders.

Heberlein, D., & Walsh, G. (1990). Corneal transplantation. In S. Smith (Ed.), *Tissue and organ transplantation: Implications for professional nursing practice* (p. 171). St. Louis: C.V. Mosby.

Hooks, M. (1990). Immunosuppressive agents used in transplantation. In S. Smith (Ed.), *Tissue and organ transplantation: Implications for professional nursing practice* (p. 15). St. Louis: C.V. Mosby.

Ignatavicius, D., & Bayne, M. (1991). *Medical-surgical nursing: A nursing process approach.* Philadelphia: W.B. Saunders.

Jackson, R. (1991). The immune system: Basic concepts for understanding transplantation. *Critical Care Nursing Quarterly, 13*(4), 83.

Kozlowski, L. (1988). Case study in identification and maintenance of an organ donor. *Heart and Lung, 17*(4), 366.

Malen, J., & Boychuk, J. (1989). Nursing perspectives on lung transplantation. *Critical Care Nursing Clinics of North America, 1*(4), 707.

Metzger, J., & Hoffman, L. (1988). Cardiac transplantation: The changing faces of immunosuppression. *Heart and Lung, 17*(4), 414.

Newell, F. (1986). *Ophthalmology principles and concepts.* St. Louis: C.V. Mosby.

Ota, B., & Bradley, M. (1984). Side effects of cyclosporine in 100 renal allograft recipients. In B. Kahan (Ed.), *Cyclosporine: Nursing and paraprofessional aspects* (p. 56). New York: Grune & Stratton.

Pezze, J. (1990). RATG: Implications for nursing care in organ transplantation. *Critical Care Nurse, 10*(9), 18.

Pillon, L. (1990). Cyclosporine: A nursing focus on immunosuppressive therapy. *Dimensions in Critical Care Nursing, 10*(2), 68.

Roitt, I. (1991). *Essential immunology* (7th ed.). Oxford: Blackwell Scientific.

Schweizer, R. (1989). Infection control and the transplant patient. *Asepsis, 11*(1), 2.

Smith, S. (1990). Immunologic aspects of transplantation. In S. Smith (Ed.), *Tissue and organ transplantation: Implications for professional nursing practice* (p. 15). St. Louis: C.V. Mosby.

Suthanthiran, M., & Garovoy, M. (1983). Immunologic monitoring of the renal transplant recipient. In A. Novick (Ed.), *The urologic clinics of North America* (p. 315). Philadelphia: W.B. Saunders.

United Network for Organ Sharing (UNOS). Richmond, VA, (804) 330-8500.

Vargo, R., & Whitman, G. (1989). Complications after cardiac transplantation. *Critical Care Nursing Clinics of North America, 1*(4), 741.

Vaska, P. (1991). OKT3 monoclonal antibody in cardiac transplant patients. *Dimensions of Critical Care Nursing, 10*(3), 126.

12

BONE MARROW TRANSPLANTATION

Bone marrow transplantation (BMT) as a curative treatment for malignancy, bone marrow aplasia, or genetic diseases is a relatively new method, with a history of success of about 20 years. Even as recently as 1986, patients undergoing bone marrow transplantation would have been seen only in major medical centers. Now, autologous bone marrow transplant units are becoming commonplace even in community hospitals. With long-term survival after transplantation increasing, nurses can expect to be caring for these individuals, if not during the actual transplantation or BMT recovery period, then during the posttransplant period in a variety of health care settings. Therefore, it is essential that all nurses have a basic understanding of the physiologic and immunologic consequences of bone marrow transplantation.

By 1970, less than 100 BMTs had been performed at fewer than 10 medical centers. By the end of 1988, over 10,000 transplants were reported by more than 100 centers (Gale & Quinn, 1989), an average of more than 500 BMTs performed each year. It is important to note that 500 BMTs per year is not indicative of the number of patients whose conditions are appropriate for BMT. There are many more people who could benefit from BMT, but the option of BMT is not widely available. The two primary reasons for this are (1) inadequate numbers of BMT units nationwide and (2) patients' lack of monetary resources. BMT is very expensive, usually costing between $100,000 and $200,000 per transplant (Schilter & Rossman, 1991). Also, for many diseases, BMT is considered experimental, and many physicians are reluctant to offer it as a treatment alternative. As long as BMT is categorized as "experimental" treatment many health insurance companies refuse to cover the costs associated with the procedure.

OVERVIEW

Many people, even health professionals, have misconceptions concerning bone marrow transplantation. For example, some people believe the actual BMT is a surgical procedure, requiring major incisions and time under anesthesia similar to a solid organ transplantation. In actuality, bone marrow transplantation is a simple procedure technically. Bone marrow is taken by needle aspiration from a donor or the actual patient and given by intravenous infusion to the patient.

The ultimate purpose of bone marrow transplantation depends on the health problem of the person receiving the transplant. The three most common purposes are to replace impaired bone marrow, to allow an increase in the intensity of conventional cancer therapies, and to cure genetic disorders.

The first and most common purpose of bone marrow transplantation is to replace a person's malignant or nonfunctional bone marrow with healthy bone marrow in the hope that the healthy marrow will grow in the patient's body in place of the malignant or nonfunctional marrow. Conditions that meet this criterion include the leukemias (Chapter 7), the myeloproliferative disorders (Chapter 8), aplastic anemia, severe combined immune deficiency syndrome, and Wiskott–Aldrich syndrome (Chapter 5) (Ammann, 1987).

Bone marrow transplantation is used as supportive therapy in the treatment of solid tumor malignancies. Many chemotherapeutic agents are cytotoxic to bone marrow cells and cause bone marrow suppression during and after treatment. This side effect is the major limitation for chemotherapy, because too much chemotherapy can permanently destroy bone marrow function, leading to the death of the patient (Chapter 10). Therefore, doses of chemotherapy are given intermittently and adjusted in the attempt to kill as many tumor cells as possible without "wiping out" the patient's normal healthy bone marrow. With the availability of BMT, very high doses of chemotherapy can be administered to the patient, killing the tumor (desirable) and the patient's bone marrow (undesirable). This treatment is followed by a BMT to "rescue" the patient from certain death as having no functional marrow would lead to profound neutropenia, anemia, and thrombocytopenia. Many solid tumor malignancies might respond to this rescue use of BMT; however, malignancies for which this treatment has demonstrated a supportive capacity include lymphoma, breast cancer, ovarian cancer, testicular cancer, neuroblastoma, malignant melanoma, multiple myeloma, and small-cell lung cancer (Armitage & Gale, 1989; Schilter & Rossman, 1991).

BMT also is being used as a treatment, in fact as a cure, for some genetic disorders with pathologies unrelated to bone marrow function. In these disorders, the bone marrow functions normally but the person has a genetic defect that makes them unable to synthesize an essential product (often an enzyme) properly. If this product is made by leukocytes, erythrocytes, or both, then transplanting bone marrow from a genetically normal individual into the person with the genetic disorder would essentially "cure" the disorder. One genetic disorder successfully treated by bone marrow transplantation is thalassemia (Ford, 1991). Other genetic disorders reportedly treated by BMT include Gaucher's disease, Hurler's syndrome, Diamond–Blackfan syndrome, Fanconi's anemia, and sickle cell anemia (Wiley & House, 1988).

TYPES OF BONE MARROW TRANSPLANTS

Even though the aspirated bone marrow is a liquid medium rather than a solid tissue, when it is transferred from one individual to another it is considered a graft. In order for the transplanted bone marrow to be functional in the recipient it must accept and be accepted by the patient's body. This acceptance or "take" is termed *engraftment*. Currently, all bone marrow for transplantation or grafting into humans is derived from humans, so all BMTs are said to be *homografts* or *homologous*. In addition, bone marrow transplantation is categorized by the donor source of the bone marrow. Preconditioning treatment, successful engraftment rates, and posttransplant complications vary significantly with the type of BMT.

Syngeneic BMT

When the donor source of bone marrow for transplantation is from a person who is genetically identical to the recipient, a perfect human leukocyte antigen (HLA) match for major and minor antigens (see Chapter 1), the graft is described as *syngeneic*. Most commonly, the donor for this type of graft is an identical twin sibling. The best rate of successful graft "take" accompanied by the fewest posttransplant complications is achieved with this type of bone marrow transplantation. This type of transplant is used primarily in the attempt to cure bone marrow malignancies.

Allogeneic BMT

Allogeneic BMT is the type of transplant in which the donor marrow comes from another human being who is not genetically identical to the recipient. Attempts are made to have the donor and recipient match HLA-A, HLA-B, HLA-C, and HLA-D types as closely as possible (Chapter 1) and the most successful transplants are those from donors who perfectly match at least three of the four major HLAs. The most common donors for this type of transplant are siblings or parents of the recipient. Individuals may be close matches for HLA type without sharing the same ABO blood type. Unrelated donors are seldom complete matches with the recipient. Diseases or conditions for which allogeneic transplantation is appropriate include asplastic anemia, leukemia, lymphomas, and genetic disorders.

Histocompatibility matching between donor and recipient is determined through two tests, actual HLA typing and response to mixed lymphocyte culture (MLC). The principle is to find a donor who most closely matches the patient. The more closely the two match, the better the odds for a successful transplant. Actual HLA typing involves using antibodies against specific HLA-A, HLA-B, and HLA-C types. HLA-D compatibility is determined by MLC. This test involves obtaining live lymphocytes from both the prospective donor and the patient and allowing these lymphocytes to mix or incubate together in a culture. If they are incompatible, the lymphocytes will react with each other, stimulating cell division (mitosis). A positive reaction to MLC is determined by an assay that measures the amount of new DNA being synthesized during mitosis. Greater mitotic activity indicates less HLA-D compatibility between donor cells and recipient cells. Total compatibility is shown if no reaction (no cell division) occurs.

Autologous BMT

Autologous BMT is the type of bone marrow transplant in which the donor and the recipient are the same person. The patient's own bone marrow is removed and is subsequently transfused back into the patient, usually after a specific treatment. This type of BMT is appropriate for support and rescue purposes necessary after high-dose or intensive chemotherapy for solid tumors. It is also being used in the treatment of leukemia. When used in the treatment of leukemia the marrow is obtained when the patient is in remission or, if complete remission has not occurred, the marrow is treated to eliminate cancer cells after it has been removed from the patient and before it is transfused back. Because this bone marrow is from the patient and therefore is identical to the patient's universal product code, whether engraftment occurs is dependent on nonhistocompatibility factors. Such factors include the amount of functional marrow transplanted and the type of medications the patient receives in the immediate posttransplantation period.

PROCEDURE OF BONE MARROW TRANSPLANTATION

After the decision to have a BMT has been made and an appropriate donor has been identified, the actual process of BMT is ready to begin. The number of steps in this process depends on the exact type of transplantation.

Donor Preparation

After determining the compatibility of a donor, bone marrow is harvested. The harvesting procedure is essentially the same whether the donor is also the patient or is a different individual. Timing of the bone marrow harvest depends on the type of transplant, the underlying disease process of the recipient, and the stage of the transplant.

All nonpatient donors must be in essentially good general health and free from infection and malignant diseases. Although no specific age limitation is placed on donors, younger people have a greater amount of functional marrow to donate than do older individuals.

In most institutions, the donor is hospitalized for the actual bone marrow harvest. The donor is prepared preoperatively just like anyone undergoing a surgical procedure. Upon being taken to the operating room the donor is placed under general anesthesia. If the donor is an averaged-sized healthy adult, approximately 600 to 1000 ml of marrow is removed from the donor's iliac crests, and occasionally from the sternum, using a large-bore needle connected to an aspirating syringe. Both the posterior and anterior aspects of the iliac crests are accessed for the aspiration. The procedure is time-consuming, as usually less than 10 ml (and often less than 5 ml) of marrow is obtained with each syringe pull.

The risks to the donor are primarily related to undergoing general anesthesia, the potential for infection related to an invasive procedure, and some blood loss. After the procedure, most donors have some pain and bruising at the aspiration sites. Usually the pain is well controlled with oral, non-aspirin-containing analgesics. To reduce the risk of infection, donors are given antibiotic prophylaxis with an oral, broad-spectrum antibiotic for 7 to 14 days following the procedure. Iron supplements are ordered to assist the donor in red-cell production. Occasionally, donors may require one to two units of blood in the early postharvest period to maintain normal red-cell counts. Usually precautions are taken to ensure that if a donor needs a blood transfusion it will be an autologous one.

Upon harvesting the donated marrow is filtered through a sterile metal screen to remove bone fragments and fat particles. An anticoagulant (usually heparin) is added, and the marrow is stored in a blood administration bag. Preservation techniques vary with the institution and the length of time between the harvest and the marrow transfusion.

Recipient Preparation

Figure 12–1 outlines the timing and steps typically involved in an allogeneic bone marrow transplantation. The day the patient actually receives the bone marrow is considered Day 0. Pretransplant conditioning days are counted in reverse chronologic order relative to the transplant day (like the countdown to the actual launch of a satellite or rocket). Posttransplant days are counted in chronologic order from day of transplant to discharge. Some of the steps depicted in Figure 12–1 are altered for syngeneic or autologous bone marrow transplantation.

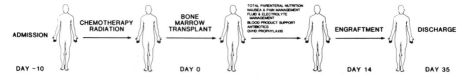

FIGURE 12-1. Timing and steps involved in allogeneic bone marrow transplantation. BMT—bone marrow transplantation; GVHD—graft-versus-host disease. (From Bone marrow transplantation by R. Ford, 1991. In S. Baird, R. McCorkle, and M. Grant [Eds.], *Cancer nursing: A comprehensive textbook* [p. 389]. Philadelphia: W.B. Saunders.)

Conditioning

Patients who are to receive the donated marrow must undergo a conditioning regimen before transplantation. The purpose of conditioning depends on the patient's diagnosis and type of transplant to be received. There are two purposes of this regimen: (1) to obliterate the patient's own bone marrow, thus preparing the patient for optimal graft take or (2) to give higher-than-normal doses of chemotherapy or radiotherapy to obliterate a malignancy, such as breast cancer.

Conditioning regimens usually require anywhere from 5 to 10 days. The conditioning regimen always includes intensive chemotherapy and sometimes includes radiotherapy, usually total body irradiation (TBI). Each conditioning regimen is tailored to the individual patient, taking into account the specific disease, overall health, and previous treatment for the condition.

A typical conditioning regimen for an adult patient receiving an allogeneic bone marrow transplant for treatment of acute myelogenous leukemia is as follows. High-dose chemotherapy is administered on Days − 7 through − 5. In this situation, the purpose of conditioning is to obliterate the patient's own bone marrow cells and to eradicate any leukemic cells still present. Specific chemotherapeutic agents used in conditioning procedures include busulfan, carmustine, cyclophosphamide, cytarabine, etoposide, and melphalan (Ford, 1991). Usually only one agent is used and the dose is many times that used for normal chemotherapy. Days − 4 through − 2 of conditioning involve delivery of fractionated TBI (smaller doses of radiation given over a time instead of one larger dose). The typical radiation dose for TBI is 1200 rad. The patient usually "rests" on Day − 1.

Bone marrow and normal tissues begin to respond to the chemotherapy and radiotherapy immediately during conditioning. The patient will experience all the expected side effects associated with both therapies. Because the chemotherapy is administered at such a high dose, the side effects are much more intense than those seen with either normal chemotherapy or TBI. These side effects include severe nausea and vomiting, diarrhea, and bone marrow suppression.

Transplantation

Day 0 is the day of bone marrow transplantation. This day is separated from the chemotherapy conditioning days by at least 2 days to ensure that the chemotherapeutic agent has been cleared and will not exert any cytotoxic effects on the transplanted bone marrow. The patient should have few if any circulating white blood cells at this point, indicating successful conditioning.

The transplant itself is a very simple procedure and is usually anticlimactic. The bone marrow is administered through the patient's central line in a fashion similar to an ordinary blood transfusion, although blood administration tubing is not used. Usually the marrow is infused over a 30-minute period, although it may also be administered by intravenous "push" directly into the central line using syringes.

Engraftment

The transfused bone marrow cells circulate only briefly in the peripheral blood. The vast majority of cells, especially the stems cells, find their way to the marrow-forming sites of the recipient's bones and establish residency there. This ability of donated marrow cells to "home in" on the appropriate sites is a property, common to other differentiated cells, to recognize like cells or cell areas, although the mechanism of recognition is not known. It is not a random event caused by the "trapping" of donated marrow cells within the microvasculature of the recipient's body. If this were the case, the donated marrow would more likely be trapped in the fine capillary meshwork of the pulmonary vasculature rather than in the bone marrow.

Engraftment is the key to this whole process. In order for the donated marrow to "rescue" patients after large doses of chemotherapy or radiotherapy obliterate their own bone marrow, the donated marrow must survive and grow in the patients' bone marrow sites. When successful, the engraftment process can take 2 to 5 weeks. Engraftment has occurred when the patient's white-cell, erythrocyte, and platelet counts begin to rise. Other engraftment indicators can be determined by changes in peripheral blood cells or bone marrow cells. If the donated marrow was obtained from a person with an ABO blood type different from the patient's, engraftment can be called successful when the patient's blood type changes to that of the donor's. Similarly, if the donated marrow was obtained from a person of the opposite sex, engraftment is successful when the sex chromosomes of the patient's blood lymphocytes change to those of the donor. For example, if a woman is transplanted with her brother's bone marrow, engraftment is successful when her peripheral blood lymphocytes have XY sex chromosomes instead of XX chromosomes.

Sometimes the donated marrow fails to engraft. This possibility should be discussed in advance with the patient and the donor. Bone marrow transplantation can result in death from infection or hemorrhage unless the patient, the donor, and the facility agree to continue to transplant until engraftment occurs. Successful transplantations have been reported among individuals who failed to engraft the first two or three times they underwent transplantation. Failure to engraft occurs more frequently with allogeneic and syngeneic transplantation than it does with autologous transplantation.

EARLY COMPLICATIONS OF BONE MARROW TRANSPLANTATION

Complications among bone marrow transplant recipients may be related to the underlying disease, the conditioning treatment, or to the transplant itself. For the purposes of this discussion, complications are categorized as nonimmunologic and immunologic.

Nonimmunologic Complications

These complications arise primarily as a consequence of the conditioning treatment or the underlying disease. Transient treatment-associated complications include nausea, vomiting, alopecia, mucositis, and diarrhea. More serious, life-threatening complications include severe toxicities of the kidneys, heart, lungs, liver, and central nervous system (Champlin & Gale, 1984). Renal insufficiency occurs in approximately half of all patients undergoing bone marrow transplantation during the acute recovery phase (Ford & Ballard, 1988). The causes of the insufficiency include renal perfusion problems, secondary to other physiologic changes, leading to hypotension/hypoperfusion as well as more direct insults to renal tubules. Cardiac toxicities, while rare, can occur secondary to high-dose chemotherapy used in the conditioning treatment, especially cyclophosphamide. Individuals with diminished cardiac function, as measured by a lower-than-normal ejection fraction, prior to the transplantation procedure are more at risk for debilitating cardiac toxicities. Liver, lung, and central nervous system toxicities appear to be related more to radiotherapy conditioning and may be a greater problem in individuals who have undergone radiation therapy (of those organs) for their malignancies before the conditioning for bone marrow transplantation.

Immunologic Complications

Bone Marrow Suppression

Until engraftment occurs, the patient has no functional bone marrow. As a result, the new bone marrow is not yet producing either erythrocytes or platelets and the patient is profoundly anemic and thrombocytopenic. Fatigue, inadequate oxygenation, and potential hemorrhage are constant problems during this period. To reduce the intensity of these problems, the patient with a transplant receives many red-cell and platelet transfusions during the early posttransplant period.

The most critical problem for the patient undergoing BMT before engraftment is immunosuppression. Because the new marrow is not yet functional the patient has no immune system and absolutely no protection against any type of infection. All three types of immunity—neutrophils, antibodies, and cell-mediated immunity—are severely deficient in these patients. This problem is common to all transplant recipients regardless of transplant type. The types of infection these patients usually get are pneumonia, cellulitis, otitis media/sinusitis, meningitis, septicemia, and skin, perirectal, and gastrointestinal infections. The different types of organisms that cause these infections are Pseudomonas, *Staphylococcus aureus,* gram-negative and gram-positive organisms, and Klebsiella. Viral organisms are cytomegalovirus (CMV) and herpes simplex virus (HSV). Other opportunistic organisms are Pneumocystis, Toxoplasma, Candida, and Aspergillus (Gurevich & Tafuro, 1986).

Ironically, most of the infections these patients acquire are caused by the patient's own (endogenous) flora (Gurevich & Tafuro, 1986). This is a time when meticulous personal hygiene becomes of utmost importance, and when the patients are less likely to be able to provide it for themselves. In addition, relatives and caretakers may believe that the patients should be allowed to rest rather than be "bothered" with bathing and other personal hygiene measures.

There are other opportunistic organisms that come from outside sources. Aspergillus and other molds can be found whenever construction is in progress. *Pseudomonas aeruginosa* grows in stagnant water. A major problem for patients with new transplants is CMV infection. Before transplantation, each potential candidate should be tested to determine if they carry CMV. Transplant patients who are CMV-negative before transplantation can be protected (to some degree) against CMV infection by ensuring that the marrow donor is also CMV-negative. In addition, CMV-negative patients ideally should receive only CMV-negative blood products.

Essentially, during the early posttransplant period the patient is at risk for anything and everything. It is the nurse's responsibility to maintain a protective environment for these patients to minimize risk of nosocomial infections. The care plan in Chapter 15 provides specific interventions for the patient at risk for infection and sepsis.

Extreme precautions are necessary to prevent or limit infections in this population of patients. Most BMT units are in areas of the hospital physically separated from common areas. Some units use laminar airflow rooms (LAF) or bed units to limit transferring exogenous infectious organisms to the patient with a transplant. The principle behind an LAF room is to create an extremely clean, almost sterile, air supply for the room. All care for the patient becomes a sterile procedure. Supplies are sterilized, food is made as germ-free as possible, all invasive procedures are aseptic, minimal direct contact with the patient is made possible through a special wall with gloves, and anyone who comes into direct contact with the patient must scrub and wear protective clothing similar to that of people who work in surgery.

Graft-versus-Host Disease

Graft-versus-host disease (GVHD) is an immunologic complication unique to the allogeneic patient with BMT. "GVHD occurs in 40 per cent–50 per cent of all allogeneic transplants. GVHD or complications arising from GVHD, such as opportunistic infections, are responsible for 8 per cent of all BMT deaths. Patients at highest risk are those over age 30, those with an opposite sex donor, and those who are not perfectly matched with their donors" (Ford & Ballard, 1988, p. 17).

GVHD does not begin to manifest until engraftment is initiated. Mild GVHD can be taken as a positive sign that the transplant is a technical success: Because the allogeneic bone marrow recipient essentially receives someone else's immune system, and often that someone else is less than a perfect HLA match, the new immune system cells can recognize the patient's (host's) body cells as foreign to the immune system cells. In GVHD, the new immune system cells (the graft) initiate actions to destroy the "foreign" body cells of the patient (host). This situation is exactly the reverse of that in solid organ transplantation, in which the host's own immune system cells recognize the newly transplanted kidney (or other solid organ) as foreign and initiate cytotoxic actions to destroy the kidney cells (even though the transplanted kidney cells are very beneficial to the host).

GVHD can be seen as a "no-win" situation. If the graft succeeds in eliminating important host body cells, the host will die. If the host completely succeeds in eliminating the graft (the new immune system cells) the host will also die. T cells, specifically the cytotoxic T cells, together with the natural killer cells appear to be responsible for GVHD reactions. Although in theory all host body cells are at risk of damage during GVHD, the tissues primarily involved in this reaction are the liver, the skin, and the gastrointestinal system (Ford & Ballard, 1988).

Often the first system to show clinical manifestations of GVHD is the skin. The symptoms may start out as a rash followed by extreme generalized dry desquamation of the skin.

Gastrointestinal manifestations of GVHD may be hard to discern from the side effects of the conditioning treatment. Most commonly, the patient has a persistent watery diarrhea with abdominal cramping and pain.

Liver GVHD first manifests with serum elevations of liver enzyme levels. Patients may also experience upper-right-quadrant pain, liver enlargement and jaundice. A severe associated complication is venooclusive disease (VOD) of the liver blood vessels. It is unclear how much of the pathophysiology of VOD is a sequala of conditioning therapy or is an actual type of GVHD. This complication is more likely to occur among individuals who have preexisting liver disease or damage and those who have had liver irradiation. Immune cell re-actions within blood vessels of the liver cause fibrin to build up inside the ves-sels, occluding the lumen. When sufficient vessels have been occluded, pres-sure within the liver vasculature increases, causing ascites formation and impaired liver function. Significant liver dysfunction from VOD in this patient population is a major cause of death in the early posttransplantation period.

In addition to symptomatic and supportive treatment during GVHD, some control can be achieved with drug therapy aimed at either slowing the rate of engraftment or depressing T-cell function. Both types of treatments endanger the success of transplantation and increase the patient's risk for infection. Methotrexate and corticosteroids have been shown to slow the rate of engraft-ment (Ford, 1991). As described in Chapter 11, cyclosporine and antithymocyte globulin can specifically depress T-cell function (Sullivan et al., 1984).

LATE COMPLICATIONS OF BONE MARROW TRANSPLANTATION

Late complications of bone marrow transplantation are considered to be those that either manifest more than 100 days after transplantation or become chronic. These complications usually can be attributed to conditioning treat-ment, immunologic changes, or both.

Nonimmunologic Complications

Relapse of Initial Disease

A primary nonimmunologic complication after transplantation is recur-rence of the initial malignancy. This complication, obviously, is associated only with individuals who underwent transplantation in the hope of a cure for a malignant disease.

Pulmonary Complications

Pulmonary complications are relatively common in the late posttransplant period, occurring in approximately 10 per cent of transplant survivors (Nims & Strom, 1988). This complication is seen more among individuals with allo-geneic transplants. The bases for the pulmonary complications are infectious and secondary fibrosis related to tissue damage.

During the first year after transplantation the patient is not fully immu-nocompetent and is at risk for infection. Upper respiratory infections among these individuals can easily lead to life-threatening pneumonia.

Some fibrosis and scarring of pulmonary epithelium occur as a consequence of high-dose chemotherapy, especially when combined with TBI. This fibrosis and scarring thicken some areas of the alveolar membrane, diminishing the tissue available for gas exchange. This increase in the physiologic dead space may not be a problem at basal metabolic levels. However, when patients attempt to increase their physical activity, inadequate oxygenation may place significant limits on the type and duration of activity. In addition, interstitial fibrosis and scarring can decrease the amount of elastic tissue present in the lungs, limiting pulmonary compliance and causing restrictive pulmonary disease (Sullivan et al., 1984).

Reproductive Complications

Reproductive complications are a major long-term and usually permanent consequence of allogeneic bone marrow transplantation. For men, the chemotherapy conditioning together with the total body irradiation lead to permanent sterility. Sperm banking (for later artificial insemination) prior to initiating treatment is an option that should be discussed with the patient and his significant other. Obviously, this option is only viable for males who have reached puberty.

This topic is extremely sensitive, as are many reproductive issues. Sperm banking involves masturbation to obtain the semen specimens. Not only do many men consider masturbation wrong or repugnant, the practices of masturbation and artificial insemination violate the tenets of some religions. When the patient is a teenaged boy, his parents may object to this procedure. In theory, sperm frozen in liquid nitrogen has an indefinite "shelf-life." In practice, the consequences of very-long-term sperm storage are not known. In addition, the quantity of semen (as well as the quality) that can be obtained in a relatively short time may not be sufficient.

Females also have major and probably permanent long-term consequences from the conditioning treatment for bone marrow transplantation. Although the ovary is less sensitive to many chemotherapeutic agents than are the testes, radiation can render the ovarian follicular cells useless and damage the chromosomes in the oocytes. Young women may enter menopause within a short time after transplantation because the ovarian cells cannot respond to hormonal stimulation by producing estrogen. Without estrogen influences, any oocytes that have survived radiation fail to mature to the point at which fertilization can occur. In addition, should fertilization and pregnancy occur, the potential for birth defects secondary to radiation-induced gene damage cannot be underestimated.

Depending on the underlying reason for the transplant, women can be treated with estrogen–progesterone replacement therapy to prevent early menopause and decrease the health risks thought to be associated with diminished estrogen levels. These health risks include osteoporosis and arteriosclerosis (Cotran, Kumar, & Robbins, 1989).

Cataracts

Cataracts form, at a relatively early age (as compared with cataract formation in the general population), in approximately 10 per cent of patients who undergo TBI as part of their conditioning therapy (Ford, 1991). The incidence is higher among individuals who receive TBI as a single intensive dose than among those who receive TBI in smaller fractionated doses. Treatment for cataracts involves surgical removal, with or without lens replacement, when the cataracts significantly impair the patient's vision.

Immunologic Complications

Although all three components of immunity are initially affected by the bone marrow transplantation, the three components do not recover at an equal rate or to an equal degree. Within a few weeks of engraftment, the patient with a transplant usually has a normal granulocyte count and normal inflammatory responses. Antibody-mediated and cell-mediated immunity have much longer recovery periods.

Compromised Antibody-Mediated Immune Status

Even though most recipients of bone marrow transplants are usually transplanted with marrow from a fully immunocompetent donor, antibody-mediated immunity is not completely transferred with allogeneic transplantation, and the patient remains immunocompromised for at least 1 year after transplantation.

The consequence of this problem is that the patient does not have antibodies directed against any of the viruses and bacteria already encountered by the donor either by infection or by vaccination and therefore remains at risk for infection by these organisms. For instance, even though the donor had the chickenpox and therefore is fully immune against getting the chickenpox a second time, this immunity is not passed on to the marrow recipient. Not only are few antibodies present in the bone marrow directly (as opposed to the donor's serum), but the sensitized B cells are not present in the marrow to any great extent either (see Chapter 3 for a more detailed explanation of acquisition and maintenance of antibody-mediated immunity).

Patients are at increased risk for infection during the first year after transplantation. Prophylaxis for this susceptibility includes regularly scheduled doses of intravenous immune globulin (see Chapter 3) and continuous maintenance doses of an oral, broad-spectrum antibiotic. Over time, the surviving patients will develop good antibody-mediated immunity through the actions of their transplanted immune systems. This immunity will reflect what the patient has been exposed to and not what the donor had been exposed to.

Compromised Cell-Mediated Immune Status

Deficits in cell-mediated immunity appear to be treatment-related and have been documented as persisting for as long as 10 years after high-dose chemotherapy (see Chapter 10). Deficits are seen not in a deficiency of T-cell and natural-killer-cell numbers but in their functional capacities. Function of T helper/inducer cells and natural killer cells appears most impaired. It is possible that such impairment may put the patient with a transplant at an increased risk for the development of second malignancies. Currently, the actual incidence of second malignancies among transplant recipients is not greater than among individuals treated with conventional cancer therapies (Nims & Strom, 1988). This problem may become more apparent as the numbers of long-term survivors of bone marrow transplantation increase.

Chronic Graft-versus-Host Disease

Chronic GVHD, similar in pathophysiology to GVHD in the more acute phase after transplantation, manifests later and affects different sites in approximately 30 per cent (Sullivan et al., 1984). Whereas early GVHD is totally a cell-mediated response, chronic GVHD includes an antibody-mediated response similar to autoimmune disease. Some patients with early GVHD go on subsequently to develop chronic GVHD. In addition, some patients who did not have early GVHD do develop chronic GVHD in the later posttransplant period.

The skin and other dermal areas are common sites of chronic GVHD activity. Instead of the desquamation seen with early GVHD, manifestations of chronic GVHD include dermal thickening, epidermal atrophy, decreased keratinization, and telangiectasia. The dermal thickening may be so severe that joint contractures form, limiting mobility in these patients. Areas exposed to the sun appear to experience a more severe involvement than do areas not exposed to the sun.

According to Nims and Strom (1988), other sites manifesting changes related to chronic GVHD include skeletal muscles (characterized by a polymyositis), the eye (corneal wasting and keratoconjunctivitis), the lining of the entire gastrointestinal tract (xerostomia, dysphagia, increased development of caries, malabsorption, and weight loss), and the liver (jaundice, elevated liver enzymes, and intolerance to dietary fats). GVHD-induced changes in these areas have been shown to persist for years after transplantation and may lead to significant disabilities along with diminished quality of life. Treatment of chronic GVHD is titrated suppression of immune function. The agents most commonly used for this purpose are methotrexate, cyclosporine, and prednisone.

CASE PRESENTATION

Mr. Young was diagnosed 2 years ago with acute myelogenous leukemia (AML) and underwent aggressive chemotherapy at that time (see Chapter 7). Remission was achieved after induction therapy followed by consolidation therapy. Mr. Young started maintenance therapy with follow-up every 3 months. At 2 years after the initial diagnosis, Mr. Young's routine bone marrow aspiration showed a return of blast cells and emergence of cells with tumor markers. Even though Mr. Young had no subjective symptoms of the disease at this time, he was diagnosed as having a relapse of the AML.

At this time the option of bone marrow transplantation was discussed with Mr. Young. Mr. Young was the second oldest of a family of six children. HLA typing and MLC revealed his 16-year-old brother to be a perfect match with Mr. Young. Because research has shown that getting the patient into a second remission before transplantation does not enhance long-term survival and may in fact endanger the patient's life before transplantation (Appelbaum, 1988), it was decided that Mr. Young should undergo transplantation as soon as was safely possible.

Mr. Young's brother Brian and his parents were approached about Brian's being a marrow donor for Mr. Young. Brian was anxious to be the donor and was considerably relieved to hear that the marrow would be taken under anesthesia.

After consents were obtained, Brian underwent physical and psychologic examinations to determine his suitability as a bone marrow transplant donor. After ascertaining that Brian was physically and emotionally ready for the transplant procedure, he donated two units of blood 2 weeks apart. Brian also agreed to donate platelets on a biweekly basis for the next 6 weeks.

Mr. Young was admitted to the medical center's bone marrow transplant unit, and a double-lumen central venous catheter was placed. He was started on total parenteral nutrition at that time. The day after the catheter was placed Mr. Young began conditioning with high-dose cyclophosphamide (Cytoxan) at 50 mg/kg/day for 4 days and placed in reverse isolation in a laminar airflow room. The chemotherapy was followed by total body irradiation of 1200 rad fractionated into four doses over a 2-day period. Mr. Young was allowed to rest for 2 days following the TBI.

On the second resting day, Brian was admitted to the hospital, and 800 ml of bone marrow was harvested. Although his brother was in reverse isolation and very uncomfortable with nausea and vomiting, Brian was glad to be hospitalized on the same unit as Mr. Young. Brian experienced no complications and was discharged to home the day after donating the marrow.

The day Brian was discharged Mr. Young's white-cell count was 200/cu mm. His marrow was acellular and the conditioning was deemed successful. Mr. Young received his brother's marrow at that time by intravenous infusion into his central line over a 20-minute period. His temperature increased to 101°F immediately following the transfusion but he had no other indications of a reaction to the transfusion. He continued to be supported with antiemetics and intravenous fluid and electrolytes. Because he had a history of herpes simplex viral infection, Mr. Young was started on acyclovir.

By the next day Mr. Young's white-cell count was 0 and his hematocrit was 19 per cent. He received two units of packed red cells from his brother on Day 2 after transplantation. During the next week Mr. Young received several units of random donor platelets that had been obtained from CMV-negative donors.

On Day 7 after transplantation Mr. Young had a white-cell count of 50 cells/ cu mm of blood. A fever developed. Bacterial/fungal cultures were drawn peripherally and from his central line; a urine culture was sent; and an immediate portable chest x-ray film was taken. After the cultures and chest x-ray film were obtained, he was started immediately on ticarcillin 3 gm IVPB (administered by intravenous piggy-back infusion) every 4 hours and tobramycin 100 mg IVPB every 8 hours. A maintenance intravenous infusion of supplemental potassium (K +) also was started.

Over the next 2 weeks Mr. Young's blood counts gradually increased and he began having frequent episodes of watery diarrhea. The stool was initially guaiac-negative but became positive on the fifth day of diarrhea. Intravenous fluid replacement was continued as was the total parenteral nutrition because of Mr. Young's anorexia. A tentative diagnosis of GVHD was made, and Mr. Young was started on oral prednisone and cyclosporine. The diarrhea gradually diminished, and Mr. Young did not manifest any other symptoms of GVHD.

By the 36th day after transplantation Mr. Young's white-cell count was 550, with 75 per cent segmented neutrophils, 4 per cent band forms, 18 per cent lymphocytes, and 3 per cent monocytes. His vital signs, including temperature, had been within normal limits for 4 days. Cultures of skin at the catheter site, blood, stool, oral mucosa, and urine obtained on Day 32 were all negative and he was discharged to home with outpatient follow-up.

SELECTED BIBLIOGRAPHY

Abbas, A., Lichtman, A., & Pober, J. (1991). *Cellular and molecular immunology.* Philadelphia: W.B. Saunders.

Ammann, A. (1987). Immunodeficiency diseases. In D. Stites, J. Stobo, & J. Wells (Eds.), *Basic and clinical immunology* (6th ed.) (p. 317). Norwalk, CT: Appleton & Lange.

Appelbaum, F. (1988). Marrow transplantation for hematologic malignancies: A brief review of current status and future prospects. *Seminars in Hematology, 25*(3, Suppl. 3), 16.

Armitage, J., & Gale, R. (1989). Bone marrow autotransplantation. *American Journal of Medicine, 86*, 203.

Canellos, G., Nadler, L., & Takvorian, T. (1988). Autologous bone marrow transplantation in the treatment of malignant lymphoma and Hodgkin's disease. *Seminars in Hematology, 25*(2, Suppl. 2), 58.

Carlson, A. (1985). Infection prophylaxis in the patient with cancer. *Oncology Nursing Forum, 12*(3), 56.

Champlin, R., & Gale, R. (1984). Role of bone marrow transplantation in the treatment of hematologic malignancies and solid tumors: Critical review of syngeneic, autologous, and allogeneic transplants. *Cancer Treatment Reports, 68*(1), 145.

Corcoran-Buchsel, P., & Ford, R. (1988). Introduction. *Seminars in Oncology Nursing, 4*(1), 1.

Corcoran-Buchsel, P. (1986). Long-term complications of allogeneic bone marrow transplantation: Nursing implications. *Oncology Nursing Forum, 13*(6), 61.

Cotran, R., Kumar, V., & Robbins, S. (1989). *Robbins pathologic basis of disease* (4th ed.). Philadelphia: W.B. Saunders.

Ford, R. (1991). Bone marrow transplantation. In S. Baird, R. McCorkle, & M. Grant (Eds.), *Cancer nursing: A comprehensive textbook* (p. 385). Philadelphia: W.B. Saunders.

Ford, R., & Ballard, B. (1988). Acute complications after bone marrow transplantation. *Seminars in Oncology Nursing, 4*(1), 15.

Ford, R., & Eisenberg, S. (1990). Bone marrow transplantation: Recent advances and nursing implications. *Nursing Clinics of North America, 25*(2), 405.

Freedman, S. (1988). An overview of bone marrow transplantation. *Seminars in Oncology Nursing, 4*(1), 3.

Gale, R., & Quinn, S. (1989). The management of acute leukemias. Part I: bone marrow transplants. *Clinical Advances in Oncology Nursing, 1*(2), 1.

Gurevich, I., & Tafuro, P. (1986). The compromised host: Deficit-specific infection and the spectrum of infection. *Cancer Nursing, 9*(5), 263.

Hughes, C. (1985). Interpreting the white blood cell count in the cancer chemotherapy patient: Nursing responsibilities. *National Intravenous Therapy Association, 8,* 279.

Nims, J., & Strom, S. (1988). Late complications of bone marrow transplant recipients: Nursing care issues. *Seminars in Oncology Nursing, 4*(1), 47.

O'Quin, T., & Moravec, C. (1988). The critically ill bone marrow transplant patient. *Seminars in Oncology Nursing, 4*(1), 25.

Ruggiero, M. (1988). The donor in bone marrow transplantation. *Seminars in Oncology Nursing, 4*(1), 9.

Schilter, L., & Rossman, E. (1991). Bone marrow transplantation. In S. Baird, M. Donehower, V. Stalsbroten, & T. Ades (Eds.), *A cancer source book for nurses* (p. 91). Atlanta: American Cancer Society.

Sullivan, K., Deeg, J., Sanders, J., Shulman, H., Witherspoon, R., Doney, K., Appelbaum, F., Schubert, M., Stewart, P., Springmeyer, S., McDonald, G., Storb, R., & Thomas, E. (1984). Late complications after marrow transplantation. *Seminars in Hematology, 21*(1), 53.

Thomas, E. (1988). The future of marrow transplantation. *Seminars in Oncology Nursing, 4*(1), 74.

Wiley, F., & House, K. (1988). Bone marrow transplant in children. *Seminars in Oncology Nursing, 4*(1), 31.

Ziegfeld, C. (1987). *Core curriculum for oncology nursing.* Philadelphia: W.B. Saunders.

Miscellaneous Conditions Causing Immunosuppression

13

IMMUNODEFICIENCY ASSOCIATED WITH AGING

It is well known that a variety of changes in immune function accompany the normal aging process. It is likely that these changes, to some extent, contribute to an increased frequency of bacterial and viral infections and an increased incidence of cancer seen with advancing age. However, the underlying mechanisms that result in altered immune function in the elderly are not well understood. This age-associated decline in immune responsiveness is referred to as immunosenescence.

In a review of current research in immunosenescence, Saltzman and Peterson (1987) identified five factors to be considered when interpreting research findings. First, there is no universally accepted definition of "aged." Physiologic aging and chronologic aging do not always occur at the same rate. Second, it is difficult to separate the effect of age on the immune system from the effects of other health-related conditions. Chronic diseases, medications, nutritional problems, and environmental factors all have an impact on immune function. Third, alterations in nonspecific defense mechanisms will alter the incidence of infection in the elderly. Fourth, methodologic differences among studies are frequently encountered and may contribute to contradictory results. Finally, many studies are performed using animal models, which may not accurately reflect changes in immune function in elderly humans.

To complicate matters further, research results are often conflicting, particularly when reporting lymphocyte number and function. Differences may be attributable to the fact that the distribution of lymphocytes throughout the body is constantly changing. Evaluating one lymphoid compartment (for example, peripheral blood) may yield results that are not representative of the whole (Weksler, 1986).

BIOLOGY OF IMMUNOSENESCENCE

Involution of the thymus gland has long been linked to changes observed in immune function in aging humans and research animals. The thymus reaches its maximum cellular mass during childhood. The mass of the thymus remains stable until sexual maturity is reached. At this time, the mass begins to decrease rapidly until the age of 45 to 50, when only about 10 per cent of the original total mass is retained.

The involution of the thymus gland results in a decrease in thymic hormone concentrations. By approximately 60 years of age, these hormones are no longer detectable. Moreover, the aging thymus apparently loses its ability to promote the maturation or differentiation of T-lymphocyte precursors. With increasing age, fewer precursors enter the thymus and fewer still emerge as mature T lymphocytes. The result is an increase in the number of immature lymphocytes in the peripheral circulation and in the thymus gland.

Research has demonstrated that lymphocytes from aged humans and laboratory animals are more sensitive to conditions that damage DNA, including ionizing radiation and mutagenic drugs. This observation may explain in part the increased incidence of cancer with aging.

Nonspecific defense mechanisms also undergo alterations with normal aging that further diminish the ability to mount a successful response to invasion. These changes will be reviewed on a system-by-system basis.

Inflammatory Response

Bacterial infections in the elderly, particularly those involving the respiratory tract, are not always easy to identify in their early stages because of minimal or absent symptoms. Sputum production, leukocytosis, and temperature elevation rarely reach levels demonstrated in younger adults. These observations have led researchers to question the competence of the inflammatory response in older adults, particularly the action of polymorphonuclear leukocytes (PMNs).

Although there is no evidence of granulocytopenia in aging, studies reporting a variety of PMN functions in the elderly provide conflicting results. There is no consensus among the studies reviewed by Saltzman and Peterson (1987) regarding chemotaxis, phagocytosis, or bactericidal activity in the elderly. Moreover, even when defects in PMN function were noted, there was no associated increase in the incidence of bacterial infections (Laharrague et al., 1983).

Lack of a febrile reaction to bacterial invasion may play a part in an impaired immune response. In a study reported by Gleckman and Hilbert (1982), afebrile bacteremia occurred in 25 of 192 elderly subjects as compared with 5 of 128 nonelderly subjects ($p < 0.01$). Leukocytosis was absent in eight of the 25 elderly patients. There is evidence to suggest that the febrile response augments immune reactions. A limited febrile response may have a role in compromising the ability of the aging immune system to mount an effective reaction to invasion (Rudd & Banerjee, 1989; Schwab, Walters, & Weksler, 1989).

Antibody Mediated Immunity

Clinical investigations have shown subtle changes in antibody mediated or humoral immunity occurring with age. Although the total number of B cells in the marrow appears to increase with age, the number in peripheral blood remains stable. However, the number of colony-forming B cells lessens with age, along with a decline in maturation to antibody-producing cells (Fox, 1985).

Many studies have attempted to clarify changes in antibody production and response in the elderly. Total concentration of serum immunoglobulin changes only slightly with age, although minor shifts in distribution have been documented. IgG and IgA concentrations gradually increase, while IgM levels decrease or remain stable.

Increased levels of autoantibodies and monoclonal immunoglobulins are also noted in aging humans. Production of these proteins is thought to reflect a disorder in regulation of normal B cells and is not associated with neoplastic transformation. The significance of autoantibodies and benign monoclonal immunoglobulins is unclear; however, it has been suggested that circulating autoantibodies produce physiologic changes associated with aging by damaging tissue and organs (Weksler, 1986; Fox, 1985; Adler & Nagel, 1985). There is no correlation between the incidence of autoimmune disease and the presence of these autoantibodies.

Other changes in humoral immunity related to the aging process include a decline in natural antibodies, decreased response to foreign antigens, and a reduction in the length of time the antibody response is maintained.

There is evidence for a possible link between thymic involution and changes in antibody response. Administration of thymic hormones in old mice augmented the response of IgG, IgA, and antibody (Weksler, 1986). It has also been noted that T-cell dependent antibody responses are impaired to a greater degree than T-cell independent responses (Saltzman and Peterson, 1987; Weksler, 1986). In fact, impaired humoral immunity associated with aging is now thought to be the result of alterations in T-cell function, a defect in the interaction between T and B cells, or both.

Cell-Mediated Immunity

The major defect in cell-mediated immunity is probably related to the decrease in the number of responsive T cells and an impaired capacity of stimulated T cells to proliferate. The number of T cells that can be stimulated to divide in culture is reduced by 50 to 80 per cent among elderly donors (Inkeles et al., 1977). Cells that are still able to respond are unable to divide more than once or twice (Hefton, Darlington, Casazza, & Weksler, 1980). Studies of inter-leukin-2/(T-cell growth factor) have shown that the number of T-cell receptor sites for interleukin-2 and the synthesis of interleukin-2 by T cells decreases with age. Based on these findings, it has been hypothesized that the decreased capacity of T cells from elderly donors to divide repeatedly in culture is due to an impaired ability of the cells to produce and respond to interleukin-2. Pre-liminary studies suggest that the proliferative defect lies in the failure of the nucleus to carry out DNA replication following an otherwise normal cellular and cytoplasmic stimulation (Weksler, 1986).

CLINICAL CONSEQUENCES OF IMMUNOSENESCENCE

Infectious Complications

Skin and Mucous Membranes

A variety of changes occur in the skin over time, predisposing to infection. The epidermis becomes thin, dry, and fragile, with a decreased rate of epider-mal turnover and collagen synthesis. In the dermal and subcutaneous regions, there is a loss of vascularity, connective tissue, and fat. As a result, the skin is prone to injury by tearing, shearing, and ulceration. The same physiologic changes predispose the elderly to infection and delayed wound healing. Other complicating factors include dehydration, malnutrition, anemia, and periph-eral vascular disease. Conditions associated with altered mentation—immo-bility, incontinence, and poor personal hygiene—further increase the risk of disrupted skin integrity and subsequent infection.

BACTERIAL INFECTIONS. Bacterial infections are common at any site where the skin has been damaged. Postoperative wound infections are far more likely to develop in the elderly than in younger patients. Chronic skin ulcers and pressure sores commonly become secondarily infected with a variety of pathogens.

Prevention of bacterial skin infections is almost exclusively the domain of nursing, particularly in the hospitalized or institutionalized older adult. Pro-tective measures to reduce risk of injury include strategies to prevent skin breakdown due to pressure and irritating agents, such as excreta, wound drain-age, and dressing supplies. Consultation with an enterostomal therapist is often helpful in identifying specific skin care products and procedures that minimize trauma and facilitate healing.

SUPERFICIAL FUNGAL INFECTIONS. Superficial fungal infections, particu-larly Candida, are a common mucocutaneous problem in the elderly. Sites in-volved usually include the oropharynx, genitalia, and areas where moist skin surfaces are in close contact with each other (e.g., under the breasts, in the groin). Assessment for evidence of oral Candida (thrush) should include in-spection of the mouth with the dentures removed, as a common site in the elderly is under the upper denture. Topical antifungal agents are effective in treating Candida infections, with nystatin most commonly prescribed.

VIRAL INFECTIONS. Viral infections of the skin are relatively uncommon, with the exception of herpes or varicella–zoster virus (VZV) ("shingles"). The incidence of VZV infection increases with age. In the general population, the incidence is approximately 1.3 cases per 1000 persons per year. However, among those between the ages of 60 and 79, the rate is 6.5 per 1000 per year and nearly 10 per 1000 per year over age 80. Risk is not associated with gender, race, or season of the year (Bentley, 1986).

In reviewing the role of interferons in host defenses against viral infection, Rytel (1987) reported certain preliminary observations that could explain the dramatic increase in the rate of VZV infection associated with age. Interferon functions in a variety of direct and indirect ways to protect against viral infection. By studying the immune response of elderly subjects to VZV and two herpes viruses, a significant decrease was noted in the interferon response to viral antigens. Rytel suggested that "failure to inhibit viral replication by suboptimal amounts of interferon and inadequate cytotoxic reaction would lead to sufficient concentrations of VZV to cause clinical zoster" (Rytel, 1987, p. 1097).

VZV infection is caused by reactivation of latent virus residing in the dorsal-root ganglia. Once it is reactivated, VZV proceeds along the nerve axon and produces characteristic skin lesions along involved dermatomes. The lesions are usually limited to one or two dermatomes, most commonly in the thoracic region (50 to 60 per cent). Other areas of involvement, in order of frequency, are the trigeminal (10 to 20 per cent), cervical (10 to 20 per cent), lumbar (5 to 10 per cent), and sacral (<5 per cent) regions (Bentley, 1986; Fretwell & Lipsky, 1985). Although the reason for reactivation is generally unknown, it may be precipitated by stress, trauma, treatment with immunosuppressive agents, local irradiation, or development of a malignancy, particularly leukemia or lymphoma.

The frequency and severity of complications, like the incidence of VZV, correlate directly with the age of the patient. The most common complication of VZV infection is postherpetic neuralgia (PHN), defined as "pain in the involved dermatome lasting for more than one month following the acute episode" (Bentley, 1986, p. 460). The underlying mechanism of PHN is unclear, although it may be related to postinflammatory fibrosis in the dorsal-root ganglia. PHN occurs in 25 to 40 per cent of those over age 60 and up to half of those over age 70. It is more frequently associated with trigeminal distribution.

Trigeminal involvement is also more likely to result in ophthalmic complications, including conjunctivitis and corneal ulceration. Ophthalmologic consultation is warranted when ocular complications occur.

Other less common neurologic complications of VZV infection include motor neuropathies, encephalitis, myelitis, and peripheral neuropathy. Lumbosacral involvement is associated with constipation, urinary retention, and impotence.

Treatment of uncomplicated VZV infection is primarily symptomatic, consisting of wet compresses of aluminum acetate (Burrow's solution) and analgesia. Pain management is frequently achieved with aspirin or other mild analgesics.

For complicated VZV, systemic corticosteroids, although somewhat controversial, are most often recommended. The usual course of therapy begins with doses of oral prednisone at 40 to 60 mg per day for 1 week, decreasing to 20 to 30 mg per day during the second week, 10 to 15 mg per day the third week, and discontinuing the drug at the fourth week. This treatment plan has resulted in a significant reduction in PHN—15 to 30 per cent in treated patients versus 65 to 75 per cent treated by analgesics or placebo (Bentley, 1986). Concern about the use of steroids in VZV infection is based on the potential risk of disseminated infection, the progression of local dermatome lesion, and secondary bacterial infection (Garagusi, 1989). However, these complications have not been observed (Eaglstein, Katz, & Brown, 1970; Keczkes & Basheer, 1980).

VZV treatment using DNA inhibitors, such as idoxuridine, vidarabine, and acyclovir, has been successful in shortening the period of pain and improving the rate of healing. Vidarabine also reduces the total duration of PHN and the frequency of cutaneous and visceral dissemination. Acyclovir administration results in decreased dissemination; in addition, duration of viral shedding is significantly reduced. However, acyclovir has no demonstrated effect on the incidence or severity of PHN.

Respiratory Tract

Pulmonary infections, specifically pneumonia and influenza, comprise the fourth leading cause of death among adults age 65 and over (Bentley, 1986). A variety of physiologic changes reduce the ability of the elderly to clear secretions and aspirated microorganisms from the lung. Loss of elasticity around the alveoli, increased chest diameter, and weakening of respiratory muscles combine to produce a less effective cough and a tendency for collapse of lower airways. In addition, changes have been observed in mucociliary function, including a slowing of transport of foreign material out of the lung. Colonization of the respiratory tract by gram-negative organisms is relatively common among those who are debilitated or seriously ill. It has been postulated that alterations in mucosal defense barriers in the tracheobronchial tree may increase bacterial adherence and facilitate infection (Phair et al., 1978; Valenti, Trudell, & Bentley, 1978; Verghese & Berk, 1983; Haddy, 1988). An intrinsic defect in alveolar macrophages and PMNs, impaired T-cell function, or both have also been suggested as contributing factors (Bentley, 1986).

Other conditions compromising pulmonary function in the elderly include chronic disease (e.g., bronchitis, emphysema, congestive heart failure, vertebral arthritis), dehydration, malnutrition, history of smoking, and alcoholism. Factors that increase risk of aspiration include diminished or absent cough and gag reflexes (e.g., cerebrovascular accident, treatment with sedatives or tranquilizers), esophageal disorders (e.g., decreased relaxation of the esophageal sphincter, reduced peristalsis, large hiatal hernia), endotracheal intubation, nasogastric tubes, and tracheostomy (Verghese & Berk, 1983).

BACTERIAL PNEUMONIAS. Bacterial pneumonias occur frequently and with significant morbidity and mortality among the aged. The incidence is highest for those who are institutionalized, probably a reflection of disability and severity of other chronic health problems. Rates of community-acquired bacterial pneumonia range from 20 to 40 cases per 1000 per year, depending on specific population or community characteristics (Bentley, 1986). Among the institutionalized elderly, incidence may be as high as 70 to 115 per 1000 per year (Bentley et al., 1981). The incidence of hospital-acquired pneumonias among those over age 65 is twice the rate for persons between 18 and 50 (Schwartz, 1982).

Although *Streptococcus pneumoniae* accounts for the majority of diagnosed cases, the etiologic agent varies according to the setting in which the infection is acquired (Table 13–1). Determining the causative agent is not always possible, however, because of difficulty in obtaining an adequate and reliable specimen for culture. Commonly, aspiration of oropharyngeal secretions results in multiple organisms potentially either contributing to or confounding the diagnosis.

The majority of elderly patients with bacterial pneumonia will present with classic symptoms: fever, productive cough, and leukocytosis. However, in a considerable number of cases, symptoms are more subtle. Temperature elevation and abnormal breath sounds may be absent, and chest x-ray films unremarkable. Most common among atypical presentations are lethargy and altered mental status, particularly confusion. In addition, preexisting chronic cardio-

TABLE 13–1. Estimated Prevalence (%) of Etiologic Agents Causing Bacterial Pneumonia in the Elderly According to Setting.

	Setting		
Agent	Community Acquired	Institution Acquired	Hospital Acquired
Streptococcus pneumoniae	55	35	20
Haemophilus influenzae and other Haemophilus species	10	5	5
Staphylococcus aureus	1	1	5
Gram-negative bacilli	5	15	35
Mixed flora*	25	40	30
Other†	4	4	5

(From Bacterial pneumonia in the elderly by A. Verghese and S.L. Berk, 1983, *Medicine* 62:271. Copyright © Williams & Wilkens, 1983.)
*Two or more respiratory pathogens, normal oropharyngeal commensals, or both.
†Other: Legionella pneumophilia, anaerobes, fungi, unknown.

pulmonary disorders may worsen, progressing to acute cardiac or respiratory failure.

Although in some cases, treatment can be managed on an outpatient basis using oral antimicrobial agents, pneumonia in the older adult complicated by volume depletion, nausea and vomiting, dyspnea, or altered mental status requires hospitalization. Every effort should be made to obtain a reliable sputum specimen for culture. Blood cultures may also be requested, especially when the patient is severely ill, when Gram stains of sputum reveal the presence of gram-positive cocci, or when sputum specimens are nondiagnostic.

Nurses have an important role in prevention of bacterial pneumonia due to aspiration in the elderly adult. Strict attention must be paid to positioning, feeding, suctioning, and other aspects of care, particularly in patients with a preexisting health problem that increases the risk of aspiration.

Availability of the polyvalent pneumococcal vaccine may offer some protection to the elderly. The antibody response to the vaccine, although somewhat diminished as compared with young, healthy adults, has reached adequate levels in most studies with few, if any, serious side effects noted. However, results of clinical trials have failed to demonstrate a reduction in the incidence, morbidity, or mortality of pneumococcal pneumonia in elderly subjects (Schwartz, 1982; Roghmann, Tabloski, Bentley, & Schiffman, 1987). Additional studies are needed to clarify the role of the pneumococcal vaccine for older persons.

In addition to administration of appropriate antibiotic regimens to those who are infected, nursing care measures include monitoring oxygen therapy, maintaining body temperature within normal range, assisting with chest physiotherapy, encouraging cough and deep-breathing exercises, and promoting adequate hydration and nutrition. When there is no observable improvement in patient status after 48 to 72 hours of antibiotic therapy, the physician should be notified, so that specimens for repeat culture can be obtained and changes in antimicrobial agents prescribed.

VIRAL PNEUMONIA. As with bacterial pneumonia, viral pneumonia accounts for significant morbidity and mortality among the elderly. Whereas persons over age 65 comprise about 13 per cent of the total population and only 10 per cent of all reported cases of influenza, they make up at least 50 per cent of the hospitalizations and 75 to 80 per cent of deaths attributed to the disease. The presence of certain underlying diseases has been associated with increased risk of morbidity and mortality: cardiovascular disease, pulmonary disease, metabolic disorders (e.g., diabetes), renal dysfunction, anemia, and immunosuppression. A history of any one of these disorders is likely to increase the risk of death by at least 39-fold. When more than one is present, the risk may increase as much as 870-fold (Barker & Mullooly, 1982).

The influenza virus attacks and destroys the ciliated epithelial lining of the respiratory tract, causing epithelial sloughing, fluid extravasation, submucosal inflammation, and alveolar collapse. Damage to the integrity of epithelium enables the virus and other organisms to invade the alveoli.

The infection is transmitted from one infected host to another by an airborne route—coughing, sneezing, or, in some cases, talking—and by physical contact. Following an incubation period of 24 to 48 hours, infected persons note an abrupt onset of fever, chills, myalgia, headache, and malaise. Systemic symptoms are frequently accompanied by respiratory complications, including cough, nasal congestion, and pharyngitis.

Unlike the pneumococcal vaccine, evidence is available regarding efficacy of the influenza vaccine in the elderly. A significant reduction in influenza-related hospitalizations and deaths has been reported in a variety of studies. Overall, the results suggest that the vaccine is about 70 per cent effective in preventing influenza, with few minimal adverse reactions (Fretwell & Lipsky, 1985). Contraindications to the vaccine include history of Guillain-Barré syndrome following prior vaccination or allergy to eggs (Centers for Disease Control, 1984).

Treatment in uncomplicated cases is primarily symptomatic: rest, adequate fluid intake, antipyretics and analgesics, and over-the-counter "cough-and-cold" remedies, according to patient preference. Amantadine hydrochloride (Symmetrel) may be used as an antiviral agent in documented cases of influenza A; it has no effect on influenza B. Although the mechanism of action is unclear, it is thought that amantadine inhibits an early stage of the viral replication cycle (Consensus Development Panel Conference, 1984; Hayden & Douglas, 1985). The currently recommended dose is 100 mg twice daily for 3 to 5 days. Plasma half-life increases in those with renal dysfunction who may note adverse reactions more frequently.

The most commonly encountered complications of influenza in the elderly are bronchitis, secondary bacterial pneumonia, and congestive heart failure. Recommendations for treatment are the same as those for bacterial pneumonia.

TUBERCULOSIS. Tuberculosis continues to be a problem, especially for the debilitated elderly. The incidence of a positive purified protein derivative (PPD) test ranges between 10 and 40 per cent, depending on the characteristics of the population studied (Fretwell & Lipsky, 1985). Reactivation of latent infection is the most common presentation of the disease, although many who were successfully treated for tuberculosis in the past will now be susceptible to new primary disease.

Signs and symptoms may be very subtle in elderly patients. Some with active disease will not react to the PPD and chest x-ray films are not always helpful. Tuberculosis should be considered in cases of biapical pulmonary disease, acute lower lobe pneumonia that does not respond to conventional therapy (Garibaldi, Neuhaus, & Nurse, 1988), or fever of undetermined origin (Garagusi, 1989).

Tuberculosis can be a particularly serious problem in nursing homes because of the potential number of asymptomatic carriers of active infection. It is recommended that all nursing home residents undergo chest roentgenography and have a PPD test on admission to identify as many cases as possible (Garagusi, 1989). Surveillance should extend to personnel who are likely to demonstrate a reliable response to PPD testing (Fretwell & Lipsky, 1985).

Treatment of tuberculosis in the elderly is generally similar to that for younger adults. However, caution should be used when administering isoniazid, in view of its hepatic toxicity.

Genitourinary System

Physiologic changes associated with aging contribute to the frequency of genitourinary infections. In postmenopausal women, mucosal changes in the bladder and urethra occur because of the decline in estrogen production. Relaxation of the pelvic floor, a consequence of reduced muscle mass and tissue elasticity, decreases bladder emptying and promotes the accumulation of residual urine. Muscle relaxation also functionally reduces the length of the urethra and, as a result, limits its effectiveness as a barrier to ascending organisms (Fretwell & Lipsky, 1985). Perineal contamination develops with physical impairments that compromise personal hygiene and especially with fecal incontinence.

In men, prostatic hypertrophy obstructs urine flow and reduces bladder emptying. Other prostatic problems that increase the risk of urinary tract infection include surgical interventions, instrumentation, chronic prostatitis, and alterations in prostatic secretions that may interfere with antiinfective properties. Neurogenic bladder, diabetes, indwelling urinary catheters, and incontinence due to confusion are common complicating factors for members of both sexes.

THE URINARY TRACT. The urinary tract is the most common site of bacterial infection in the elderly; its incidence is related to age, level of care required, and declining functional capacity (Table 13–2). The majority of older adults with urinary tract infections (UTIs) remain asymptomatic. For them, the significance of UTI and recommendations for treatment remain controversial. Research results defining the natural history of asymptomatic UTIs are conflicting, with some reporting increased morbidity and mortality while others do not. In most cases, it appears that long-term success in eradicating asymptomatic UTI is very limited. In one series, up to 50 per cent of successfully treated patients experienced recurrence. Moreover, treatment predisposes to the development of and colonization by resistant organisms (Alling et al., 1975). Frequent problems with adverse reactions to drug therapy and concerns about cost, in addition to lack of proven benefit, have convinced most physicians not to treat asymptomatic UTI.

There is agreement, however, that use of indwelling catheters poses a definite risk, with significant bacteriuria developing in nearly all patients after about 1 week (Fretwell & Lipsky, 1985). For the institutionalized patient who

TABLE 13-2. Estimated Prevalence (%) of Bacteriuria According to Age and Level of Care.

Age	Women	Men
<65 Home	5	<1
65–79	20	10
Over 80	40	20
Over 65		
Nursing home	25	20
Acute hospital	30	30
Chronic disease hospital	40	35

(Modified from Kaye D.: Urinary tract infections in the elderly. Bull NY Acad Med 56:209, 1980. In I. Rossman [Ed.], *Clinical geriatrics* [p. 447]. Philadelphia: J.B. Lippincott.)

is incontinent and possibly bedridden, the potential risk of urosepsis must be weighed against the potential benefit of maintaining skin integrity when the use of an indwelling catheter is considered.

Although classic presentation of symptomatic UTI may occur in the aged, more often than not, symptoms are difficult to interpret. Urinary frequency, dysuria, and incontinence may be attributable to a chronic disease or to medication. Unusual progression to a markedly confused state may be the only indication of infection. Pyelonephritis or sepsis (or both) is more likely to result in patients with obstructive uropathies or recent invasive procedures of the urinary tract.

The laboratory data that may be most useful is the microscopic examination of urinary sediment. Pyuria (presence of 10 white blood cells per high-power field), while absent in asymptomatic UTI, is usually present in the majority of symptomatic UTIs. Confirmation of the causative agent in women is complicated by frequent contamination of midstream specimens. Obtaining a valid culture specimen by straight catheterization, using the smallest catheter possible, may facilitate an accurate diagnosis and appropriate treatment.

When antibiotic therapy is indicated, the agents chosen should concentrate in the urine yet have a low risk of adverse reaction. Considerations in antimicrobial selection for the elderly are summarized in Table 13-3. Relapses are to be expected and usually occur within 2 weeks. Treatment is withheld unless the infection again becomes symptomatic (Fretwell & Lipsky, 1985).

Fungal infections of the urinary tract are frequently found in patients requiring long-term indwelling urinary catheters or who have undergone antibiotic therapy. Colonization by *Candida albicans* or *Torulopsis glabrata* in the lower urinary tract requires treatment with an antifungal agent to prevent the development of pyelonephritis.

TABLE 13-3. Toxicity Considerations in Antibiotic Selection for Infections in the Elderly.

Agent	Renal	Hepatic	Other
Aminoglycosides Amikacin Gentamicin Kanamycin Netilmicin Tobramycin	Not to exceed recommended dose; may require lower daily doses in accordance with decreased renal function. Monitor renal function carefully during therapy.		Hearing loss may develop even in patients with normal renal function.
Penicillins	May require dosage adjustment with age-related decline in renal function		Antibiotic-associated pseudomembranous colitis
Amdinocillin Amoxacillin + clavulanate Ampicillin + sulbactam			
Azlocillin	Hypokalemia	Cholestatic jaundice	
Bacampicillin			
Carbenicillin	Alterations in serum Na$^+$ and K$^+$		Platelet dysfunction
Cyclacillin	Hypokalemia	Cholestatic jaundice	
Mezlocillin	Hyperkalemia, hypernatremia		
Penicillin G	Hypokalemia		
Piperacillin	Alterations in serum Na$^+$ and K$^+$	Cholestatic jaundice	Platelet dysfunction
Ticarcillin + clavulanate			
Cephalosporins	May require dosage adjustment with age-related decline in renal function		Antibiotic-associated pseudomembranous colitis
Cefaclor Cefadroxil			
Cefamandole			Hypoprothrombinemia

Drug	May require dosage adjustment	Adverse reactions
Cefazolin		
Cefonicid		
Cefoperazone	May require dosage adjustment with severe liver disease	Hypoprothrombinemia
Ceforanide		
Cefotaxime		
Cefotetan		Hypoprothrombinemia
Cefoxitin		
Ceftazidime		
Ceftizoxime		
Ceftriaxone		
Cefuroxime		
Cephalexin		
Cephalothin		
Cephapirin		
Cephradine		
Moxalactam		Hypoprothrombinemia
Sulfonamides		
Sulfamethoxazole + phenazopyridine	May require dosage adjustment with age-related decline in renal function	
+ trimethoprim		Skin reactions, bone marrow depression, thrombocytopenia
Sulfisoxazole + phenazopyridine	May require dosage adjustment with age-related decline in renal function	
Other		
Cinoxacin		
Ciprofloxacin	May require dosage adjustment with age-related decline in renal function; May require dosage adjustment with liver disease	Neurotoxicity
Nitrofurantoin		
Norfloxacin		

(Adapted from *Drug information for the health care professional*, 1990. Rockville, MD: United States Pharmacopeial Convention. Copyright 1992, The USP Convention, Inc. Used by permission.)

PROSTATITIS. Prostatitis often accompanies UTI in elderly men and may present as either a chronic or an acute problem. While most acute cases are the result of noninfectious processes (e.g., carcinoma, prostatic stones), the pathogen involved in a bacterial prostatitis is usually identified by routine urine culture. When acute bacterial prostatitis is present, placement of indwelling urinary catheters is contraindicated. Antibiotic therapy is prescribed based on the pathogen involved.

Chronic bacterial prostatitis is the most common cause of UTI in elderly males and is frequently complicated by the presence of prostatic stones. Although antimicrobial treatment is quite effective in clearing the infection, relapse may occur in up to two thirds of patients (Fretwell & Lipsky, 1985). Eradication of infection may be achieved by excision of the involved tissue via transurethral prostatectomy.

Cardiovascular System

Atherosclerosis and valvular disease pose additional risks for infection in older adults. Specific defects of concern include degenerative valvular disorders, history of rheumatic heart disease of long duration, calcified aortic stenosis, atheromatous plaques, and prosthetic heart valves. Any alteration of the vascular endothelium leads to an accumulation of platelet aggregates and fibrin. These deposits, or vegetations, tend to be colonized by organisms that result from transient bacteremia secondary to an infection elsewhere in the host. The bacteria are protected from phagocytic leukocytes by the fibrin meshwork and are thereby able to proliferate.

INFECTIVE ENDOCARDITIS. *Infective endocarditis* is the term currently used to denote infection of the endocardial surface of the heart and is increasingly seen as a disease of aging. Factors influencing the shift to an older population include the prolonged survival of the very old, improvements in the treatment of rheumatic heart disease, and an increase in the number of hospital-acquired bacteremias resulting from invasive procedures.

Symptoms of infective endocarditis are not always consistent with the classic clinical picture of fever, heart murmurs, splenomegaly, and petechiae. As many as 25 per cent of cases in the elderly may be afebrile at the time of presentation, although rectal temperatures have been reported to demonstrate at least a low-grade fever in nearly 100 per cent of cases (Ries, 1976). Heart murmurs may be absent or mistakenly thought to be benign. Congestive heart failure due to secondary valve dysfunction, cardiac arrhythmia, and heart block have been observed more frequently in the elderly than in the general population (Weksler, 1986).

Laboratory findings of significance include an elevated erythrocyte sedimentation rate, leukocytosis, positive latex-agglutination test, and hematuria. Blood cultures reveal streptococci in about 50 per cent of cases and staphylococci in another third.

The mortality rate for infective endocarditis in patients over age 65 is 45 per cent, as compared with 25 per cent in the general population. The insidious onset in the elderly probably accounts for most of the difference, as morbidity and mortality in older adults diagnosed and treated early more closely approximates that of younger adults (Fretwell & Lipsky, 1985). Other factors and complications influencing prognosis include the organism involved, extent of valvular or myocardial injury, presence of renal failure, and development of large emboli with subsequent infarctions in major organs (Bentley, 1986; Gantz, DeMaria, & Miller, 1980).

Treatment for infective endocarditis requires intravenous antibiotics administered for 4 to 6 weeks. Specific agents are selected based on blood culture reports, although empirical therapy will be started in seriously ill patients.

Prevention of infective endocarditis may be achieved through antibiotic prophylaxis for at-risk individuals undergoing certain procedures. Cardiac conditions associated with increased risk for infective endocarditis are listed in Table 13–4. High-risk procedures include: oral/dental surgical procedures resulting in gingival bleeding; gynecologic and urologic surgical procedures, particularly in the presence of infection; drainage of abscesses; surgery involving soft tissues; and open heart surgery. Procedures of low risk include: dilation and curettage in the absence of infection, pacemaker insertions, cardiac catheterizations, and coronary artery surgery.

VASCULITIS. Vasculitis develops in the elderly population in the same fashion as infective endocarditis and often involves an atherosclerotic aneurysm. The abdominal aorta appears to be particularly vulnerable. *Staphylococcus aureus* and gram-negative bacilli, especially Salmonella species, are the primary pathogens involved. The risk of bacteremia with subsequent vasculitis in the elderly has led some physicians to prescribe more aggressive treatment for patients with Salmonella gastroenteritis (Fretwell & Lipsky, 1985).

TABLE 13–4. Underlying Cardiac Conditions and Risk of Infective Endocarditis.

High Risk
    Prosthetic heart valves
    Atrial/mitral-valve disease
    Mitral stenosis/insufficiency
    Prior infective endocarditis
Intermediate risk
    Mitral-valve prolapse
    Calcific degenerative changes
Negligible risk
    Atherosclerotic plaques
    Coronary artery disease
    Cardiac pacemakers

(Data from Infectious diseases by D.W. Bentley, 1986. In I. Rossman [Ed.], *Clinical geriatrics* [p. 438]. Philadelphia: J.B. Lippincott. Copyright 1986 by J.B. Lippincott.)

BACTEREMIA. Bacteremia in the elderly is usually secondary to an uncontained infection elsewhere in the body. The most frequently identified sources are the urinary tract (34 per cent), biliary tract (20 per cent), and lungs (13 per cent) (Esposito et al., 1980). Organisms commonly isolated include *Escherichia coli*, *Klebsiella* species, and *Streptococcus pneumoniae*.

The mortality rate for secondary bacteremia is around 25 per cent, highlighting the importance of early identification of primary infections and prompt initiation of treatment.

Gastrointestinal System

A variety of changes in nonspecific defenses place the elderly at risk of a gastrointestinal (GI) infection. These infections are more common and more serious in the older adult than in any other age group, with the exception of infants.

Production of GI secretions diminishes with increasing age. Decreased salivation results in lower levels of protective enzymes and immunoglobulins and in a more alkaline pH in the mouth. The evidence of achlorhydria (reduced production of hydrochloric acid in the stomach) exists in up to 30 per cent of those over age 60 (Gorbach et al., 1967). Achlorhydria has been associated with an increase in incidence and severity of gram-negative infections of the GI tract, including Salmonella, Shigella and *E. coli*.

Chronic diseases, such as diabetes, and administration of certain medications, including antacids and antibiotics, may delay intestinal motility, thereby increasing susceptibility to infection.

GASTROENTERITIS. Gastroenteritis may result from either viral or bacterial infection. Viral agents are probably the most frequent cause, although the specific organism is rarely identified. Patients with viral gastroenteritis experience frequent loose stools, sometimes progressing to watery diarrhea. However, abdominal pain and systemic symptoms are unlikely.

Bacterial pathogens include Salmonella, Shigella, and Campylobacter. Although they account for only about 15 per cent of cases, diarrhea due to infection with these organisms poses more serious problems for the fragile elderly. Patients may present with bloody diarrhea, abdominal pain, and fever. Treatment requires replacement of fluid and electrolytes, with the addition of antibiotic therapy when there is a risk of systemic infection. Antidiarrheal agents are not recommended, as these may prolong the duration of infection and, by delaying expulsion of the infecting organism, increase the likelihood of invasion (Raudin and Guerrant, 1983).

BILIARY-TRACT INFECTIONS. Biliary-tract infections are among the principle sources of intraabdominal sepsis in the elderly (Garibaldi et al., 1988). Over 90 per cent of cases develop as a result of obstruction of the cystic duct by gallstones. Other less common causes of obstruction include stricture and malignancy. Trapped bile acids produce inflammation (cholangitis) and infection eventually develops. Pathogens most often implicated are *E. coli*, enterococci, and, particularly in the elderly, anaerobic organisms. Complications of an un-corrected obstruction include impaired circulatory and lymphatic flow, tissue necrosis, and perforation of the gallbladder with secondary peritonitis and ab-scess formation.

Clinical manifestations of biliary-tract infection include right-upper-quad-rant pain, nausea and vomiting, fever, and chills; however, these symptoms may be absent in as many as 35 per cent of the elderly (Garibaldi et al., 1988). Typically, laboratory data will reveal leukocytosis and elevations in bilirubin and hepatic enzymes. Ultrasound examination is most helpful in verifying the presence of stones (90 per cent accuracy) and abscesses.

In addition to antibiotic therapy, treatment requires adequate pain man-agement and hydration. Cholecystectomy is usually performed as soon as the patient is stable enough to undergo the surgical procedure. Cholecystostomy may be considered in cases where the patient is unable to tolerate the more extensive procedure.

DIVERTICULITIS. Diverticulitis develops when fecal matter occludes the lu-men of diverticuli in the intestinal wall. Diverticular formation originates when increased intraluminal pressure and weakening of the bowel wall forces an "outpouching" in the intestine. Evidence of diverticulosis is present on au-topsy in nearly 40 per cent of patients over age 70 (Garibaldi et al., 1988). Fecal obstruction of the diverticulum results in irritation, erosion, leakage, and in some cases, perforation into the pericolic fat. When intestinal perforation oc-curs, subsequent complications include intraabdominal abscesses, fistulae, bowel obstructions, peritonitis, and sepsis.

Initial complaints in cases of diverticulitis include abdominal pain, partic-ularly in the left lower quadrant; change in bowel pattern, with constipation more frequent than diarrhea; and fever. Nausea and vomiting may also be present. Diagnosis is made on the basis of sigmoidoscopy and barium enema.

Treatment is determined by the severity of the illness. Mild cases of di-verticulitis are managed with liquid diet and mineral oil to soften fecal ma-terial during recovery. When fever and leukocytosis are present, intravenous fluids and antibiotics are usually added. Bowel resection may be recommended to prevent recurrence of infection.

Neurologic System

BACTERIAL MENINGITIS. Although bacterial meningitis is not commonly seen in the elderly, it is associated with a high degree of morbidity and mortality when it does occur. Age-specific incidence rates in older adults are exceeded only by those for neonates and children (Fretwell & Lipsky, 1985). *Streptococ-cus pneumoniae* is the pathogen most commonly encountered, associated with almost half of the cases. Other organisms are considered "unusual" causes of meningitis: *Listeria monocytogenes, Staph. aureus,* Enterobacteriaceae, Pseu-domonas, and Streptococcus (Fretwell & Lipsky, 1985; Garibaldi et al., 1988). Predisposing health problems include regional infections (sinusitis, otitis media, mastoiditis), head trauma (including surgery), diabetes, malignancy (particularly lymphomas), and infections of the respiratory and urinary tract (Fretwell & Lipsky, 1985; Garibaldi et al., 1988).

In general, presenting signs and symptoms of bacterial meningitis in the aged do not differ significantly from the classic picture—headache, stiff neck, fever, nausea and vomiting, and altered mental status. However, some elderly patients may have few symptoms, while still others have none. Diagnosis is made on the basis of cerebrospinal fluid studies performed following lumbar puncture. Gram stain, culture, and cell counts are critical in obtaining evidence of meningitis. Other helpful studies include chest roentgenography and cultures of blood, urine, and sputum to identify the potential source of infection. Choice of an antimicrobial agent for treatment is determined by the pathogen involved.

Even when promptly treated, morbidity and mortality from bacterial meningitis remain high. Long-term neurologic sequelae include deafness, hemiparesis, cranial-nerve paralysis, and dementia. Mortality rates range between 44 and 80 per cent (Garibaldi et al., 1988).

TETANUS. Tetanus is a serious problem for older adults who become infected with the causative agent *Clostridium tetani*. Although the overall incidence in the United States is low, persons over age 60 account for over 50 per cent of reported cases, with a 75 per cent case-fatality rate. One study reported less than 20 per cent of cases resulting from farm injuries, while over half of the infections developed following accidents at home. Surgery may also increase risk, particularly with amputations of gangrenous extremities or abdominal procedures. Other factors include chronic skin ulcers, infected pressure sores, and varicose veins (LaForce, Young, & Bennett, 1969).

Tetanus occurs almost exclusively in individuals who have not been immunized, who are inadequately immunized, or whose immunization history is not known. Currently available vaccines have a high efficacy rate; however, evidence of a protective effect can be demonstrated in only 25 per cent of older adults immunized 8 years previously. Booster doses yield an adequate response in 93 per cent of cases (Solomonova & Vizev, 1973). The vaccine is inexpensive and safe; it is contraindicated only in those with a prior hypersensitivity reaction.

It may be argued that immunization programs for the elderly are not cost effective in light of the low incidence of infection. However, the increased frequency and severity of tetanus in older adults in addition to the increased likelihood of conditions predisposing to tetanus support the need for maintaining adequate antibody titers in the elderly.

Musculoskeletal System

The changes in the skeleton that accompany aging may directly or indirectly increase the risk of infection. Unstable ambulation and osteoporosis frequently result in fractures of the hip and the spine. Hospitalization, surgical procedures, and immobilization are well known to increase susceptibility to infection among the elderly. Intraarticular steroid injections and orthopedic prosthetic devices are commonly employed for patients with arthritis. Both interventions are associated with increased risk of infection.

SEPTIC ARTHRITIS. Septic arthritis is increasingly seen among the elderly, with between one third and one half of all cases diagnosed in those over age 60. Predisposing risk factors for older adults include preexisting joint disease, such as rheumatoid arthritis, degenerative joint disease, or prosthetic surgery; recent or recurrent infection not involving the joint; compromised immune system, including use of immunosuppressive agents; underlying chronic disease, such as diabetes; and recent trauma to the joint (Yoshikawa & Norman, 1987). When a prosthetic device is involved, removal of the prosthesis may be necessary. Replacement of the prosthesis is not always possible in these cases.

Joints most often involved are the knee, hip, wrist, and shoulder. On assessment, the joint is usually warm, swollen, and tender and range of motion is decreased. Fever and chills may or may not be present. Diagnosis is made by aspirating and culturing synovial fluid from the affected joint.

Hematogenous spread is thought to be the route of transmission for most cases of septic arthritis (Yoshikawa & Norman, 1987). Special attention should be given to older adults with preexisting joint disease and extraarticular infection so that septic arthritis, when it develops, is identified and treated promptly.

OSTEOMYELITIS. Osteomyelitis occurs as a result of hematogenous spread (e.g., gram-negative bacteriuria), contiguous infection (e.g., infected pressure sore) or vascular insufficiency (Yoshikawa & Norman, 1987). Physical manifestations include localized tenderness over the affected site, erythema, and possibly fever. Osteomyelitis secondary to peripheral vascular disease may also present with local ulceration.

Diagnosis is usually made by ruling out other possible causes of symptoms, such as malignancy or fracture, through the use of radiologic procedures. Bacterial, fungal, and mycobacterial cultures are commonly obtained. Biopsy of the involved site may also be performed.

Fever of Undetermined Origin

Fever of undetermined origin (FUO) is defined as an illness of at least 3 weeks' duration associated with a temperature of 101°F or higher, with no established diagnosis following appropriate clinical evaluation (Fretwell & Lipsky, 1985). The primary causes of FUO are infection, connective tissue disorders, and malignancy. The most common infectious etiologies associated with FUO are intraabdominal abscesses, infective endocarditis, and tuberculosis; giant-cell arteritis is the most frequent cause among connective-tissue disorders. The longer the fever is present in the older adult, the more likely it is to be attributed to malignancy, particularly lymphoma.

The prognosis for the elderly with FUO is poorer than with younger adults.

TABLE 13-5. Average Annual Cancer Incidence Rates per 100,000 Population, Surveillance, Epidemiology & End Results, All Races, Both Sexes, 1983 to 1987.

	<5	5-9	10-14	15-19	20-24	25-29	30-34	35-39	40-44	45-49	50-54	55-59	60-64	65-69	70-74	75-79	80-84	85+
Oral cavity & pharynx	0.0	0.2	0.3	0.4	0.6	1.1	2.1	3.8	7.1	14.5	22.9	34.4	42.0	49.5	50.6	47.2	45.3	45.1
Digestive system	0.9	0.2	0.2	0.5	0.9	2.2	5.1	10.4	23.3	49.1	92.5	157.7	245.0	354.6	484.1	621.6	758.0	801.0
Esophagus	—	—	—	0.0	0.0	0.0	0.1	0.3	1.3	2.9	6.0	10.9	15.8	19.2	21.1	21.1	20.7	20.1
Stomach	—	—	0.0	0.1	0.1	0.4	0.8	1.3	2.8	5.9	9.5	15.8	24.1	34.7	47.9	63.2	82.0	88.8
Small intestine	0.0	—	0.0	—	0.0	0.0	0.2	0.2	0.7	1.4	1.7	2.5	3.1	3.9	6.0	6.5	7.0	6.0
Colon/rectum	—	—	0.0	0.1	0.5	1.2	2.7	6.1	12.9	28.1	56.0	96.6	152.6	226.1	314.7	412.0	501.5	525.4
Colon	—	—	0.0	0.1	0.3	0.8	2.0	4.3	8.6	18.1	36.0	64.1	101.4	158.6	227.1	310.7	384.4	413.2
Rectum	—	—	—	0.0	0.2	0.4	0.7	1.8	4.3	10.0	20.0	32.5	51.2	67.5	87.6	101.3	117.1	112.2
Anus & anal canal	—	—	—	0.0	0.0	0.0	0.2	0.2	0.4	0.9	1.4	2.2	3.1	3.2	3.7	4.2	5.2	5.0
Liver & intrahepatic	0.5	0.1	0.1	0.2	0.1	0.3	0.3	0.8	1.2	1.9	3.8	5.6	8.4	11.7	13.3	16.4	18.0	16.8
Liver	0.5	0.1	0.1	0.1	0.1	0.2	0.3	0.7	1.1	1.8	3.6	5.1	7.9	10.8	12.3	14.5	16.1	13.9
Gallbladder	0.0	—	—	—	0.0	—	0.0	0.1	0.3	0.4	1.1	2.0	2.9	4.9	7.2	11.4	14.9	17.8
Other biliary	0.0	—	—	—	0.0	0.1	0.1	0.1	0.3	0.6	1.3	1.8	3.3	4.7	6.6	9.8	13.9	13.7
Pancreas	0.0	—	—	0.0	0.0	0.1	0.5	1.0	2.6	6.1	10.7	18.3	29.8	43.0	59.3	71.6	89.2	100.2
Retroperitoneum	0.4	0.1	0.0	0.0	0.1	0.1	0.1	0.2	0.5	0.6	0.5	0.8	0.8	1.1	1.5	2.2	1.5	1.7
Respiratory system	0.4	0.1	0.1	0.3	0.5	0.8	2.1	6.5	21.0	49.6	100.7	176.0	250.3	325.3	370.8	362.7	310.6	209.0
Nasal cavity, sinuses, ear	0.1	0.1	—	0.0	0.1	0.1	0.1	0.3	0.3	0.9	1.0	1.6	2.0	2.5	3.0	3.2	3.7	3.1
Larynx	—	—	—	—	0.0	0.1	0.1	0.6	1.8	4.4	10.0	15.8	21.4	23.6	22.8	18.7	14.7	9.1
Lung & bronchus	—	—	0.1	0.1	0.3	0.5	1.6	5.3	18.4	43.5	88.8	156.7	224.1	294.8	339.9	334.3	285.9	193.2
Pleura	—	—	—	—	0.0	0.0	0.0	0.1	0.3	0.5	0.7	1.5	2.3	3.5	4.4	5.8	5.3	3.0
Bones & joints	0.1	0.6	1.3	1.5	0.7	0.5	0.5	0.6	0.6	0.6	0.6	0.8	1.3	1.3	1.7	1.8	1.9	1.1
Soft tissue	1.4	0.4	0.7	1.0	1.0	1.2	1.3	1.6	2.2	2.1	3.0	3.4	4.3	5.7	6.9	7.1	10.5	11.5
Melanoma of skin	0.1	0.1	0.2	1.2	3.3	6.2	9.6	13.7	15.7	16.9	20.1	22.4	23.9	25.8	27.6	28.5	31.1	29.8
Breast	—	—	—	0.0	0.5	3.9	13.6	33.6	64.2	93.4	109.4	136.9	171.6	207.5	232.9	265.7	286.6	291.1
Female genital system	0.0	0.1	0.4	1.2	2.4	5.5	9.8	14.7	21.9	33.3	45.4	63.1	88.0	106.5	116.7	116.8	116.9	115.9
Cervix uteri	0.0	—	0.2	0.2	1.0	3.4	6.0	7.8	8.7	8.9	8.6	9.1	9.6	10.1	11.7	12.1	12.6	14.0
Corpus	—	—	0.0	0.0	0.0	0.3	1.2	2.8	6.3	11.9	20.6	32.3	49.1	62.1	64.2	58.4	52.1	42.6
Uterus, not otherwise specified	—	0.0	0.0	0.0	0.0	—	0.0	0.1	0.1	0.2	0.2	0.3	0.3	0.5	0.9	1.2	1.7	3.0

Site																		
Ovary	—	0.1	0.3	0.8	1.1	1.4	1.9	3.3	5.7	10.8	13.7	18.7	24.7	28.3	32.6	33.6	36.8	35.1
Vagina	—	—	—	—	0.0	0.0	0.1	0.2	0.3	0.3	0.5	0.7	1.3	1.4	1.9	2.6	3.7	4.0
Vulva	0.0	—	0.0	0.0	0.1	0.1	0.2	0.4	0.5	0.8	1.2	1.4	1.9	2.7	4.2	7.0	8.3	15.4
Male genital system	0.2	0.0	0.1	1.6	4.3	5.8	5.9	5.2	4.3	5.9	17.0	47.2	107.0	204.6	299.3	372.3	393.8	324.5
Prostate gland	0.1	—	0.0	0.0	0.0	0.0	0.0	0.1	0.7	3.0	14.8	45.2	105.0	202.2	296.5	369.0	390.9	321.0
Testis	0.2	0.0	0.1	1.5	4.3	5.7	5.8	4.9	3.3	2.3	1.7	1.2	0.7	0.7	0.5	0.4	0.5	0.2
Penis	—	—	—	—	0.0	0.0	0.1	0.1	0.2	0.4	0.5	0.7	0.9	1.4	1.8	2.0	1.5	2.3
Urinary system	2.0	0.7	0.1	0.4	0.5	0.9	2.1	4.5	10.2	18.3	33.8	55.5	84.2	117.3	147.1	179.0	194.5	185.9
Urinary bladder	0.0	0.0	0.0	0.2	0.3	0.6	1.2	2.4	5.4	9.7	20.0	34.2	53.7	79.1	102.1	124.9	144.2	145.7
Kidney & renal pelvis	1.9	0.7	0.1	0.1	0.2	0.3	0.8	2.0	4.5	8.3	12.9	19.9	27.9	34.5	39.1	46.5	42.0	34.4
Ureter	—	—	—	—	—	—	0.0	0.0	0.1	0.2	0.4	1.0	1.6	2.7	4.3	4.8	6.0	3.3
Eye & orbit	1.3	0.1	0.0	0.0	0.0	0.1	0.2	0.2	0.4	0.8	0.7	1.4	1.4	2.0	2.5	2.6	3.2	3.0
Brain & nervous system	3.5	3.2	1.9	2.1	2.0	2.5	3.4	4.1	4.9	6.4	8.7	11.9	14.9	19.6	19.9	20.5	18.6	10.2
Thyroid	0.0	0.1	0.5	1.7	3.3	4.6	6.0	6.6	7.2	7.8	8.0	7.4	8.1	8.5	8.1	6.5	8.4	7.0
Other endocrine	1.2	0.2	0.2	0.2	0.2	0.2	0.2	0.4	0.4	0.4	0.8	1.0	1.5	1.2	1.4	1.2	0.7	0.6
Hodgkin's disease	0.0	0.5	1.4	3.8	5.2	4.3	3.7	3.3	2.7	2.4	2.8	3.3	3.2	3.6	3.9	4.1	4.5	3.3
Non-Hodgkin's lymphomas	0.5	1.0	1.2	1.4	1.8	2.5	4.3	6.4	10.0	13.5	18.1	25.6	35.8	47.7	60.4	73.0	84.0	74.9
Multiple myeloma	—	—	—	—	0.0	0.0	0.2	0.6	1.5	2.6	4.8	8.6	12.5	19.4	24.2	34.5	37.1	35.3
Leukemias	6.6	3.4	2.8	2.3	1.7	1.9	2.5	3.8	4.4	6.8	10.2	15.6	22.7	31.4	45.0	60.7	81.8	89.6
Lymphocytic leukemia	5.3	2.8	1.8	1.3	0.6	0.6	0.5	0.8	1.1	2.0	3.6	6.2	9.7	13.2	19.7	24.2	32.7	37.9
Acute lymphocytic	5.3	2.8	1.8	1.3	0.5	0.5	0.4	0.6	0.5	0.7	0.6	0.6	0.7	1.1	0.9	1.2	2.3	1.9
Chronic lymphocytic	—	—	—	—	0.0	0.0	0.0	0.2	0.6	1.3	2.9	5.4	8.8	12.0	18.4	22.0	29.1	33.6
Granulocytic leukemia	0.7	0.4	0.7	0.8	0.9	1.1	1.6	2.4	2.3	3.2	4.8	6.6	9.1	12.5	17.3	25.8	33.8	33.9
Acute granulocytic	0.5	0.4	0.4	0.5	0.5	0.7	0.9	1.4	1.3	1.9	2.9	3.8	5.8	7.3	10.6	15.1	19.0	18.4
Chronic granulocytic	0.1	0.1	0.1	0.2	0.2	0.3	0.5	0.9	0.9	1.3	1.6	2.4	2.7	4.0	5.6	8.7	12.1	12.5
Monocytic leukemia	0.2	0.0	0.1	0.1	0.0	0.1	0.1	0.1	0.1	0.3	0.2	0.5	0.7	0.8	0.8	1.2	3.0	2.0
Acute monocytic	0.2	0.0	0.1	0.1	0.0	0.1	0.1	0.1	0.1	0.2	0.2	0.4	0.5	0.7	0.7	0.9	1.9	1.3
Chronic monocytic	—	—	—	—	—	—	—	—	—	0.0	—	0.1	0.1	—	0.0	0.1	0.4	0.2
Other leukemia	0.4	0.1	0.2	0.1	0.2	0.2	0.3	0.5	0.8	1.2	1.6	2.3	3.3	4.9	7.0	9.5	12.5	15.8
Ill-defined/unknown	0.4	0.1	0.1	0.2	0.3	0.4	0.8	1.8	3.6	6.3	12.0	20.5	29.3	39.9	60.3	75.6	106.6	137.1
All sites	18.8	11.1	11.4	20.0	30.3	47.7	79.1	129.1	211.0	335.0	514.3	795.3	1148.9	1574.2	1967.2	2286.6	2500.5	2383.3

(From *Cancer Statistics Review* by LAG Ries, BF Hankey and BK Edwards, *1973–1987*, 1990. Bethesda, MD: National Cancer Institute, NIH Publication No. 90-2789.)

TABLE 13–6. Nursing Interventions Related to Immunosenescence.

Site	Risk Factors	Nursing Interventions
Skin and mucous membranes	Fragile epidermis Loss of vascularity, connective tissue, and fat Dehydration, malnutrition Anemia Immobility Incontinence Poor personal hygiene	Caution in turning, moving patient to prevent skin injury. Promote adequate fluid, nutritional intake. Schedule time to walk with patient or for him or her to sit in chair, as condition permits. Establish plan for toilet patterning, bowel retraining. Develop comprehensive plan for skin care, including cleansing procedures, assessment for evidence of breakdown and treatment of open areas.
Respiratory tract	Loss of alveolar elasticity Weakened chest muscles Chronic illness History of smoking, alcoholism Immobility Absent/altered cough, gag reflexes Reduced peristalsis Esophageal disorders	Assess breath sounds and respiratory effort on a regular basis, depending on risk factors and current health status. Encourage cough and deep breathing during periods of increased risk. Offer influenza vaccine. Monitor results from chest x-ray, purified protein derivative. Obtain sputum specimen for routine and acid-fast bacillus cultures when productive cough is present. Schedule exercise regimen: range of motion, ambulation, sitting in chair, as condition permits. Assist patient to sitting position at minimum 60-degree angle when eating, drinking.
Genitourinary system	Decreasing bladder emptying	Encourage adequate fluid intake. Monitor for evidence of infection: urinary frequency, dysuria, incontinence; onset or progression of confusion; pyuria; complaints of perineal itching, white discharge.

System	Risk Factors	Nursing Interventions
	Poor personal hygiene Fecal incontinence	Avoid use of indwelling catheters as much as possible. Provide thorough cleansing of perineum daily and after each episode of fecal incontinence.
Cardiovascular system	Degenerative valvular disorders Aortic stenosis Prosthetic heart valves History of rheumatic heart disease	Observe for signs, symptoms of infection: new onset or progression of congestive heart failure, arrhythmia, leukocytosis, temperature elevation. Consult physician about administration of prophylactic antibiotics when high-risk procedures are planned. Report evidence of suspected infection promptly to physician.
Gastrointestinal system	Decreased salivation, gastrointestinal secretions Diminished intestinal motility	Monitor for adequate fluid intake to prevent constipation and to reduce dehydration secondary to diarrhea. Encourage increased intake of fiber. Offer stool softeners if chronic constipation is present. Assess for evidence of infection: diarrhea, abdominal pain, temperature elevation, decreased bowel sounds, nausea, vomiting, abdominal distention.
Neurologic system	Infection of head, neck, respiratory system, urinary tract Inadequate immunization for tetanus	Monitor for evidence of infection: headache, stiff neck, fever, nausea, vomiting, altered mental status. Offer tetanus vaccine; repeat every 5 to 7 years.
Musculoskeletal system	Risk of fracture Orthopedic prosthetic devices Intraarticular steroid injections Immobilization	Minimize risk of falls for those with osteoporosis or unsteady ambulation: well-fitting shoes, use of cane or walker for stability; eliminate environmental hazards: slippery throw rugs, electric/telephone cords across floor, etc. Observe for evidence of infection: inflamed joint or extremity; decreased range of motion.

225

One study reported mortality rates of 15 per cent for those under 35, 42 per cent for those between 35 and 54, and 62 per cent for those over 55 (Fretwell & Lipsky, 1985).

HEMATOLOGIC AND NEOPLASTIC COMPLICATIONS

The increased incidence of cancers among the elderly is thought to be, to some extent, the result of immunosenescence. Neoplasms commonly encountered among the elderly will not be addressed in depth here, as a complete discussion may be found elsewhere in this text.

Multiple myeloma (see Chapter 9) is a progressive disease characterized by proliferation of a malignant B-cell clone and production of an abnormal monoclonal protein. Incidence increases with age, peaking between 60 and 70 years.

Non-Hodgkin's lymphomas (NHL) (Chapter 10) also demonstrate an increased incidence with increasing age. NHL represent a diverse family of lymphoid neoplasms, ranging from indolent to very aggressive. Widespread disease at time of presentation is not uncommon.

The incidence of Hodgkin's lymphoma has a bimodal distribution, with the second peak occurring after age 65 (Hyams, 1985). Response rate and duration of remission is less among the elderly.

Chronic lymphocytic leukemia (CLL) (Chapter 7) is a slowly progressing disorder of B-cell lineage, although increased numbers of both T and B cells may be present, most often occurring after age 60. Although most patients with CLL are asymptomatic at the time of diagnosis, some may present with fatigue, weight loss, and night sweats. Lymphadenopathy and splenomegaly may also be noted.

Acute myelomonocytic leukemia is a variant of acute myeloid leukemia and is characterized by a primarily monocytic component in the peripheral blood and a primarily myelocytic component in the bone marrow (Hyams, 1985).

Over half of all solid tumors occur in adults over the age of 65. Immunosenescence has been considered to be a contributing factor (Jurivich and Cohen, 1988), although long exposure to a variety of carcinogenic agents is likely to have a critical role. Age-specific incidence rates according to primary site can be found in Table 13–5.

IMPLICATIONS OF IMMUNOSENESCENCE FOR NURSING

Although the actual mechanisms contributing to immunosenescence are not entirely clear, the fact that the elderly are at increased risk for certain infections is well established. Nursing's primary responsibilities for elderly clients involve identification of those at highest risk and implementation of disease-prevention strategies.

All problems listed in the care plan for the immunocompromised patient (Chapter 15) are applicable for the elderly patient. Interventions specific to immunosenescence are listed in Table 13–6.

SELECTED BIBLIOGRAPHY

Adler, W.H., & Nagel, J.E. (1985). Clinical immunology. In R. Andres, E.L. Bierman, & W.R. Hazzard (Eds.), *Principles of geriatric medicine.* New York: McGraw-Hill.

Alling, B, et al. (1975). Effect of consecutive antibacterial therapy on bacteriuria in hospitalized geriatric patients. *Scandinavian Journal of Infectious Diseases, 7,* 201.

Barker, W.H., & Mullooly J.P. (1982). Pneumonia and influenza deaths during epidemics: Implications for prevention. *Archives of Internal Medicine, 142,* 85.

Bentley, D.W. (1986). Infectious diseases. In I. Rossman (Ed.), *Clinical geriatrics* (p. 438). Philadelphia: J.B. Lippincott.

Bentley, D.W., Ha, K., Mamot, K., et al. (1981). Pneumococcal vaccine in the institutionalized elderly: Design of a nonrandomized trial and preliminary results. *Reviews of Infectious Diseases, 3,* S71.

Centers for Disease Control (1984). Prevention and control of influenza: Recommendations of the immunization practices advisory committee. *Annals of Internal Medicine, 101,* 218.

Consensus Development Conference Panel (1980). Amantadine: Does it have a role in the prevention and treatment of influenza? *Annals of Internal Medicine, 92,* 256.

Eaglstein, W.H., Katz, R., & Brown, J.A. (1970). The effects of early corticosteroid therapy on the skin eruption and pain of herpes zoster. *Journal of the American Medical Association, 211,* 1681.

Esposito, A.L., et al. (1980). Community-acquired bacteremia in the elderly: Analysis of one hundred consecutive episodes. *Journal of the American Geriatrics Society, 28,* 315.

Fox, R.A. (1985). Immunology of aging. In J.C. Brocklehurst (Ed.), *Textbook of geriatric medicine and gerontology* (3rd ed.) (p. 82). New York: Churchill-Livingstone.

Fretwell, M., & Lipsky B.A. (1985). Infectious agents: The compromised host. In R. Andres, E.L. Bierman, & W.R. Hazzard (Eds.), *Principles of geriatric medicine* (p. 477). New York: McGraw-Hill.

Gantz, N.M., DeMaria, A., & Miller, M. (1980). Infective endocarditis in the elderly. *Southern Medical Journal, 73*(10), 1335.

Garagusi, V.F. (1989). Infectious disease problems in the elderly. In W. Reichel (Ed.), *Clinical aspects of aging* (p. 199). Baltimore: Williams & Wilkins.

Garibaldi, R.A., Neuhaus, E.G., & Nurse, B.A. (1988). Infections in the elderly. In J.W. Rowe & R.W. Besdine (Eds.), *Geriatric medicine* (2nd ed.) (p. 302). Boston: Little, Brown.

Gleckman, R., & Hilbert, D. (1982). Afebrile bacteremia: A phenomenon in geriatric patients. *Journal of the American Medical Association, 248*(12), 1478.

Gorbach, SL, et al. (1967). Studies of intestinal microflora. I: Effects of diet, age and periodic sampling on numbers of fecal microorganisms in man. *Gastroenterology, 53,* 845.

Haddy, R.I. (1988). Aging, infections, and the immune system. *Journal of Family Practice, 27*(4), 409.

Hayden, F.G., & Douglas, R.G. (1985). Antiviral agents. In G.L. Mandell, R.G. Douglas, & J.E. Bennett (Eds.), *Principles and practice of infectious diseases* (p. 270). New York: John Wiley.

Hefton, J.M., Darlington, G.J., Casazza, B.A., & Weksler, M.E. (1980). Immunologic studies of aging V: Impaired proliferation of PHA responsive. *Journal of Immunology, 125,* 1007.

Hyams, D. (1985). The blood. In J.C. Brocklehurst (Ed.), *Textbook of geriatric medicine and gerontology* (p. 835). New York: Churchill-Livingstone.

Inkeles, B., Innes, J.B., Kuntz, M.M., et al. (1977). Immunological studies of aging III. Cytokenetic basis for the impaired response of lymphocytes from aged humans to plant lectins. *Journal of Experimental Medicine, 145,* 1176.

Jurivich, D.A., & Cohen, H.J. (1988). Immune system and immunoproliferative disorders. In J.W. Rowe & R.W. Besdine (Eds.), *Geriatric medicine* (2nd ed.) (p. 276). Boston: Little, Brown.

Keczkes, K., & Basheer, A.M. (1980). Do corticosteroids prevent post-herpetic neuralgia? *British Journal of Dermatology, 102,* 551.

LaForce, F.M., Young, L.S., & Bennett, J.V. (1969). Tetanus in the United States 1965–1966. *New England Journal of Medicine, 280,* 479.

Laharrague, P., Corberand, J., Fillola, G., Nguyen, F., Fantanilles, A.M., et al. (1983). Impairment of polymorphonuclear functions in hospitalized geriatric patients. *Gerontology, 29*, 325.

Phair, J.P., Kauffman, C.A., Bjornson, A., et al. (1978). Host defenses in the aged: Evaluation of components of the inflammatory and immune system. *Journal of Infectious Diseases, 138*(1), 67.

Raudin, J.I., & Guerrant, R.L. (1983). Infectious diarrhea in the elderly. *Geriatrics, 38*, 95.

Ries, K. (1976). Endocarditis in the elderly. In D. Kaye (Ed.), *Infective endocarditis* (p. 143). Baltimore: University Park Press.

Roghmann, K.J., Tabloski, P.A., Bentley, D.W., & Schiffman, G. (1987). Immune response of elderly adults to pneumococcus: Variation by age, sex, and functional impairment. *Journal of Gerontology, 42*(3), 265.

Rudd, A.G., & Banerjee, D.K. (1989). Interleukin-1 paroduction by human monocytes in aging and disease. *Age and Aging 18*, 43.

Rytel, M.W. (1987). Effect of age on viral infections: Possible role of interferon. *Journal of the American Geriatrics Society, 35*, 1092.

Saltzman, R.L., & Peterson, P.K. (1987). Immunodeficiency of the elderly. *Reviews of Infectious Diseases, 9*(6), 1127.

Schwab, R., Walters, C.A., & Weksler, M.E. (1989). Host defense mechanisms and aging. *Seminars in Oncology, 16*(1), 20.

Schwartz, J.S. (1982). Pneumococcal vaccine: Clinical efficacy and effectiveness. *Annals of Internal medicine, 96*, 208.

Solomonova, K., & Vizev, S. (1973). Immunological reactivity of senescent and old people actively immunized with tetanus toxoid. *Zeitschrift für Immunitäts for schung Experimentelle und Klinische Immunologie, 146*, 81.

Valenti, W.M., Trudell, R.G., & Bentley, D.W. (1978). Factors predisposing to oropharyngeal colonization with gram-negative bacilli in the aged. *New England Journal of Medicine, 298*, 1108.

Verghese, A., & Berk, S.L. (1983). Bacterial pneumonia in the elderly. *Medicine, 62*(5), 271.

Weksler, M.E. (1986). Biologic basis and clinical significance of immune senescence. In I. Rossman (Ed.), *Clinical geriatrics* (p. 57). Philadelphia: J.B. Lippincott.

Yoshikawa, T.T., & Norman, D.C. (1987). *Aging and clinical practice: Infectious disease.* New York: Igaku-Shoin.

14

INFECTIONS IN THE IMMUNOCOMPROMISED HOST

Infection and sepsis constitute the primary causes of morbidity and mortality among immunocompromised persons. In up to 80 per cent of deaths among persons with acute leukemia and in 90 per cent of those with acquired immunodeficiency syndrome (AIDS), infectious processes are the ultimate cause of death (Young, 1985; Kovacs & Masur, 1988). The advent of more aggressive forms of cancer treatment, the development of methicillin-resistant strains of Staphylococcus, and the emergence of AIDS have presented new challenges in infection control. Problematic microorganisms may be opportunistic, although many are acquired in the hospital environment.

The primary goal of nursing care relative to infection is prevention. The nature of the immune disorder determines specific strategies and potential for achieving goals. Opportunistic pathogens and latent infections predispose immunocompromised patients to overwhelming infections that cannot always be predicted or prevented. Reduction of environmental pathogens, however, remains a critical factor in protecting the patient during granulocytopenic episodes. Regardless of the primary disease causing immunodeficiency, health promotion can be encouraged through adequate nutrition and fluid intake, diligent personal hygiene, and activity within the limits imposed by the disease.

Evidence of infection may be very subtle on presentation, mandating thorough and regular physical assessments. Any indication, no matter how slight, that infection may be present must be communicated promptly to the physician.

Comprehensive assessments continue through periods of antimicrobial therapy and monitoring for determinants of response. If there is no evidence of improvement within 5 to 7 days of starting initial therapy, the treatment regimen should be reviewed and consideration given to modifying the agents prescribed (Pizzo & Meyers, 1989).

Assessment criteria will be reviewed here for each system; however, specific nursing interventions are addressed elsewhere in this book. Please refer to the appropriate chapter discussing the primary immune disorder. Common infections seen in the immunocompromised host and factors associated with those infections are listed in Table 14–1.

PREDOMINANT PATHOGENS

Bacteria

Improvements in antibiotic therapy have resulted in shifting patterns in bacterial infections. During the 1950s and 1960s, *Staphylococcus aureus* was the most commonly isolated organism in immunocompromised patients. Development of beta-lactamase-resistant penicillins provided highly effective therapy for *Staph. aureus,* leading to the emergence of gram-negative pathogens as predominant isolates. The use of empirical antibiotic combinations, incorporating third-generation cephalosporins, has effectively reduced the incidence of gram-negative infections. However, a recent resurgence of infections caused by gram-positive organisms has been observed and is believed to be related to the prevalence of methicillin-resistant strains of Staphylococcus and to the increased use of central-venous-access catheters (Pizzo & Meyers, 1989; Lazarus, Creger, & Gerson, 1989).

Uncommon bacterial organisms more recently isolated in immunocompromised patients include Legionella, Nocardia, and Listeria. The incidence of mycobacterial infections, particularly *Mycobacterium tuberculosis* and *M. avium–intracellulare,* have also increased, with AIDS a prominent risk factor.

Fungi

Fungal infections constitute the most frequent source of secondary infection in immunocompromised patients. Those at highest risk are those who experience prolonged granulocytopenia and extended courses of antibiotic therapy. Persistent fever or a new or progressive pulmonary infiltrate in spite of the administration of broad-spectrum antibiotics is often the first clue that a fungal infection is present.

Candida remains the most common source of fungal infection; however, Histoplasma, Torulopsis, Cryptococcus, and Aspergillus have increasingly been encountered. The Phycomycetes Mucor and Rhizopus are less commonly isolated.

Diagnosis of fungal infection is often difficult to establish and may require

TABLE 14–1. Infectious Complications in the Immunocompromised Host.

Site	Organism(s)	Associated Factors	Presenting Signs/ Symptoms	Comments
Disseminated infection/sepsis	Bacteria Staphylococcus Streptococcus Escherichia coli Klebsiella 　pneumoniae Pseudomonas 　aeruginosa Fungi Candida Histoplasmosis Cryptococcus Torulopsis	Neutropenia Concurrent respiratory infection (accounts for 25% of septic episodes), perianal/perioral infection, GI-tract infection, GU-tract infection	In neutropenic patient, classic symptoms of sepsis (fever, chills) are usually absent; more common complaints of malaise, anorexia	Endotoxin shock most often associated with gram-negative sepsis; shock may also develop with some gram-positives. Disseminated candidiasis is associated with endophthalmitis, causing white moundlike retinal lesions. Histoplasmosis may involve the reticuloendothelial system, causing lymphadenopathy and hepatosplenomegaly, which may be confused with progressive malignancy. Disseminated Torulopsis produces endotoxiclike shock.
Implanted vascular access catheter	Bacteria Staphylococcus Streptococcus Gram-negative bacilli Fungi Candida	Degree of catheter use Compliance with catheter care procedures	Positive blood culture (obtained via all ports/lumens and peripherally)	"Tunnel infection" along subcutaneous catheter track requires removal of catheter to ensure complete resolution of infection.
Respiratory system	Bacteria Streptococcus 　pneumoniae Haemophilus 　influenzae	Obstruction secondary to primary or metastatic lesions	Frequently nonspecific: productive/ nonproductive cough, dyspnea; with/without fever	

TABLE 14–I. Infectious Complications in the Immunocompromised Host. *(continued)*

Site	Organism(s)	Associated Factors	Presenting Signs/ Symptoms	Comments
	Pseudomonas aeruginosa Klebsiella Enterobacter			
	Legionella pneumophila	Aerosolization of contaminated water (air conditioners, shower heads)	Fever, nonproductive cough, pulse deficit, neurologic dysfunction, diarrhea	
	Nocardia	Renal dialysis/transplant Lymphoreticular neoplasm Long-term corticosteroid use HIV seropositive		Concurrent cutaneous and/or CNS infection in one third of cases.
	Mycobacteria *Mycobacterium tuberculosis*	Latent TB IV drug abuse Resident of/emigrant from region with endemic disease	Fever, night sweats, weight loss, anorexia, chills, productive cough, dyspnea Extrapulmonary: regional lymphadenopathy, headaches, meningismus	Positive PPD test in HIV-seropositive patient requires isoniazid prophylaxsis to prevent progression to active TB. Extrapulmonary TB is thought to indicate a greater degree of cellular immune dysfunction.
	Mycobacterium avium–intracellulare	Hairy-cell leukemia		
	Fungi Aspergillus	Construction dust, ventilation problems Hematologic malignancies Organ transplants Corticosteroids	Hemoptysis	Aspergillus invades blood vessels, resulting in pulmonary hemorrhage and thrombosis of pulmonary arteries.
	Histoplasma Phycomycetes (Mucor, Rhizopus)	Hematologic malignancies		

Organism	Predisposing Factors	Clinical Manifestations	Comments
Viruses			
Herpes simplex	Endotracheal intubation		Rare
Cytomegalovirus	Allogeneic bone marrow transplant, especially with total body irradiation and GVHD; hematologic malignancies; solid organ transplants		Infection usually disseminated at time of diagnosis. Primary site of infection is alveolar lining.
Varicella zoster	Immunocompromised children; Cutaneous varicella infection		In children, pneumonitis appears 3 to 7 days after development of typical skin lesions.
Protozoa			
Pneumocystis carinii	AIDS; Intensive chemotherapeutic regimens; Prolonged corticosteroid therapy; Hematologic malignancy	Mild to severe dyspnea; With/without fever; Bilateral diffuse infiltrates or normal chest x-ray film	Most common cause of diffuse pulmonary infiltrate in non-neutropenic patients; more indolent course in AIDS.
Gastrointestinal system **Oral**			
Bacteria			
Staphylococcus aureus *Staphylococcus epidermidis* *Pseudomonas aeruginosa*	Mucositis/gingivitis due to chemotherapy, radiation; Acute leukemia; Preexisting periodontal disease	Pain, erythema in oral mucous membranes; Bleeding from gums	
Fungi			
Candida	Diabetes; Antibiotic; Corticosteroids; HIV-seropositivity	White plaques on buccal mucosa, tongue, palate	Oral cavity may serve as major portal of entry for disseminated candidiasis.
Viruses			
Herpes simplex	Acute leukemia; Chemotherapy; Radiation therapy to oral cavity	Erythema, pain; With/without cutaneous and/or intraoral vessicles	Oral HSV infection may be confused with treatment-related mucousitis; frequently masked by Candida overgrowth.

Table continued on following page.

TABLE 14–I. Infectious Complications in the Immunocompromised Host. *(continued)*

Site	Organism(s)	Associated Factors	Presenting Signs/Symptoms	Comments
Esophageal	Fungi Candida	AIDS Mediastinal radiation Neutropenia Corticosteroids Broad-spectrum antibiotics	Pain on swallowing Burning retrosternal chest pain	Diagnosis to confirm fungal versus viral etiology may require endoscopy and/or biopsy. Biopsy is not always safe to perform during thrombocytopenic episodes.
	Viruses Herpes simplex Cytomegalovirus	AIDS Bone marrow transplant		
Intestinal Necrotizing enterocolitis	Bacteria Gram-negative bacteria (especially Pseudomonas)	Prolonged granulocytopenia Broad-spectrum antibiotics Acute leukemia	Right-lower-quadrant pain, acute or subacute onset; Watery or bloody diarrhea	Mortality, despite aggressive therapy, is 30 to 50 per cent.
Antibiotic-associated colitis	*Clostridium difficile* with toxin production	Recent treatment with clindamycin, ampicillin, broad-spectrum β-lactam antibiotics	Acute generalized abdominal pain; fever; leukocytosis; foul-smelling, watery or mucoid diarrhea	Toxin production, in addition to stool culture positive for *C. difficile*, is required for diagnosis.
Gastroenteritis	Salmonella	AIDS	Nonspecific GI complaints	High incidence in patients with AIDS; common cause of bacteremia.
	Viruses Cytomegalovirus	AIDS	Abdominal cramping; large-volume watery/bloody diarrhea; rectal discharge	Infection may progress to intestinal hemorrhage or perforation.
	Parasitic Cryptosporidium	AIDS, particularly in homosexual/bisexual males and in areas with poor sanitary conditions	Severe watery diarrhea; abdominal cramping; nausea, occasional vomiting; profound weight loss	

Hepatic	Fungi Candida	Preexisting Candida infection	Persistent fever after resolution of neutropenia; right-upper-quadrant discomfort; nausea; elevated alkaline phosphate levels	Hepatic candidiasis is characterized by appearance of "bull's-eye" lesions on ultrasound or CT scan following granulocyte recovery.
	Viruses Hepatitis A virus Hepatitis B virus	Multiple transfusions Immunosuppressive therapy AIDS History of IV drug abuse	Hepatomegaly, jaundice; elevated liver function studies; clay-colored stools; anorexia; right-upper-quadrant pain/discomfort	Hepatitis non-A, non-B currently accounts for 85 to 90 percent of posttransfusion cases.
	Hepatitis non-A, non-B virus Secondary infection Herpes simplex Cytomegalovirus Epstein–Barr virus Adenovirus	Preexisting infection with infectious agent		
Central nervous system	Bacteria Staphylococcus Listeria monocytogenes Other gram-positive or gram-negative organisms	Intraventricular shunts Ommaya reservoirs Hematologic malignancy Corticosteroids Concurrent infection in contiguous site History of penetrating head trauma Congenital cardiac disease Bacterial endocarditis Pulmonary infection	Fever; headache; altered mental status Some patients may be asymptomatic	
	Treponema pallidum	History of syphilis, especially in HIV seropositive patients		

Table continued on following page.

235

TABLE 14–1. Infectious Complications in the Immunocompromised Host. (continued)

Site	Organism(s)	Associated Factors	Presenting Signs/Symptoms	Comments
	Fungi *Cryptococcus neoformans*	Lymphoma AIDS	Low-grade fever; persistent headache	
	Viruses Cytomegalovirus	AIDS Disseminated CMV infection		HSV and CMV encephalitis may appear concurrently, although HSV encephalitis is more common in otherwise healthy adults.
	Human immunodeficiency virus	HIV seropositivity	Cognitive impairment (early in disease course): forgetfulness, loss of concentration, slowness of thought; motor dysfunction: loss of balance, leg weakness; behavioral symptoms: apathy, social withdrawal, depression, personality change; psychosis	HIV-related neurologic disorders may present as subacute encephalitis (65%), peripheral neuropathy (50–95%), or aseptic meningitis (5–10%).
	Protozoa *Toxoplasma gondii*	AIDS Immunocompromised children	Fever; seizures, focal motor abnormalities, altered mental status	Most common cause of CNS mass lesions in AIDS; usually requires biopsy to confirm diagnosis.
Genitourinary system	Bacteria Streptococcus *Escherichia coli* Klebsiella Proteus *Pseudomonas aeruginosa*	Local tumor obstruction; neurologic dysfunction due to cord compression or drug therapy; radiation therapy; surgery; catheterization; invasive diagnostic procedures	Dysuria, frequency, urgency, fever; foul-smelling urine; less frequently, flank pain	In symptomatic neutropenic patients, colony counts greater than 10³/ml may be considered diagnostic of infection.

Treponema pallidum	AIDS Multiple sex partners Prior syphilis	Suspicious lesion in oral, anal, or genital area	CDC recommends all HIV-seropositive patients be tested for syphilis and all patients with new cases of syphilis be tested for HIV.
Fungi Candida Torulopsis	Indwelling urinary catheters Antibiotic therapy HIV-seropositive women Concurrent oral candidiasis	White discharge Vaginal itching	
Bacteria Staphylococcus Streptococcus Gram-negative bacilli	Neutropenia Immunosuppressant therapy Disrupted skin integrity	Erythema, edema, heat, pain in involved site; may present as mild erythema and slight discomfort when neutropenia is present	
Cutaneous Fungi Candida Viruses Herpes simplex	AIDS, particularly with IV drug abuse Immunosuppressive therapy History of herpes simplex infection (asymptomatic carrier)	Characteristic vesicles, pain in involved site; occasionally fever; regional lymphadenopathy	
Varicella–zoster	Hematologic malignancy Chemotherapy ±radiation therapy Elderly Immunodeficiency disorders of childhood HIV seropositivity	Prodromal phase: fever, pain, itching, altered sensation in involved dermatome Eruption phase: erythematous patches progressing to vesicles, usually along dermatome Dissemination: generalized lesions, some becoming hemorrhagic or gangrenous	Complications more common in immunocompromised patients with zoster: postherpetic neuralgia, secondary infections, and dissemination.

Table continued on following page.

TABLE 14–1. Infectious Complications in the Immunocompromised Host. (*continued*)

Site	Organism(s)	Associated Factors	Presenting Signs/ Symptoms	Comments
	Cytomegalovirus	Solid organ transplant AIDS	Skin ulcers Maculopapular rash	Usually associated with systemic CMV infection
Cardiovascular system	Bacteria Streptococcus Staphylococcus Enterococcus Pseudomonas aeruginosa Listeria monocytogenes	Dental abscesses IV drug abuse Congenital cardiac abnormalities	Fever, chills; malaise, fatigue; night sweats; heart murmurs	Diagnosis made by isolation of organism from multiple blood cultures.
	Fungi Candida	Implanted vascular-access catheter		
	Aspergillus	Steroid therapy Prolonged antibiotic therapy Hematologic malignancy Chemotherapy AIDS	Fever; embolic phenomena; shortness of breath	Fungal endocarditis may result in large-vessel embolization.
	Cryptococcus	AIDS		
	Viruses Cytomegalovirus	AIDS	Usually asymptomatic	Rare in other immunosuppressed patients.
	Human immunodeficiency virus	AIDS	Usually asymptomatic	Evidence of left ventricular dysfunction may be present on cardiac monitoring.
	Protozoa Toxoplasma gondii	AIDS Severely immunosuppressed cancer patients		Rare; usually associated with disseminated disease.

GI = gastrointestinal; GU = genitourinary; HIV = human immunodeficiency virus; TB = tuberculosis; IV = intravenous; CNS = central nervous system; PPD = purified protein derivative; GVHD = graft-versus-host disease; AIDS = acquired immunodeficiency syndrome; HSV = herpes simplex virus; CMV = cytomegalovirus; CT = computed tomographic; CDC = Centers for Disease Control.

biopsy to confirm. Treatment options are limited to a fairly small number of antimicrobial agents, with amphotericin B the most reliable.

Viruses

Herpesviruses are among the most common sources of opportunistic infection in immunocompromised patients. This family of viruses includes herpes simplex (HSV), varicella–zoster (VZV), and cytomegalovirus (CMV), among others. Those at greatest risk are patients who have undergone bone marrow transplantation, persons with AIDS or hematologic malignancies, and the elderly.

Protozoa

In February 1981, an unusual unexplained increase in reported cases of *Pneumocystis carinii* pneumonia hinted of the massive epidemic now known as AIDS. Although also seen in patients with cancer, pneumocystis pneumonia progresses far more rapidly in those with AIDS.

Infection with *Toxoplasma gondii* is typically systemic at time of diagnosis and is commonly associated with myocarditis and encephalitis.

COMMON SITES OF INFECTION

Bacteremias and Sepsis

Early identification of infection in the immunocompromised patient is not always possible because of a diminished response to invasion. As a result, bacteremias and sepsis are commonly encountered. Most often, the primary site of infection is the lung (25 per cent), followed by perioral and perianal cellulitis, gastrointestinal tract infections, and genitourinary system infections (approximately 10 per cent each) (Pizzo & Meyers, 1989). Increased use of indwelling catheters, such as the Hickman and Broviac catheters, also contribute to the number of bacteremias seen. However, a considerable number of systemic infections occur without a source ever being identified. Organisms most often identified are bacteria and fungi.

Bacteria

Gram-negative sepsis is commonly encountered in the patient with neutropenia, probably the result of bacteria entering the bloodstream through ulcerations in the gastrointestinal tract. The predominant organisms are *Escherichia coli, Pseudomonas aeruginosa,* and *Klebsiella pneumoniae.* The most significant consequence of gram-negative sepsis is endotoxic, or septic, shock.

Endotoxin is a lipopolysaccharide found on the outer membrane of gram-negative bacteria. Effects of endotoxin include stimulation of leukocytosis and the febrile response; alteration of the vascular epithelium; release of vasoactive kinins that appear to have a role in the collapse of microvascular circulation; and initiation of the complement cascade, which, in turn, activates the coagulation and fibrinolytic systems (Rabinowitz, 1985). Without early identification and prompt treatment, endotoxic shock ultimately produces hypotension, inadequate tissue perfusion, multisystem failure, and death.

The vast majority of systemic infections related to vascular access catheters involve *Staph. aureus, Staph. epidermidis,* and Streptococcus, although gram-negative bacteria and Candida have also been implicated. Variables that influence the incidence of catheter-associated infections include primary disease process, type of catheter, frequency of use, and adherence to proper technique when accessing and performing maintenance procedures.

Fungi

Fungemia, most often caused by Candida, is commonly found in patients who are diabetic, on steroids, experiencing prolonged neutropenia or receiving broad-spectrum antibiotic therapy, receiving total parenteral nutrition, or undergoing therapy via indwelling venous catheters.

Assessment

Early identification of bacteremia in the immunocompromised patient is often complicated by an impaired response to invasion. Signs and symptoms usually relied on are diminished or absent, allowing a localized infection to become systemic before it is even recognized. Often the predominant indication is a temperature elevation of one degree that persists for 24 hours or more. The development of new fever will represent infection in at least 60 per cent of all patients with granulocytopenia (Schimpff, 1986). Occasionally, the patient will complain of "not feeling well" or will be mildly confused.

Diagnosis is typically confirmed on the basis of blood cultures and cultures of all potential sites of infection. Empirical treatment should be initiated as soon as possible after culture specimens are obtained. Sepsis, particularly in the patient with granulocytopenia, progresses rapidly and will result in death within 24 to 48 hours unless appropriate antimicrobial therapy is initiated promptly (Schimpff, 1986).

When an indwelling venous catheter is in place, blood cultures should be obtained from each lumen or port, in addition to peripheral sites, to determine if the infection is catheter-related. Subcutaneous tunnels, catheter exit sites, and subcutaneous port pockets should be carefully assessed for evidence of infection. Although administration of antibiotics through an infected catheter may be effective in resolving the infection, the presence of a fibrin sleeve around the catheter may provide sanctuary for residual organisms. Inadequate penetration of the fibrin–platelet matrix by the antimicrobial agent may result in treatment failure (Young, 1985).

Respiratory Tract

The respiratory tract is the most common site of serious infection, as well as the primary cause of sepsis, in the immunocompromised patient. Extent of infection ranges from upper respiratory tract (e.g., otitis media and sinusitis) to pneumonia. Diagnosis is often complicated by the inability to detect evidence of an infiltrate on roentgenography. Possible pathogens include bacteria, fungi, viruses, and protozoa, frequently in combination.

Upper Respiratory Tract

The upper respiratory tract is often overlooked as a source of infection in the immunocompromised patient. Mucosal erosions caused by nasotracheal or endotracheal intubation, nasogastric tubes for feeding or suction, tumor progression, or diagnostic procedures (e.g., bronchoscopy) frequently provide opportunities for invasion. Resulting infections include otitis media, otitis externa, and sinusitis.

BACTERIA. The bacterial organisms most commonly found in upper respiratory infections are *Streptococcus pneumoniae, Ps. aeruginosa,* and *Haemophilus influenzae.* However, susceptible patients may be infected by any gram-negative or gram-positive organism colonizing the oropharynx. *Ps. aeruginosa* should be suspected in cases of recurrent ear infections. Aggressive therapy is required to prevent extension of infection through the petrous bone and into the brain. Sinusitis that does not improve with 72 hours of broad-spectrum antimicrobial therapy should be evaluated further with aspiration or biopsy.

FUNGI. Paranasal sinus infections are frequently the result of fungi, including Aspergillus and Mucoraceae, among others. Aspergillus has particularly become a problem where spores have contaminated ventilation systems via construction dust. Without treatment, progressive infection will cause bony erosion; destruction of the nose, paranasal sinuses, and orbits; and extension into the brain (Pizzo & Meyers, 1989). Treatment includes debridement and administration of amphotericin B.

ASSESSMENT. The risk of upper respiratory infection is increased in patients with anatomic alterations, resulting from tumor progression or treatment (e.g., surgery and radiation) or both. These alterations often impair circulation, compromising both immunologic and pharmacologic efforts at infection control.

Physical assessment findings range from pain, swelling, erythema, discharge and fever in the patient without neutropenia to mild discomfort and minimal erythema when neutropenia is present.

Although routine culture is usually successful in identifying bacterial pathogens, diagnosis of fungal infections may require aspiration or biopsy (or both) for confirmation. Early empirical antifungal therapy is recommended for patients in whom persistent fever and granulocytopenia are seen during broad-spectrum-antibiotic treatment.

Bacterial Pneumonia

In the patient with neutropenia, bacterial pneumonia may be caused by any gram-positive or gram-negative organism. In addition, infections involving Mycobacteria, Nocardia, and Legionella are increasing in incidence among immunocompromised patients with and without neutropenia.

BACTERIA. Patients who are chronically ill are known to have increased oropharyngeal colonization with gram-negative bacilli (GNB), including Klebsiella, E. coli, and Enterobacter (Lerner, 1983). Aspiration of contaminated oropharyngeal contents is believed to be a major factor in the development of GNB pneumonia. In addition, many GNB, particularly Pseudomonas, Klebsiella, and Enterobacter, are able to multiply and reach high titers in water reservoirs used in inhalation therapy. Improvements in techniques and equipment, most notably the change from nebulizers to humidifiers, has lessened the risk of acquiring GNB pneumonia from inhalation therapy.

Legionella is an uncommon cause of respiratory infections in most centers and tends to be limited in certain geographic locales. Although the lung is the primary target organ, the disease rapidly progresses to involve many other systems. Immunocompetent patients frequently recover from Legionella infection; however, death may result in up to 80 per cent of infected immunocomprised patients (McCabe, 1988).

MYCOBACTERIA. The number of new mycobacterial infections reported to the Centers for Disease Control (CDC) had steadily declined until, in 1986, the incidence increased by 2.6 per cent. Most dramatic changes have occurred in areas with a prevalence of HIV infection (Chaisson & Slutkin, 1989; CDC, 1989). The strong association between human immunodeficiency virus (HIV) seropositivity and mycobacterial infection led the CDC to include extrapulmonary tuberculosis (TB) as an AIDS-qualifying diagnosis in HIV-infected patients (CDC, 1986a).

Mycobacterial infections are particularly common in patients with impaired cellular immunity. It is believed that the deficiency of lymphokines produced by T cells results in decreased macrophage activation and, consequently, inadequate response to mycobacterial invasion. However, it has also been noted that HIV-infected patients exhibit an independent abnormality in macrophage response, specifically, the failure to inhibit mycobacterial growth. The potential for a "double and interdependent deficiency" in response may explain the significant increase in mycobacterial infections in AIDS patients (Crowle, Cohn, & Poche, 1989).

The findings of a prospective study of TB risk among HIV-infected intravenous drug users suggest that most TB/AIDS cases represent reactivation of latent TB (Selwyn et al., 1989). This report is consistent with the observation that AIDS-associated M. tuberculosis infection is particularly problematic among ethnic minorities, in which both AIDS and TB are prevalent (Kovacs & Masur, 1988; Chaisson & Slutkin, 1989). Demographic studies have determined that Blacks and Hispanics account for 80 per cent of TB/AIDS cases in New York City, 90 per cent of cases in Florida, and 100 per cent of cases in Newark, N.J. (CDC, 1989).

The diagnosis of TB often precedes or coincides with the diagnosis of AIDS, but may follow it. Extrapulmonary TB will be noted in 40 to 75 per cent of TB/AIDS cases, with lymph nodes, bone marrow, and the central nervous system most commonly involved.

Although *M. avium–intracellulare* (MAI) may present as a pneumonia, the infection is usually disseminated at the time of diagnosis. It has been estimated that between 40 and 60 per cent of HIV-infected patients will also be infected with MAI at the time of death (Kovacs & Masur, 1988). MAI infection is also known to occur in conjunction with hairy-cell leukemia (Maurice et al., 1988; Maziarz et al., 1988).

FUNGI. Aspergillus is probably the most common cause of fungal infection of the respiratory tract. Aspergillus species is the most prominent fungi in the environment; it is abundantly present in air, water, soil, and decaying vegetation. When spores are released, they frequently become contaminants in ventilation systems and are easily inhaled. At highest risk are patients with leukemia who have an incidence of aspergillosis 20 times higher than those with lymphomas or solid organ transplants (McCabe, 1988). Aspergillus infections are rare in patients with AIDS.

Aspergillus infection typically begins in the lungs, sinuses, or both. Inhaled spores invade the pulmonary vasculature, causing localized infarction, tissue necrosis, and hemoptysis. Necrotic debris forms an ideal medium for further growth of Aspergillus (Young, 1989). Thrombosis of pulmonary veins and arteries may result from invasive infection. Death often occurs either as a result of respiratory failure or massive hemoptysis.

The Phycomycetes, particularly Mucor and Rhizopus, are far less common than Aspergillus but follow a similar pattern of infection and invasion.

Histoplasma capsulatum has been increasingly identified in patients with AIDS. The organism is endemic to the central and southern United States and has been known to cause asymptomatic pulmonary infections in immunocompetent individuals. In patients with AIDS, however, the disease is usually disseminated at the time of diagnosis. Histoplasmosis has also been identified in nonendemic areas, such as New York City, particularly among HIV-positive Hispanics. Although some cases represent new infections, reactivation of latent infection appears to have a role (Kovacs & Masur, 1988).

Cancer-related immunodeficiency also increases risk of disseminated infection with *Hist. capsulatum*. Involvement of the reticuloendothelial system may cause lymphadenopathy and hepatosplenomegaly, which may be confused with progression of the underlying malignancy (Pizzo & Meyers, 1989).

VIRUSES. Cytomegalovirus (CMV) is a frequent cause of severe interstitial pneumonia, primarily following bone marrow transplantation (BMT) or solid organ transplantation. Less commonly, the infection will be noted in patients with hematologic malignancy. Specific risk factors for CMV pneumonia following allogeneic BMT include seropositivity for CMV prior to transplant, inclusion of total-body irradiation in pretransplantation preparation, and development of graft-versus-host disease (GVHD) after transplantation (Pizzo & Meyers, 1989). CMV pneumonia is most likely to develop within the first 3 months after transplant.

Respiratory syncytial virus (RSV) is a well-known pathogen among neonates and young children; however, there is little documentation of clinical infection among adults. It has recently been observed that immunocompromised patients may be at considerable risk, particularly after BMT or solid organ transplantation (Englund et al, 1988). The virus may cause upper respiratory tract infection, most notably sinusitis, as well as pneumonia.

Other viruses that may cause severe pneumonia include herpes simplex virus (HSV) and varicella–zoster virus (VZV). HSV pneumonia is rare and may be related to endotracheal intubation in patients with local mucocutaneous infection (McCabe, 1988). VZV is a relatively common cause of viral pneumonia in immunocompromised children, with pneumonitis appearing within 3 to 7 days after development of typical skin lesions. In adults with advanced malignancy, reactivation of latent VZV ("shingles") may produce disseminated disease, including involvement of the lungs.

PROTOZOA. *Pneumocystis carinii* is the most commonly encountered protozoal pathogen producing pneumonia in immunocompromised patients. Initial infection is believed to occur early in life and then remains latent, probably in the lung, until immunodeficiency provides an opportunity for reactivation. Pneumocystis pneumonia presents as a bilateral interstitial infiltrate that progresses rapidly. Organisms fill alveolar spaces, forming inclusion cysts, which severely limit gas exchange.

Pneumocystis pneumonia is the primary life-threatening opportunistic infection in patients with AIDS. It is the initial indication of AIDS in approximately 65 per cent of HIV-infected individuals and ultimately develops in 80 per cent of all patients with AIDS (Kovacs & Masur, 1988). Other risk factors, in addition to HIV seropositivity, include hematologic malignancy and immunosuppressive therapy following solid organ transplantation.

ASSESSMENT. In view of the high incidence of pneumonia in the immunocompromised patient, thorough assessment of the respiratory tract is imperative, particularly when infection is suspected. Underlying disease process and other risk factors may provide clues regarding the specific pathogen(s) involved. When neutropenia is present, evidence of pneumonia may be limited to low-grade fever and mild dyspnea.

Diagnostic procedures vary, depending on the suspected organism involved. An excellent review of current procedures, including microbiologic and serologic studies, has been written by McCabe (McCabe, 1988).

For bacterial pneumonias, Gram stain and culture are fairly successful for identifying pathogens. Two common problems, however, compromise the reliability of routine cultures. First, obtaining a reliable sputum specimen for culture is usually not easy. A typical specimen will contain mostly saliva and very little sputum. Second, differentiating lung pathogens from organisms colonizing the oropharynx is also difficult. These same problems exist for viral, fungal, and mycobacterial cultures.

Efforts to improve the reliability of culture specimens have led to the development of transtracheal aspiration procedures. An appropriate candidate for transtracheal aspiration is an individual who cannot produce sputum or has no pathogen identified on Gram stain or who has a poor response to antibiotics selected on the basis of Gram stain and culture results (McCabe, 1988). Potential complications of the procedure include bleeding, infection, and pneumothorax, among others; therefore, the procedure should be attempted only by those skilled in the technique.

Bronchoscopy may also be considered to obtain a reliable specimen. Bronchial brushings during bronchoscopy are less helpful for bacterial pneumonias, but frequently enable confirmation of viral, fungal, and Pneumocystis infection. Bronchoalveolar lavage, also performed in conjunction with bronchoscopy, may provide additional valuable information regarding the pathogens involved. Both brushing and lavage can be performed relatively quickly and safely.

Percutaneous aspiration biopsy may be considered for evaluation of peripheral focal lesions. However, when a diffuse pneumonia is present, diagnostic yield is poor. In addition, percutaneous aspirations carry a greater risk of hemorrhage, depending on the size of the needle used for the procedure. Open lung biopsy is reserved for cases in which diagnosis could not be obtained by a less invasive procedure.

Radiographic studies have a limited role in evaluating pneumonia in the immunocompromised host. In the patient with neutropenia, evidence of an infiltrate is commonly absent.

Gastrointestinal Tract

The alimentary canal in the immunocompromised host provides ready access for multiple organisms. Routes of entry include oropharyngeal lesions due to periodontal disease or stomatitis, esophageal and intestinal lesions due to mucositis, and local trauma to the perirectal area due to hemorrhoids, constipated stool, and invasive procedures. In addition, suppression of normal anaerobic flora in the gastrointestinal (GI) tract predisposes the patient further to opportunistic infection.

Oropharyngeal Infections

Oropharyngeal infections are often the result of aggressive chemotherapy combinations that cause ulceration of the oral mucosa. In addition, the oral cavity is traumatized by chemotherapy-induced emesis. The incidence of oral infection may be as high as 32 per cent (Pizzo & Meyers, 1989), depending on disease entity and treatment regimen.

A great deal of attention has been given to treatment-related stomatitis. It has been recognized as a potential source of sepsis in the patient with neutropenia. Pain accompanying infection discourages adequate fluid and nutritional intake, thereby complicating and delaying recovery.

BACTERIA. Preexisiting periodontal disease is a major factor in the development of bacterial infections of the oropharynx. The organisms most often found on culture include *Staph. aureus, Staph. epidermidis,* and *Ps. aeruginosa,* the same organisms most often associated with systemic bacterial infection in the immunocompromised host.

FUNGI. *Candida albicans,* the causative agent in thrush, is particularly problematic in immunosuppressed patients. In patients with severe neutropenia, oral Candida may ultimately result in systemic disease. For those with AIDS, the infection may be the first indication of HIV seropositivity.

Candida is the most common cause of esophagitis in patients with AIDS. Although candidiasis rarely becomes systemic in HIV-infected individuals, the resulting pain interferes with nutrition and quality of life. In addition to AIDS, neutropenia, mediastinal radiation, and use of corticosteroids are risk factors for esophageal candidiasis.

VIRUSES. HSV is well known to cause significant oral disease in the immunocompromised host. Oral herpetic infection may not present with the typical intraoral lesions associated with HSV. Instead, the pain and inflammation arising from HSV infection may be incorrectly attributed to treatment-related mucositis and gingivitis. When HSV and Candida infections are concurrent, Candida overgrowth masks evidence of the viral component.

CMV has been recognized as a less common cause of esophagitis in patients with AIDS and those undergoing bone marrow transplantation.

ASSESSMENT. Inspection of the oral cavity should include observation for white plaques, erythema, gingival edema, bleeding gums, and open lesions. Complaints of oral pain or pain on swallowing should be noted and appropriate cultures—bacterial, fungal, and viral—promptly obtained.

An oral hygiene plan should be in place, taking into consideration specific risk factors (e.g., chemotherapy) that are likely to complicate care. Adherence to the oral hygiene protocol and frequent thorough assessment are critical in preventing complications from oral and esophageal infection.

Intraabdominal Infections

Intraabdominal infections in the immunocompromised host most commonly involve the intestine and the liver. Abdominal infections are often difficult to detect in the patient with neutropenia. During periods of granulocytopenia, abscess formation does not occur, prolonging diagnosis and allowing for progression of infection. Nonspecific symptoms of GI-tract infections include fever, weight loss, myalgias, malaise, anorexia, diarrhea, and fatigue. Abdominal pain or cramping may be absent.

BACTERIA. Necrotizing enterocolitis is an inflammatory cellulitis caused by GNB, particularly *Ps. aeruginosa*. The phenomenon that produces necrotizing lesions in the large bowel most commonly occurs in patients with acute leukemia who have pancytopenia and are undergoing intensive antibiotic therapy. Other high-risk patients are those receiving chemotherapeutic agents that damage the intestinal mucosa. Necrotizing enterocolitis presents with right-lower-quadrant pain and watery or bloody diarrhea. The high mortality rate (between 30 and 50 per cent) is due to perforation, obstruction, sepsis, or all of these (Pizzo & Meyers, 1989).

Antibiotic-associated colitis (AAC) is a well-documented complication following therapy with certain antimicrobial agents. Specifically, the condition has been observed in patients receiving clindamycin, ampicillin, and broad-spectrum beta-lactam antibiotics. AAC is the result of colonic overgrowth by *Clostridium difficile,* an anaerobic bacillus that produces large quantities of endotoxin. The endotoxin is the agent responsible for the development of diarrhea. Isolating the organism is not sufficient for diagnosis, which requires evidence of toxin production for confirmation (Young, 1985; Pizzo & Meyers, 1989).

Nontyphoid salmonellosis is a common cause of diarrhea in patients with impaired cell-mediated immunity (CMI), particularly those with AIDS, leukemia, lymphoma, and other diseases requiring immunosuppressive therapy. The notable increase in reported cases of salmonellosis in patients with AIDS and AIDS-related complex (ARC) has led the CDC to include it as an HIV-associated infection (CDC, 1986b).

In patients with AIDS, salmonellosis is of special concern because HIV infection predisposes to multiple GI disorders, which may confound definitive diagnosis. In addition, Salmonella infection in patients with AIDS usually does not present with typical GI symptoms. As a result, salmonellosis may not be detected until bacteremia develops.

In the immunocompetent patient with salmonellosis, antibiotic therapy is usually unnecessary and, in fact, should probably be avoided, as elimination of normal intestinal flora is likely to prolong infection. However, the significant risk of systemic infection creates a different scenario in the immunocompromised host. Determining appropriate treatment is complicated when the Salmonella serotype isolated is resistant to many antibiotics used for treatment of gram-negative infection. Failure to eradicate the organism is suspected as a significant factor in recurrent salmonella bacteremia in patients with AIDS (Sperber & Schlueper, 1987).

VIRUSES. CMV colitis is not a common cause of diarrhea in patients with AIDS; it affects only approximately 5 to 10 per cent (Drew, 1988). When it does occur, the infection may become life-threatening. Severe abdominal pain associated with significant weight loss may aid in differentiating CMV infection from other GI pathogens (Connolly et al., 1989). In addition to nonspecific GI symptoms, CMV colitis produces voluminous watery or bloody diarrhea. Without treatment, GI hemorrhage and perforation may develop (Kovacs & Masur, 1988).

Adenovirus infections are not often identified in immunocompromised patients. The incidence is probably underestimated for several reasons. Adenovirus infection may be misdiagnosed by physical examination and by laboratory analysis. Adenovirus infections present in a manner similar, both clinically and histopathologically, to CMV and, occasionally, HSV. It is not uncommon to find adenovirus coinfection with CMV, HSV, or both. Viral cultures may be heavily contaminated with bacterial overgrowth, making it impossible to identify the pathogen involved.

The only major risk factor that can be identified for adenovirus infection is moderate to severe GVHD (Landry et al., 1987). In a prospective study of bone marrow transplant recipients, adenovirus was identified as the most common pathogen responsible for diarrhea following the development of GVHD (Yolken et al., 1982). Indications for suspicion of adenovirus infection include diarrhea and abnormal liver function studies, both of which may also result from GVHD alone.

Hepatitis in the immunocompromised host is usually the result of primary infection by a variety of viral agents: hepatitis A, B (HBV), non-A, non-B (NANB), or delta. Chronic HBV, in both its chronic active and asymptomatic carrier states, is associated with impaired CMI, as is seen in patients who have undergone renal transplantation and are receiving immunosuppressive therapy. It is believed that cytotoxic T cells in the immunocompetent host destroy HBV-infected hepatocytes and mediate elimination of the virus (Zuckerman 1988).

Hepatitis can also occur secondarily, following infection by HSV, VZV, CMV, Epstein–Barr virus (EBV), or adenovirus. Histologic evidence of CMV hepatitis has been found in between one third and one half of patients with AIDS who have evidence of CMV infection in other sites (Drew, 1988).

NANB hepatitis is the most commonly encountered blood-transmissible hepatitis among patients with cancer (Pizzo & Meyers, 1989). With current donor screening procedures to detect HBV, 85 to 90 per cent of cases of post-transfusion hepatitis are NANB hepatitis (Dienstag, 1983; Tabor et al., 1978). The disease has an insidious onset, with relapse common. As many as 50 per cent of those infected may become chronic carriers (Tabor et al., 1978), with cirrhosis developing in 10 to 25 per cent. Treatment with interferon-alfa has been shown to be effective in NANB hepatitis.

Little is known about NANB hepatitis in patients infected with HIV. However, a report of three cases of NANB hepatitis in HIV-seropositive patients described a far more progressive form of the disease. Symptomatic cirrhosis occurred within less than 3 years of primary infection. Although the exact cause of the infection's rapid progression is unclear, it is possible that the deficient immune status resulting from HIV infection allows greater viral replication and, consequently, increased liver damage (Martin et al., 1989).

Although less common in patients with cancer, HBV infection is frequently associated with AIDS. Routes of transmission for both HBV and HIV are sexual and parenteral, so that concurrent infection is very common. Evidence of past or present HBV infection can be found in approximately 90 per cent of all patients with AIDS (Lebovics, Dworkin, Heier, & Rosenthal, 1988). Furthermore, the risk of a person with HIV infection becoming a carrier after HBV infection is approximately 20 per cent, more than three times the risk of those not infected with HIV (Taylor et al., 1988).

It appears that chronic HBV infection is less severe when accompanied by HIV infection; however, there is evidence to suggest that HBV in HIV-infected patients is both more contagious and more resistant to antiviral agents (Bodsworth, Donovan, & Nightengale, 1989). An attempt to immunize homosexually active men who were seronegative to HBV has been reported. Those who were HIV seropositive but had no evidence of AIDS experienced low antibody response or no response to immunization. It is likely that the early T-cell and B-cell defects of HIV infection are sufficient to impair antibody response to neoantigens (Collier, Corey, Murphy, & Handsfield, 1988).

Although primary routes of HBV transmission are sexual and parenteral, other routes of transmission do exist, including saliva, urine, and feces. Immunosuppressive therapy may reactivate HBV infection in those who are asymptomatic carriers (Pariente et al., 1988; Berk et al., 1976; Hoofnagle et al., 1982).

Hepatitis delta is an incomplete RNA virus that depends on HBV for its replication. Among patients with cancer, it is most likely to be diagnosed in those who have received multiple transfusions. As fewer units of HBV-infected blood are available the incidence of hepatitis delta infection will diminish (Pizzo & Meyers, 1989). Among patients with AIDS, the risk of hepatitis delta infection is directly related to participation in known high-risk behaviors for HIV infection (Solomon et al., 1988).

FUNGI. Hepatic candidiasis is being more frequently recognized as a serious problem in the patient with neutropenia following bone marrow recovery. The patient will typically experience persistent fever, nausea, and right upper-quadrant pain. In addition, an elevated level of serum alkaline phosphatase is usually observed. The presence of characteristic "bull's-eye" hepatic lesions on ultrasound or computed tomography is highly suggestive of candidiasis. However, biopsy is required to confirm diagnosis.

PROTOZOA. Cryptosporidiosis was not recognized as a human pathogen until relatively recently. It is spread by the fecal–oral route and has been shown to be present among a large number of immunocompetent adults. Although diarrhea will occur in the presence of immunocompetence, it is mild and self-limiting. However, in patients with AIDS, it is likely to produce a profound and debilitating watery diarrhea. Blood is usually absent. The diarrhea is commonly accompanied by nausea and dramatic weight loss.

ASSESSMENT. Enterocolitis frequently presents as some form of diarrhea, with the specific characteristics of the stool dependent on the pathogen involved. Fever and abdominal pain or tenderness are also common. Evaluation to determine the organism involved includes stool culture and documentation of stool frequency and character.

Invasive procedures, such as barium enema or colonoscopy, may be employed with caution but are often contraindicated because of a risk of perforation or sepsis. Abdominal ultrasound or computed tomography is generally preferred to detect abscesses or evidence of tumor involvement.

Abdominal computed tomography is also helpful in evaluating for hepatic or biliary obstruction. Liver-function studies and serologic testing aid in differentiating jaundice due to primary disease versus hepatitis.

Perirectal Infections

Perirectal infections are decreasing in frequency, probably because of the use of empirical antibiotic therapy in patients with febrile granulocytopenia. In addition to neutropenia, risk factors for perirectal or perianal infection include hemorrhoids, treatment-related mucositis, anal fissures, and any type of rectal manipulation (e.g., rectal examination, barium enema, or sigmoidoscopy).

BACTERIA. GNB are the most common pathogens responsible for the development of perirectal infections in patients with neutropenia. The use of stool softeners reduces local trauma during bowel movements and may prevent development of anal fissures and subsequent infection.

VIRUSES. The most common presentation of HSV in HIV-infected homosexual males is perirectal ulceration. Initially, there may be only erythema and tenderness prior to ulceration. Other symptoms include itching, burning, pain, hematochezia, fever, and rectal discharge (Kovacs & Masur, 1988). As with many other opportunistic infections in patients with AIDS, recurrent infection after apparently successful treatment is common.

Patients with perirectal HSV can easily spread the infection to other sites by contaminating their fingers with the virus.

ASSESSMENT. The perirectal area should be regularly inspected for evidence of inflammation or infection. The presence of other risk factors, such as hemorrhoids or fissures, should be noted. The organism involved can be determined by rectal swab or culture of drainage.

Central Nervous System

Central nervous system (CNS) infections are difficult to evaluate in the immunocompromised host. Not only are symptoms nonspecific, but many symptoms of CNS infection can also represent progression of the disease (e.g., malignancy, AIDS) responsible for the immunodeficient state. Presentation of CNS infections in the immunocompromised patient is typically accompanied by subtle changes in personality, level of consciousness, cognitive ability, or affect.

CNS infections may be classified as shunt infections, meningitis, encephalitis, or brain abscesses. In certain cases, different forms of CNS infection may present concurrently. Between 10 and 25 per cent of HIV-seropositive patients will present with neurologic symptoms, with half of all patients with AIDS acquiring encephalopathy during the end stage of their disease (Wiley & Nelson, 1988).

BACTERIA. Bacterial CNS infections are most likely to appear as shunt infections or brain abscesses. The use of intraventricular shunts and Ommaya reservoirs increases the risk of infection by organisms colonizing the skin around the point of access. Staphylococci are the most common isolate, although other organisms, including GNB and Candida, may be identified (Pizzo & Meyers, 1989; Lishner et al., 1990).

Brain abscesses are often the result of infection in a contiguous site (e.g., otitis, sinusitis, or dental abscesses) and may be caused by a variety of gram-negative or gram-positive organisms. Other predisposing factors for brain abscesses include a history of penetrating cranial trauma, congenital cardiac disease, bacterial endocarditis, and pulmonary infection (Pizzo & Meyers, 1989).

Listeria monocytogenes is a gram-positive rod that has increasingly been noted as a cause of meningitis in patients being treated for hematologic malignancy or who are receiving corticosteroid therapy (Gold, 1985; Paterson, 1985). In patients with AIDS, *L. monocytogenes* meningitis is rare, with few case reports cited (Gould, Belok, & Handwerger, 1986; Harvey & Chandrasekar, 1988; Calubiran, Horiuchi, Klein, & Cunha, 1990).

One report has described an unusually aggressive progression of neurosyphilis in four young homosexual men with AIDS (Johns, Tierney, & Felsenstein, 1987). The advent of antibiotics has made neurosyphilis a rare occurrence. However, the immunodeficiency state resulting from HIV infection may provide a survival advantage for *Treponema pallidum* that enables progression to CNS involvement.

FUNGI. *Cryptococcus neoformans* is a common cause of meningitis in patients with defects in CMI, specifically, those with AIDS or lymphomas. In some cases, cryptococcal meningitis is the initial manifestation of HIV infection (Giberson & Kalyan-Raman, 1987). The organism is acquired by inhalation and transported to the CNS by hematogenous spread. Cryptococcal meningitis is typically indolent and presentation subtle, with the majority of patients complaining of low-grade fever and persistent headache (Kovacs & Masur, 1988; Pizzo & Meyers, 1989).

VIRUS. HSV and VZV may produce viral encephalitis in immunocompromised patients, although cutaneous manifestations of infection are far more likely. Unlike HSV encephalitis, which occurs in otherwise healthy individuals, CMV encephalitis develops almost exclusively in the immunocompromised host (Laskin, Stahl-Bayliss, & Morgello, 1987). Among patients with AIDS, CMV encephalitis usually presents in association with disseminated infection. (Drew, 1988; Masdeu et al., 1988). Concurrent HSV and CMV encephalitis has also been reported in patients with AIDS (Laskin et al., 1987; Morgello et al., 1987).

There is increasing evidence that the subacute encephalitis and "aseptic" meningitis seen in HIV-seropositive patients is actually a manifestation of CNS infection by the HIV (Hollander & Stringari, 1987; Vazeux et al., 1987). In fact, primary infection with HIV appears to be the most common cause of meningitis (5 to 10 per cent) and encephalitis (90 per cent) in patients with AIDS (Gabuzda & Hirsch, 1987). The frequency of CNS coinfection by HIV and CMV may suggest a role for interaction between the viruses in the ultimate development of AIDS-related encephalopathy (Wiley & Nelson, 1988).

PROTOZOA. *Toxoplasma gondii* may present as an encephalitis in an immunosuppressed child or as a CNS lesion in a patient with AIDS or in a patient who has undergone transplantation. Pregnant women may experience activation of latent infection and transmit the organism to the fetus. Congenital infection commonly involves the CNS.

Although initial presentation may occur in the CNS, toxoplasmosis is usually disseminated at the time of diagnosis. *T. gondii* is a ubiquitous pathogen; therefore, it is most likely that infections in immunocompromised hosts are the result of reactivation, rather than primary infection.

ASSESSMENT. Patients with CNS infection will present with a variety of neurologic symptoms, depending on the type and extent of infection. Shunt infections will usually present with fever, headache, meningismus, and increased intracranial pressure. With meningitis, early symptoms include low-grade fever, personality changes, and focal neurologic signs. Patients with encephalitis complain of fever, headache, and nuchal rigidity. Altered mental status is common, with progression to stupor and coma.

In AIDS-related encephalitis, symptoms are evident early in the overall disease process. Clinical manifestations include cognitive impairment (forgetfulness, loss of concentration, slowness of thought), motor dysfunction (loss of balance, leg weakness), and behavioral symptoms (apathy, social withdrawal, depression, and personality changes) (Gabuzda & Hirsch, 1987).

Routine diagnostic testing to evaluate CNS infections includes cerebrospinal fluid analysis, computed tomographic (CT) scans, electroencephalography (EEG), magnetic resonance imaging (MRI), and biopsy.

Genitourinary Tract

Urinary-tract infections (UTIs), particularly in the patient with neutropenia, are important sources of bacteremia. Factors that contribute to the development of infection include indwelling urinary catheters, local therapeutic maneuvers (e.g., cystoscopy), local obstruction by tumor or prostatic enlargement, neurologic deficits due to medications or spinal cord compression, and physical impairments that interfere with personal hygiene.

The incidence of sexually transmitted diseases (STDs) is noted to be higher among homosexual men and intravenous drug users. In the presence of HIV infection, STDs appear to take a more aggressive course, progressing at a faster rate (Kovacs & Masur, 1988), and are less responsive to conventional therapy (Fiumara, 1989).

BACTERIA. GNB are, by far, the most common pathogens responsible for UTI. Organisms typically isolated include *E. coli, Ps. aeruginosa,* and Klebsiella and Proteus species. In the elderly, colonization of the urinary tract without UTI is common. Asymptomatic elderly patients should not be routinely treated, in spite of positive cultures or even the presence of leukocytes in the urine (Yoshikawa & Norman, 1987).

UTIs occur in 50 per cent of patients with AIDS at some time during the course of their disease. Most commonly, isolated bacterial pathogens are Salmonella and β-hemolytic Streptococcus (Benson et al., 1988).

Prior infection with *Tr. pallidum* appears to modify risk for HIV acquisition, although the precise relationship between the two pathogens is not entirely clear. Transmission of both diseases depends on the same high-risk sexual practices. In addition, it is suspected that the genital lesion caused by syphilis provides a portal of entry for HIV. The base of the genital lesion is likely to contain large numbers of activated lymphocytes, which are the target cells for HIV (Hook, 1989).

Epidemiologic studies have demonstrated a significant association between past syphilis and risk of HIV infection among homosexuals and heterosexuals. For this reason, the CDC have recommended that all patients with newly diagnosed syphilis be tested for HIV; conversely, all newly diagnosed patients with HIV should be routinely tested for syphilis (CDC, 1988). However, there may be HIV-related B-cell dysfunctions that produce a delay in serologic response (Hook, 1989). Clinical evidence of syphilis should not be ignored in the face of negative serologic testing.

FUNGI. Candida and Torulopsis are prevalent organisms among patients with indwelling urinary catheters, those who are taking broad-spectrum antibiotics, or both. Progression to life-threatening fungemia has been observed in immunocompromised patients, especially when they are undergoing treatment for hematologic malignancy (Gold, 1985; Flynn et al., 1987).

HIV-infected women are also at risk for the development of chronic vaginal candidiasis. Recurring vaginal candidiasis is not uncommon in women who have no underlying immune system disorder. Clues that may suggest the presence of HIV include temporary symptomatic improvement following treatment with intravaginal antifungal agents, a history of risk factors for HIV infection, the presence of lymphadenopathy, and concurrent oral thrush (Rhoads et al., 1987).

ASSESSMENT. As with other infections, classic symptoms of UTI may be absent in the immunocompromised patient, particularly when neutropenia is present. Observation of urine characteristics may be the most useful method of identifying the presence of pathogens. Typically, the urine will be cloudy with a strong, foul smell. Perineal pruritus may be present with Candida infections of the urinary tract. Whenever there is reason to suspect UTI, routine culture and sensitivity analysis should be performed.

For patients with suspected syphilis, serologic testing, including Venereal Disease Research Laboratory (VDRL) and fluorescent treponemal antibody absorption (FTA–ABS) should be performed. If the validity of serologic test results is questionable, darkfield microscopy of lesion exudate or biopsy of suspicious lesions may be helpful in confirming the diagnosis (Hook, 1989).

Cutaneous Infections

Disruption of the skin and mucous membrane interferes with the primary line of defense against invasion. Cutaneous infections may either be a contributing factor in or the result of systemic infection. Multiple and frequent assaults to skin and mucous membrane integrity present an often preventable risk for infection in the immunocompromised host.

BACTERIA. Essentially any bacterial agent can produce a cutaneous infection in the immunocompromised patient. Most common organisms include Staphylococcus, Streptococcus, and GNB. The infections will present as cellulitis, impetigo, or abscess.

FUNGI. Candida represents the most common fungal cause of cutaneous infection, although fungemia due to Candida, Aspergillus, and Cryptococcus may produce secondary infection (Pizzo & Meyers, 1989).

VIRUSES. HSV and VZV are well-known agents in the development of both primary and secondary cutaneous infection. HSV lesions are usually limited to the oral area, with progression of infection involving the GI tract and, less often, the lung. Rare cases of cutaneous CMV have been reported in association with AIDS (Bournerias et al, 1989).

VZV, however, is far more common and is more likely to result in disseminated disease. Primary infection is a significant problem among immunocompromised children, with a mortality rate of 7 per cent (Pizzo & Meyers, 1989). Reactivation of latent virus residing in a dermatome is the most likely cause of VZV infection in adults. Incidence of reactivation ranges from 5 to 10 per cent among patients treated for solid tumors to 35 to 50 per cent for those with Hodgkin's disease or a bone marrow transplant (Pizzo & Meyers, 1989). The elderly are also a known risk group, with the incidence increasing with advancing age (Yoshikawa & Norman, 1987). The likelihood of reactivation also depends on defects in cellular more so than humoral immunity.

Long-term problems associated with VZV reactivation include postherpetic neuralgia (PHN) and ophthalmic zoster. PHN is more common in the elderly, with a reported incidence as high as 45 per cent (Pizzo & Meyers, 1989). Viral involvement of either the nasociliary or trigeminal nerves may result in corneal scarring and subsequent blindness.

ASSESSMENT. Skin integrity should be routinely evaluated in immunocompromised patients. Special attention should be given to sites where skin integrity has already been disrupted (e.g., IV and venipuncture sites, biopsy and other surgical wounds) or is at greatest risk of breakdown (e.g., pressure areas, skinfolds in groin and buttocks, under breasts).

Plans to minimize the risk of cutaneous infection include coordination of blood sampling, selection of skin-care products to reduce drying, and promotion of adequate nutritional and fluid intake.

Cardiovascular Infections

Newer antibiotics and improved antimicrobial treatment plans have made cardiovascular infections relatively infrequent among immunocompromised patients. Predisposing factors include dental abscesses, history of intravenous drug use, and congenital cardiac abnormalities. The incidence and mortality of infective endocarditis is higher among the elderly. The use of indwelling vascular-access catheters increases the risk of endovascular infections. Eradicating pathogens, especially those involved with an endovascular infection, is difficult.

BACTERIA. Gram-positive organisms, primarily Staphylococcus and Streptococcus, are the most common cause of endocarditis and endovascular infections. GNB have also been isolated, particularly in endovascular infections. Rare cases of Listeria endocarditis have been reported (Riancho, Echevarria, & Napal, 1988).

FUNGI. By colonizing the skin around a vascular-access catheter, Candida and Aspergillus may find easy entry into the cardiovascular system. In addition to endovascular infection, Candida is known to cause myocardial microabscesses (Pizzo & Meyers, 1989). Fungal endocarditis predisposes the patient to embolization and thrombosis. Valve replacement may be considered following Candida or Aspergillus endocarditis.

VIRUSES. Although the evidence to date is limited, HIV may be a cardiac pathogen. In a prospective study of 60 HIV-seropositive patients with little evidence of cardiac dysfunction, more than half demonstrated some abnormality by noninvasive testing. Findings were not related to the presence of opportunistic infection, although the prevalence of abnormality was higher in patients with advanced disease. The degree of immunosuppression, determined by absolute CD4 lymphocyte counts, correlated directly with the presence of an echocardiographic abnormality (Levy et al., 1989). Additional research will determine what role, if any, HIV infection has in cardiac disease.

PROTOZOA. *T. gondii* may result in myocarditis in severely immunosuppressed patients with cancer or in patients with AIDS (Kovacs & Masur, 1988; Pizzo & Meyers, 1989). Although relatively uncommon, when it does occur, it is usually a manifestation of disseminated disease.

ASSESSMENT. Symptoms of cardiovascular infection in the immunocompromised host are usually nonspecific: fever, chills, malaise, fatigue, and night sweats. Evidence to suggest cardiac involvement includes new or changing murmurs, splenomegaly, thromboemboli, unexplained heart failure, and arrhythmias. Diagnosis is usually confirmed by isolation of the involved pathogen from multiple blood cultures.

Ocular Infections

Eye infections are common complications among immunocompromised individuals. These infections can occur as a result of minor exposure to specific pathogenic organisms or may be opportunistic in nature.

Any break in the normally intact corneal epithelium can provide an entrance for bacteria, viruses, and fungi. The integrity of the corneal epithelium can be destroyed by inflammation, corneal drying, or chemical or mechanical injury. An ulcer may involve the epithelium, stroma, or endothelium. If the lesion extends into the stroma or beyond, the healing process is slow and accompanied by scar formation.

BACTERIA. Factors that predispose an immunocompromised individual to a bacterial ulcer include dry eyes, ineffective disinfection of contact lenses, and recent history of eye surgery, injury, or abrasion. Symptoms commonly reported by clients include pain, tearing, mucopurulent discharge, reduced visual acuity, photophobia, and iridescent vision (seeing halos around lights).

The most common microorganisms causing bacterial ulcers include Pneumococcus, Pseudomonas, and Staphylococcus.

Pneumococcal ulcers are the most common bacterial ulcers (Ignatavicius & Bayne, 1991). After entering through the nonintact cornea, it produces a dirty green ulcer with definitive edges. A *hypopyon,* a collection of inflammatory cells, macrophages, and pus may be present in the anterior chamber. The ulcer spreads from the site of infection toward the center of the cornea, away from the corneal–scleral margin. The ulcer moves away from the margin since the margin contains blood vessels and white blood cells that could destroy the bacteria. In addition to the general symptoms of bacterial ulcers noted previously, corneal thinning and mild to severe pain may also be present.

Pseudomonas ulcers frequently occur from using contaminated multidose bottles of medications used for the diagnosis of corneal abrasions. An example of such a medication is fluorescein. This ulcer may also result from injury or from wearing contact lenses. A gray or yellow area will be noted at the site of the epithelial break, accompanied by severe pain. The lesion spreads rapidly because of the enzyme produced by the organism that damages the fibers of the cornea. A blue-green discharge resulting from a pigment produced by the organism is common.

Staphylococcal ulcers are caused by *Staph aureus* and *Staph epidermidis.* These ulcers are being seen with increasing frequency as a complication of the treatment of exposure keratitis or corneal abrasions with corticosteroids. The treatment of minor ocular conditions with topical steroids may create an environment in which staphylococcal ulcers can develop.

PRINCIPLES OF ANTIMICROBIAL THERAPY

Bacterial Infections

The widespread use of empirical antibiotic therapy, particularly during periods of granulocytopenia, has contributed significantly to overall survival of immunocompromised patients. Antibiotic agents of choice must be broad-spectrum and as nontoxic as possible. Combination therapy has been proven to be superior in most cases to the single agents currently available (Lazarus et al., 1989).

Selection of specific agents depends on a variety of factors, including the probable source of infection (i.e., community-acquired vs. nosocomial), sensitivity of suspected or proven organisms at the individual institution, severity and anticipated length of the episode of neutropenia, and the overall health status of the patient. Primary consideration has been given to gram-negative organisms; however, the increase in gram-positive isolates is an additional factor to be addressed in drug selection.

Mycobacterial Infections

Isoniazid, alone or in combination with rifampin, is effective in treating *M. tuberculosis* infections in immunocompromised patients. To date, there is no known curative therapy for *M. avium–intracellulare;* however, combination therapy including amikacin, rifampin, ciprofloxacin, ethambutol and clarithromycin have been successful in controlling the infection (Young & Inderlied, 1990).

Fungal Infections

Although multiple effective antibacterial agents are available, the number of antifungals remains limited. The severity of immune dysfunction is the principle factor in determining the drug of choice.

The imidazoles are broad-spectrum antifungal agents that do not carry the same toxicity and cost associated with amphotericin. Although the imidazoles may be effective in eradicating fungal infection in certain patients undergoing therapy for solid tumors, amphotericin is often required for those with acute leukemias and with AIDS.

FUNGI. Fungal ulcers occur from the overgrowth of fungi resulting from immunosuppression, from the long-term use of corticosteroids or antibiotics, or as a result of injury from vegetable matter. Examples of vegetable matter include tree branches, grass, corn stalks, and leaves.

The patient usually presents with a history of a recent ocular injury or irritation. The eye is reddened and a dirty gray ulcer is present. Satellite lesions may be noted in other areas of the cornea. Most fungal ulcers are opportunistic organisms. These include Candida, Aspergillus, Penicillium, Cephalosporium, and Fusarium.

VIRUSES. Herpes simplex keratitis is the most commonly occurring corneal ulcer; it is caused by herpes simplex Type I virus (Boyd-Monk & Steinmetz, 1987). The patient usually reports symptoms of ocular irritation, photophobia, and tearing. When questioned, the client may also relate a recent history of an upper respiratory infection, "cold sores," or both. Visual acuity may be reduced. The course of herpes simplex keratitis is self-limiting in the immunologically stable patient; however, in the immunocompromised patient, it can invade the stroma and cause formation of opacities in the subepithelium. These opacities, called *ghost cells,* can take up to 1 year to resolve, and scars may be left.

Herpes zoster ophthalmicus is caused by varicella, the same virus responsible for chickenpox. This disorder is believed to be due to the activation of a virus that lies dormant in the dorsal-root ganglia of affected patients. The virus may lie dormant for years until triggered by immunosuppression.

The most common ocular opportunistic infection among immunocompromised individuals is CMV retinitis (Fay, Freeman, Wiley, Hardy, & Bozzette, 1988). The cytomegalovirus is a member of the herpes family. Direct invasion of retinal cells by the virus occurs, causing damage and necrosis.

CMV retinitis presents with granular white dots on the retina that somewhat resemble cotton wool spots. However, they are deeper and represent an increased density. These lesions tend to occur in proximity to blood vessels and coalesce to form patches of opacification. Left untreated, the patches of opacification expand, affecting large portions of the retina. Blood vessel occlusion occurs in the involved retinal areas. Changes in the optic nerve such as atrophy and papilledema can also occur (Rao & Biswas, 1988). Hemorrhages in the shapes of dots, blots, and flames are also present.

The diagnosis of CMV retinitis is based on ocular findings. These findings create a characteristic clinical appearance. If left untreated, the CMV retinitis can progress to acute retinal necrosis. Atrophic areas of white retinal tissue peel off and flake into the vitreous. Other indications of this sight-threatening disorder include ocular pain, marked vision loss, and retinal edema.

PARASITES. *Acanthamoeba Keratitis* is caused by the living amoeba present in water, soil, and air. This organism feeds on bacteria and can be found in contaminated distilled water. This form of keratitis can be found with increasing frequency in patients who prepare their own saline solution from distilled water and salt tablets for use in cleaning, disinfecting, and storing contact lenses. It is unclear if the contamination occurs after the solution is prepared or if it is due to preexisting contamination of the distilled water.

ASSESSMENT. Evaluating for possible eye infection in the immunocompromised patient begins with review of potential risk factors, including history of recent eye injury and use of contact lenses. The patient should be asked to describe any changes noted in visual acuity and symptoms indicative of altered visual status (e.g., photophobia, pain, tearing, "floaters," etc.).

Inspection for evidence of infection includes observing for erythema, periorbital edema, tearing, discharge, and changes in the appearance of the sclera.

Viral Infections

Acyclovir is effective in the treatment of HSV and VZV infections. Patients with AIDS and HSV are commonly maintained indefinitely on acyclovir because of the inevitable recurrence of infection after the drug is discontinued. Vidarabine may also be used in treatment of VZV and HSV infections, although it is less effective when viral infection is disseminated.

Ganciclovir is a virostatic agent used to suppress CMV replication. It is available only in parenteral form and is generally administered via intravenous (IV) route. However, certain patients with CMV retinitis may undergo intravitreal administration if ganciclovir toxicity precludes continued systemic therapy (USPC, Inc., 1991).

Foscarnet, another virostatic agent, may be prescribed for CMV infections that are resistant to ganciclovir (Minor & Baltz, 1991).

Protozoal Infections

Initial therapy for *P. carinii* infection is trimethoprim–sulfamethoxazole or pentamidine (or both). Dapsone may be substituted for persons with a known allergy to sulfonamides (Bartlett, 1991).

Toxoplasmosis is commonly treated with pyrimethamine and sulfadiazine or "triple sulfa" therapy (sulfamethazine, trisulfapyrimidines–sulfamerazine, and sulfadiazine). Pyrimethamine and clindamycin may also be employed.

There is no therapy known to be effective for the treatment of cryptosporidiosis; however, spiramycin is an investigational agent which may be considered (Kovacs & Masur, 1988; Bartlett, 1991).

SUMMARY

The pathobiology of immunodeficiency places the patient at significant risk of infection. Some of these infections can, to some degree, be prevented; however, many cannot.

The nursing goals specifically related to infection in the immunocompromised host include:

prevention of infection whenever possible by reducing exposures to environmental pathogens and by assisting the patient to maximize current health status;

early identification of infection by diligent monitoring of patient condition; and

prompt initiation of interventions designed to eliminate infection when it occurs.

SELECTED BIBLIOGRAPHY

Bartlett, J.G. (1991). *Pocketbook of infectious disease therapy.* Baltimore: Williams & Wilkins.

Benson, M.C., Kaplan, M.S., O'Toole, K., et al. (1988). A report of cytomegalovirus cystitis and a review of other genitourinary manifestations of the acquired immune deficiency syndrome. *Journal of Urology, 140,* 153.

Berk, P.D., Jones, A., Plotz, P.H., et al. (1976). Corticosteroid therapy for chronic active hepatitis. *Annals of Internal Medicine, 85,* 523.

Bodsworth, N., Donovan, B., & Nightengale, B.N. (1989). Effect of concurrent human immunodeficiency virus infection on chronic hepatitis B: A study of 150 homosexual men. *Journal of Infectious Diseases, 160,* 577.

Bournerias, I., Boisnic, S., Patey, O., et al. (1989). Unusual cutaneous cytomegalovirus involvement in patients with acquired immunodeficiency syndrome. *Archives of Dermatology, 125,* 1243.

Boyd-Monk, H., & Steinmetz, C. (1987). *Nursing care of the eye.* Norwalk, CT: Appleton & Lange.

Calubiran, A.V., Horiuchi, J., Klein, N.C., & Cunha, B.A. (1990). Listeria monocytogenes meningitis in a human immunodeficiency virus-positive patient undergoing hemodialysis. *Heart and Lung, 19*(1), 21.

Centers for Disease Control (1986a). Tuberculosis and acquired immunodeficiency syndrome—Florida. *Morbidity and Mortality Weekly Report, 35,* 587.

Centers for Disease Control (1986b). Classification system for human T-lymphotropic virus type III/lymphadenopathy-associated virus infections. *Morbidity and Mortality Weekly Report, 35,* 334.

Centers for Disease Control (1988). Recommendations for diagnosing and treating syphilis in HIV-infected patients. *Journal of the American Medical Association, 260,* 2488.

Centers for Disease Control (1989). Tuberculosis and human immunodeficiency virus: Recommendations of the advisory committee for the elimination of tuberculosis. *Morbidity and Mortality Weekly Report, 38,* 236.

Chaisson, R.E., & Slutkin G. (1989). Tuberculosis and human immunodeficiency virus infection. *Journal of Infectious Diseases, 159,* 96.

Collier, A.C., Corey, L., Murphy, V.L., & Handsfield, H.H. (1988). Antibody to human immunodeficiency virus (HIV) and suboptimal response to hepatitis B vaccination. *Annals of Internal Medicine, 109,* 101.

Connolly, G.M., Shanson, D., Hawkins, D.A., et al. (1989). Non-cryptosporidial diarrhea in human immunodeficiency virus (HIV) infected patients. *Gut, 30,* 195.

Crowle, A.J., Cohn, D.L., & Poche, P. (1989). Defects in sera from acquired immunodeficiency syndrome (AIDS) patients and from non-AIDS patients with Mycobacterium avium infection which decrease macrophage resistance to M. avium. *Infection and Immunity, 57,* 1445.

Dienstag, J.L. (1983). Non-A, non-B hepatitis. I. Recognition, epidemiology, and clinical features. *Gastroenterology, 85,* 439.

Drew, W.L. (1988). Cytomegalovirus infection in patients with AIDS. *Journal of Infectious Diseases, 158,* 449.

Englund, J.A., Sullivan, C.J., Jordan, M.C., et al. (1988). Respiratory syncytial virus infection in immunocompromised adults. *Annals of Internal Medicine, 109,* 203.

Fay, M., Freeman, W., Wiley, C., Hardy, D., & Bozzette, S. (1988). Atypical retinitis in patients with acquired immunodeficiency syndrome. *American Journal of Ophthalmology, 105,* 483.

Fiumara, N. (1989). Human immunodeficiency virus infection and syphilis. *Journal of the American Academy of Dermatology, 21*(1), 141.

Flynn, P., Feldman, S., Lenoir, A., et al. (1987). Torulopsis glabrata infection in immunocompromised children. *Southern Medical Journal, 80,* 237.

Freeman, W., & Gross, J. (1988). Management of ocular disease in AIDS patients. *Ophthalmology Clinics of North America, 1,* 91.

Gabuzda, D.H., & Hirsch, M.S. (1987). Neurologic manifestations of infection with human immunodeficiency virus. *Annals of Internal Medicine, 107,* 383.

Giberson, T.P., & Kalyan-Raman, K. (1987). Cryptococcal meningitis: Initial presentation of acquired immunodeficiency syndrome. *Annals of Emergency Medicine, 16,* 802.

Gold, J.W.M. (1985). Infectious complications of neoplastic diseases in the critical care unit. In

W.S. Howland, & G.C. Graziano (Eds.), *Critical care of the cancer patient.* Chicago: Year Book, 261.

Gould, I.A., Belok, L.C., & Handwerger, S. (1986). Listeria monocytogenes: A rare cause of opportunistic infection in the acquired immunodeficiency syndrome (AIDS) and a new cause of meningitis in AIDS. A case study. *AIDS Research, 2,* 231.

Harvey, R.L., & Chandrasekar, P.H. (1988). Chronic meningitis caused by Listeria in a patient infected with human immunodeficiency virus. *Journal of Infectious Diseases, 157,* 1091.

Henderly, D., Freeman, W., Smith, R., Causey, D., & Rao, N. (1987). Cytomegalovirus retinitis as the initial manifestation of acquired immune deficiency syndrome. *American Journal of Ophthalmology, 103,* 316.

Hollander, H., & Stringari, S. (1987). Human immunodeficiency virus-associated meningitis. *American Journal of Medicine, 83,* 813.

Hoofnagle, J.H., Dusheiko, G.M., Schafer, D.F., et al. (1982). Reactivation of chronic hepatitis B virus infection by cancer chemotherapy. *Annals of Internal Medicine, 96,* 447.

Hook, E.W. (1989). Syphilis and HIV infection. *Journal of Infectious Diseases, 160,* 530.

Ignatavicius, D., & Bayne, M. (1991). *Medical-surgical nursing: A nursing process approach.* Philadelphia: W.B. Saunders.

Johns, D.R., Tierney, M., & Felsenstein, D. (1987). Alteration in the natural history of neurosyphilis by concurrent infection with the human immunodeficiency virus. *New England Journal of Medicine, 316,* 1569.

Kovacs, J.A., & Masur, H. (1988). Opportunistic infections. In V.T. DeVita, S. Hellman, & S.A. Rosenberg (Eds.), *AIDS: Etiology, diagnosis, treatment, and prevention* (p. 199). Philadelphia: J.B. Lippincott.

Landry, M.L., Fong, C.K.Y., Neddermann, K., et al. (1987). Disseminated adenovirus infection in an immunocompromised host. *American Journal of Medicine, 83,* 555.

Laskin, O.L., Stahl-Bayliss, C.M., & Morgello, S. (1987). Concomitant herpes simplex virus type 1 and cytomegalovirus ventriculoencephalitis in acquired immunodeficiency syndrome. *Archives of Neurology, 44,* 843.

Lazarus, H.M., Creger, R.J., & Gerson, S.L. (1989). Infectious emergencies in oncology patients. *Seminars in Oncology, 16,* 543.

Lebovics, E., Dworkin, B.M., Heier, S.K., & Rosenthal, W.S. (1988). Hepatobiliary manifestations of human immunodeficiency virus infection. *Gastroenterology, 83,* 1.

Lerner, A.M. (1983). Gram negative bacillary pneumonias. In L. Weinstein, & B.N. Fields (Eds.), *Seminars in infectious disease* (p. 159). New York: Thieme-Stratton.

Levy, W.S., Simon, G.L., Rios, J.C., et al. (1989). Prevalence of cardiac abnormalities in human immunodeficiency virus infection. *American Journal of Cardiology, 63,* 86.

Lishner, M., Perrin, R.G., Feld, R., et al. (1990). Complications associated with Ommaya reservoirs in patients with cancer. *Archives of Internal Medicine, 150,* 173.

Martin, P., Di Bisceglie, A.M., Kassianides, C., et al. (1989). Rapidly progressive non-A, non-B hepatitis in patients with human immunodeficiency virus infection. *Gastroenterology, 97,* 1559.

Masdeu, J.C., Small, C.B., Weiss, L., et al. (1988). Multifocal cytomegalovirus encephalitis in AIDS. *Annals of Neurology, 23,* 97.

Maurice, P.D.L., Bunker, C., Giles, F., et al. (1988). Mycobacterium avium-intracellulare infection associated with hairy-cell leukemia. *Archives of Dermatology, 124,* 1545.

Maziarz, R.T., Teepler, I., Antin, J.H., et al. (1988). Reversal of infection with Mycobacterium avium intracellulare by treatment with alpha-interferon in a patient with hairy cell leukemia. *Annals of Internal Medicine, 109,* 292.

McCabe, R.E. (1988). Diagnosis of pulmonary infections in immunocompromised patients. *Medical Clinics of North America, 72,* 1067.

Minor, J.R., & Baltz, J.K. (1991). Foscarnet sodium. *DICP, 25,* 41.

Morgello, S., Cho, E.S., Nielsen, S., et al. (1987). Cytomegalovirus encephalitis in patients with acquired immunodeficiency syndrome. *Human Pathology, 18,* 289.

Newell, F. (1986). *Ophthalmology principles and concepts.* St. Louis: C.V. Mosby.

Pariente, E.A., Goudeau, A., Dubois, F., et al. (1988). Fulmanant hepatitis due to reactivation of chronic hepatitis B virus infection after allogeneic bone marrow transplant. *Digestive Disease and Sciences, 33,* 1185.

Paterson, P.Y. (1985). Infection in the immunocompromised host. In G.P. Youmans, P.Y. Paterson, & H.M. Sommers (Eds.), *The biologic and clinical basis for infectious disease,* (3rd ed.) (p. 733). Philadelphia: W.B. Saunders.

Pizzo, P.A., & Meyers, J. (1989). Infections in the cancer patient. In V.T. DeVita, S. Hellman, S.A. Rosenberg (Eds.), *Cancer: Principles and practice of oncology* (3rd ed.) (p. 2088). Philadelphia: J.B. Lippincott.

Rabinowitz, S.G. (1985). Bacterial sepsis and endotoxic shock. In G.P. Youmans, P.Y. Paterson, H.M. Sommers (Eds.), *The biologic and clinical basis for infectious disease* (3rd ed.) (p. 436). Philadelphia: W.B. Saunders.

Rao, N., & Biswas, J. (1988). Ocular pathology in AIDS. *Ophthalmology Clinics of North America, 1,* 63.

Rhoads, J.L., Wright, C., Redfield, R.R., et al. (1987). Chronic vaginal candidiasis in women with human immunodeficiency virus infection. *Journal of the American Medical Association, 257,* 3105.

Riancho, J.A., Echevarria, S., & Napal, J. (1988). Endocarditis due to Lisertia monocytogenes and human immunodeficiency virus infection. *American Journal of Medicine, 85,* 737.

Schimpff, S.C. (1986). Infections in patients with cancer. In A.R. Moossa, M.C. Robson, S.C. Schimpff (Eds.), *Comprehensive textbook of oncology* (p. 367). Baltimore: Williams & Wilkins.

Selwyn, P.A., Hartel, D., Lewis, V.A., et al. (1989). A prospective study of the risk of tuberculosis among intravenous drug users with human immunodeficiency virus infection. *New England Journal of Medicine, 320,* 545.

Solomon, R.E., Kaslow, R.A., Phair, J.P., et al. (1988). Human immunodeficiency virus and hepatitis delta virus in homosexual men. *Annals of Internal Medicine, 108,* 51.

Sperber, S.J., & Schlueper, C.J. (1987). Salmonellosis during infection with human immunodeficiency virus. *Reviews of Infectious Diseases, 9,* 925.

Tabor, E., Gerety, R.J., Drucker, J.A., et al. (1978). Transmission of non-A, non-B hepatitis from man to chimpanzee. *Lancet, 1,* 463.

Taylor, P.E., Stevens, C.E., Rodriguez de Cordoba, S., et al. (1988). Hepatitis B virus and human immunodeficiency virus: Possible interactions. In A.J. Zuckerman (Ed.), *Viral hepatitis and liver disease* (p. 198). New York: Alan R. Liss.

United States Pharmacopeial Convention, Inc. (1991). *Drug Information for the Health Care Professional.* Rockville, MD: USPC, Inc.

Vazeux, R., Brousse, N., Jarry, A., et al. (1987). AIDS subacute encephalitis. *American Journal of Pathology, 126,* 403.

Wiley, C.A., & Nelson, J.A. (1988). Role of human immunodeficiency virus and cytolomegalovirus in AIDS encephalitis. *American Journal of Pathology, 133,* 73.

Yolken, R.H., Bishop, C.A., Townsend, T.R., et al. (1982). Infectious gastroenteritis in bone marrow transplant recipients. *New England Journal of Medicine, 306,* 1009.

Yoshikawa, T.T., & Norman, D.C. (1987). *Aging and infectious diseases.* New York: Igaku-Shoin.

Young, L.S. (1985). Treatment of established bacterial and fungal infections in patients with hematologic malignancies. In P.H. Weirnik, G.P. Canellos, R.A. Kyle, C.A. Schiffer (Eds.), *Neoplastic diseases of the blood* (p. 943). New York: Churchill-Livingstone.

Young, L.S. (1989). Aspergillus infection in the neutropenic host. *Hospital Practice, 24*(5A), 37.

Young, L.S. & Inderlied, C. B. (1990). Mycobacterium avium complex infections. *AIDS Patient Care, 4,* 10.

Zuckerman, A.J. (1988). Viral Hepatitis. In D.J.M. Wright (Ed.) *Immunology of Sexually Transmitted Diseases* (p. 51). Boston: Kluwer Academic Publishers.

15

NURSING CARE PLAN FOR THE IMMUNOCOMPROMISED PATIENT

Nursing Care Plan for the Immunocompromised Patient (continued)

Problem	Expected Outcome	Nursing Care
1. Potential for systemic infection related to disease process and/or treatment.	1A. Patient remains free of systemic infection. 1B. Patient and significant other (S.O.) verbalize understanding of risk factors for infection, strategies to minimize risk, signs and symptoms to report to health care professionals. 1C. Patient and S.O. demonstrate appropriate measures to prevent systemic infection.	**Assessment:** 1a. Obtain patient history, including factors that affect immunocompetence (e.g., chemotherapy, steroids, radiation, nutritional status, HIV [human immunodeficiency virus] seropositivity, chronic infections). 1b. Calculate absolute granulocyte count daily and initiate appropriate protective measures according to institutional guidelines (e.g., private room, protective isolation, dietary restrictions). 1c. Monitor vital signs every 2 to 4 hours; note minor temperature elevation, which may be indicative of early sepsis. 1d. Perform comprehensive physical assessment every 2 to 4 hours during granulocytopenic periods and communicate changes promptly to physician (see below for body-system-specific assessment guidelines). Give special attention to venipuncture, IV, and vascular-access catheter sites. 1e. Observe patient response to medical plan of care (e.g., lack of improvement after 3 to 5 days of antibiotic therapy: patient remains febrile, chest x-ray unchanged or worsening). **Intervention:** 1a. Implement strict handwashing measures for all persons who have physical contact with patient. 1b. Encourage adequate nutritional and fluid intake. Consult dietician for specific caloric/hydration needs. 1c. Coordinate patient care assignment to avoid exposing patient to those with recent infections or immunizations.

1d. Organize patient care activities to allow for adequate periods of rest.

1e. Perform all invasive and wound care procedures using aseptic technique.

1f. Administer antibiotics and medications to stimulate immunocompetence (e.g., colony-stimulating factors) as directed.

Patient/S.O. Teaching:

1a. Caution patient about the importance of handwashing by others entering his/her room.

1b. Discuss rationale for protective measures during periods of risk.

1c. Explain importance of optimizing health status and reducing risk through diet, rest, and meticulous personal hygiene, particularly during periods of neutropenia.

1d. Inform regarding signs and symptoms of infection that should be reported promptly to MD or nurse (e.g., fever, chills, cough, mild erythema and/or tenderness at wound sites).

1e. Assure that patient and/or S.O. are able to read a thermometer. Investigate availability of digital thermometer for visually impaired.

Assessment:

2a. Obtain history of recent trauma to skin (e.g., abrasions, bruises, cuts, lacerations, burns) or conditions that predispose to disrupted skin integrity (e.g., age, bone marrow transplantation, allergy to dressing products).

2b. Inspect skin thoroughly, with special attention to skin folds (breasts, buttocks, axillae), wound sites (surgical, IV, venipuncture, vascular-access catheters, bony prominences).

2c. Evaluate for evidence of skin lesions suspicious for primary or recurrent malignancy.

Intervention:

2a. Initiate plan for meticulous personal hygiene with special attention to high-risk areas (e.g., groin, axillae, perianal area).

2. Potential for disrupted skin integrity related to disease process and/or treatment.

2A. Skin integrity is maintained.

2B. Patient remains free of skin infection.

2C. Patient and S.O. verbalize understanding of risk factors for infection, strategies to minimize risk, signs and symptoms to report to health care professionals.

2D. Patient and S.O. demonstrate appropriate measures to prevent disruption of skin integrity.

Table continued on following page.

NURSING CARE PLAN FOR THE IMMUNOCOMPROMISED PATIENT (continued)

Problem	Expected Outcome	Nursing Care
		2b. Encourage use of electric razors to minimize skin trauma.
		2c. Select dressing supplies that are less likely to result in skin abrasions. Consult enterostomal therapist for specific products.
		2d. Provide moisturizing lotion to prevent drying, chapping, and cracking of skin. Discuss with physician or enterostomal therapist specific products to be used if microbial contamination is a concern.
		2e. Encourage adequate fluid and nutritional intake. Consult dietician for specific caloric/hydration needs.
		2f. Use caution when moving bedridden patient to prevent skin shearing and abrasion.
		2g. Coordinate lab procedures to minimize venipunctures.
		2h. Encourage patient to ambulate or sit in chair to minimize risk of pressure areas; if bedfast, reposition at least every 2 hours.
		2i. Obtain cultures of all suspicious areas and promptly notify physician.
		2j. Initiate use of special mattress (e.g., "egg crate," air) to reduce trauma to pressure areas.
		Patient/S.O. Teaching:
		2a. Provide self-care information for maintaining skin integrity, including avoidance of exposure to sun and use of sun screens.
		2b. Discuss rationale for protective measures during periods of risk.
		2c. Inform regarding signs and symptoms of infection that should be reported promptly to physician or nurse.
		Assessment:
		3a. See Assessment 2a–2c above.
3. Disrupted skin integrity related to disease process and/or treatment.	3A. Patient exhibits evidence of restored skin integrity.	

3B. Patient/S.O. demonstrate ability to perform prescribed skin care procedures.

3C. Patient/S.O. identify factors that impair and restore skin integrity.

3b. Note size, depth, color of open area; also presence of associated odor or drainage.

Intervention:

3a. See Interventions 2a–2j above.

3b. Perform dressing changes using aseptic technique.

3c. Consult with enterostomal therapist regarding plan of care for complex wounds.

3d. Initiate referral to home care agency as appropriate (e.g., to reinforce teaching, supervise performance of wound care procedures, or to provide direct patient care).

Patient/S.O. Teaching:

3a. See Patient/S.O. Teaching 2a–2c above.

3b. Instruct in proper technique for wound care and dressing changes to be performed at home.

4. Potential for pulmonary dysfunction related to disease process and/or treatment.

4A. Patient maintains optimal pulmonary function.

4B. Patient and S.O. verbalize understanding of risk factors for pulmonary dysfunction, strategies to minimize risk, signs and symptoms to report to health care professionals.

4C. Patient and S.O. demonstrate appropriate measures to maintain optimal pulmonary function.

Assessment:

4a. Obtain patient history, including risk factors that affect pulmonary function (e.g., dysphagia, diminished gag reflex, smoking, asbestos or other occupational exposure, chronic lung disease, HIV seropositivity, radiation therapy to chest or mediastinum, chemotherapeutic agents associated with pulmonary toxicity).

4b. Observe respiratory effort, noting rate, rhythm, and use of accessory muscles.

4c. Evaluate cervical lymph nodes for tenderness, enlargement.

4d. Perform chest auscultation, noting presence of rales, rhonchi, or friction rubs.

Intervention:

4a. Assist patient in performing cough and deep breathing exercises.

4b. Encourage activity at appropriate level for current health status.

4c. Ensure adequate hydration, either oral or parenteral. Consult physician or dietician for specific hydration needs.

Table continued on following page.

NURSING CARE PLAN FOR THE IMMUNOCOMPROMISED PATIENT (continued)

Problem	Expected Outcome	Nursing Care
		4d. Implement protective measures as indicated by patient health status (e.g., restricting visitors and staff with respiratory infections).
		4e. Monitor test results (e.g., chest x-ray films, arterial blood gases).
		4f. Consult physician regarding need to administer PPD (purified protein derivative).
		Patient/S.O. Teaching:
		4a. Instruct in proper performance of coughing and deep breathing.
		4b. Discuss strategies for smoking cessation.
		4c. Inform regarding signs and symptoms to be reported to physician or nurse (fever, cough, sputum production).
5. Impaired pulmonary function related to disease process and/or treatment.	5A. Patient exhibits evidence of restored pulmonary function.	**Assessment:**
	5B. Patient and S.O. demonstrate ability to perform prescribed therapy.	5a. See Assessment 4a to 4c above.
	5C. Patient and S.O. identify factors that impair and restore pulmonary function.	5b. Identify recent changes in pulmonary status: cough, sputum production, pain, dyspnea on exertion or at rest, wheezing.
		5c. Examine sputum and document amount, color, character.
		Intervention:
		5a. See Intervention 4a to 4c above.
		5b. Obtain sputum cultures as indicated.
		5c. Perform suctioning procedures using aseptic/sterile technique.
		5d. Provide oxygen therapy as prescribed.
		Patient/S.O. Teaching:
		5a. See Patient/S.O. Teaching 4a to 4c above.
		5b. Describe safety precautions in use of home oxygen therapy.
		5c. Provide information about community resources and support agencies (e.g., American Lung Association, American Cancer Society).

6.		
Potential for disrupted integrity of oral mucosa related to disease process and/or treatment.	6A. Oral cavity remains free of ulceration and inflammation. 6B. Patient and S.O. verbalize understanding of risk factors for ulceration/infection, strategies to minimize risk, signs and symptoms to report to health care professionals. 6C. Patient and S.O. demonstrate appropriate measures to prevent/minimize trauma to oral mucosa.	**Assessment:** 6a. Obtain patient history, including factors influencing integrity of oral mucosa (e.g., advanced age, chemotherapeutic agents causing mucous membrane toxicity, radiation therapy to the head, neck, or mediastinum, HIV seropositivity, use of tobacco and/or alcohol, current prescription and over-the-counter [OTC] medications, periodontal disease, nutritional status). 6b. Inspect oral cavity daily while hospitalized and on each nursing visit at home, including gums, lips, tongue, palate, teeth, floor of the mouth, and oropharynx. Note color, moisture, and presence of lesions or ulcerations. 6c. Observe amount and character of saliva. 6d. Evaluate patient's routine procedure for oral hygiene. 6e. Inquire about presence of oral pain. **Intervention:** 6a. Initiate plan for oral hygiene, including use of a soft toothbrush and nonabrasive toothpaste after meals and at bedtime and use of dental floss daily. Avoid the use of solutions with high alcohol content. Acceptable alternatives: normal saline, ¼ to ½ strength; hydrogen peroxide, ½ strength; sodium bicarbonate. 6b. Obtain bacterial, fungal, and viral cultures if oral pain is present. 6c. Encourage adequate fluid intake. Consult physician or dietician about specific hydration needs. 6d. Consult physician regarding topical and/or systemic analgesic for pain in mouth or esophagus that could interfere with adequate fluid and nutritional intake and compliance with performance of oral hygiene procedures. 6e. Provide water-soluble lip lubricant.

Table continued on following page.

NURSING CARE PLAN FOR THE IMMUNOCOMPROMISED PATIENT (continued)

Problem	Expected Outcome	Nursing Care
		Patient/S.O. Teaching: 6a. Discuss appropriate dietary selections to minimize trauma to oral mucosa (e.g., avoiding spicy foods, items with high acid content, temperature extremes). 6b. Emphasize importance of consistent and thorough oral hygiene. 6c. Encourage avoidance of tobacco and alcohol products. 6d. Outline signs and symptoms to be reported to physician or nurse (e.g., pain, erythema, bleeding, ulceration, white patches on tongue or palate or inside cheeks).
7. Disruption of oral mucous membrane integrity related to disease process and/or treatment.	7A. Patient exhibits evidence of restored oral mucous membrane integrity. 7B. Patient and S.O. demonstrate ability to perform prescribed therapy. 7C. Patient and S.O. identify factors that impair and restore integrity of oral mucous membrane.	**Assessment:** 7a. See Assessment 6a to 6e above. 7b. Evaluate extent and severity of changes observed, including condition of teeth, gums, lips, palate, and inside cheeks and presence of bleeding. **Intervention:** 7a. See Intervention 6a to 6e above. 7b. Establish plan for care of oral mucosa. For mild to moderate alterations (generalized erythema, small ulcerated patches): use soft toothbrush with nonabrasive toothpaste, normal saline mouth rinses. Include rinses with ¼ strength peroxide or 1 teaspoon of sodium bicarbonate in 8 oz of water if crusts and debris are present. For severe changes, where pain and/or bleeding preclude use of a toothbrush, substitute cotton swabs or Toothettes®, followed by rinses as described above. Perform mouth care every 2 to 4 hours while awake and every 6 hours while asleep (Goodman and Stoner, 1991).

7c. Encourage use of dentures for meals only until adequate healing has taken place.

Patient/S.O. Teaching:

7a. See Patient/S.O. Teaching 6a to 6d above.

7b. Provide verbal and written instructions for oral care and administration of analgesics and antimicrobial agents.

8. Potential for disrupted integrity of rectal mucosa related to disease process and/or treatment.

8A. Anorectal area remains free of ulceration and inflammation.

8B. Patient and S.O. verbalize understanding of risk factors for ulceration/infection, strategies to minimize risk, signs and symptoms to report to health care professionals.

8C. Patient and S.O. demonstrate appropriate measures to prevent/minimize trauma to rectal mucosa.

Assessment:

8a. Obtain patient history, including factors influencing integrity of rectal mucosa (e.g., advanced age, chemotherapeutic agents causing mucous membrane toxicity, HIV seropositivity, current prescription and OTC medications, nutritional status, change in bowel habits).

8b. Inspect rectal area for erythema, ulcerations, bleeding, hemorrhoids.

8c. Monitor stools for color, consistency, and presence of blood or mucous.

Intervention:

8a. Identify modifiable lifestyle factors that may reduce trauma to intestinal mucosa (e.g., diet, sexual practices, OTC medications).

8b. Modify diet to include foods that are low-residue. Eliminate items that increase intestinal motility (e.g., high acid content, high fiber, temperature extremes).

8c. Avoid rectal temperature, enemas, suppositories, or other invasive procedures.

8d. Establish hygiene plan to prevent excoriation, infection (e.g., sitz baths).

Patient/S.O. Teaching:

8a. Discuss factors that increase risk of infection and inflammation (e.g., hemorrhoids, rectal trauma).

8b. Instruct regarding measures to limit trauma to rectal mucosa (e.g., dietary modification, avoiding invasive activities such as enemas, suppositories, and anal intercourse).

Table continued on following page.

NURSING CARE PLAN FOR THE IMMUNOCOMPROMISED PATIENT (continued)

Problem	Expected Outcome	Nursing Care
		8c. Inform regarding signs and symptoms to be reported to physician or nurse (perirectal pain or itching, rectal bleeding, pain with defecation).
9. Disruption of rectal mucosal integrity related to disease process and/or treatment.	9A. Patient exhibits evidence of restored rectal mucous membrane integrity.	**Assessment:** 9a. See Assessment 8a to 8c above. **Interventions:** 9a. See Intervention 8a–8d above.
	9B. Patient and S.O. demonstrate ability to perform prescribed therapy.	9b. Consult with physician regarding possible need for stool softener or antidiarrheal agent, as appropriate.
	9C. Patient and S.O. identify factors that impair and restore integrity of rectal mucosa.	9c. Refer to enterostomal therapist as indicated for assistance in establishing skin care regime.
		Patient/S.O. Teaching: 9a. See Patient/S.O. Teaching 8a to 8c above.
10. Potential for genitourinary infection related to disease process and/or treatment.	10A. Patient remains free of genitourinary infection.	**Assessment:** 10a. Obtain patient history, including factors that increase risk of genitourinary infection (e.g., benign prostatic hypertrophy, incomplete bladder emptying, HIV seropositivity, chemotherapeutic agents with known bladder toxicity).
	10B. Patient and S.O. verbalize understanding of risk factors for infection, strategies to minimize risk, signs and symptoms to report to health care professionals.	10b. Evaluate for symptoms of genitourinary infection: dysuria, urinary frequency, urgency, hematuria, etc; vaginal/penile discharge, pruritus.
	10C. Patient and S.O. demonstrate appropriate measures to prevent genitourinary infection.	10c. Inspect genitalia for lesions, ulcerations, discharge.
		10d. Note color, character, and odor of urine.
		Intervention: 10a. Encourage adequate hydration. Consult physician or dietician for specific hydration needs.
		10b. Obtain clean catch or catheterized urine specimen for culture and routine analysis.

Nursing Diagnosis	Outcome Criteria	Nursing Interventions
		10c. Culture genital lesions and discharge. Consult physician regarding prescription for antispasmodic/analgesic as indicated.
		10d. Avoid use of indwelling urinary catheters unless absolutely necessary. If indwelling catheter is to be used, select smallest size possible.
		Patient/S.O. Teaching:
		10a. Discuss rationale and importance of adequate hydration.
		10b. Outline signs and symptoms to be reported to physician or nurse (pain, urgency, frequency; discharge, genital lesion).
11. Potential for inadequate tissue oxygenation due to disease process and/or treatment.	11A. Hematologic evaluation of qualitative and quantitative red blood cell parameters remains within normal limits.	**Assessment:**
	11B. Patient and S.O. verbalize understanding of risk factors for anemia, strategies to minimize risk, signs and symptoms to report to health care professionals.	11a. Obtain patient history, including factors that increase risk of anemia (e.g., nutrition, OTC and prescription medications [including chemotherapy, antimicrobials and biologic response modifiers], radiation therapy to bone marrow, occupational exposures, recent surgery, malabsorption, symptoms of gastrointestinal bleeding).
	11C. Patient and S.O. demonstrate appropriate measures to prevent anemia.	11b. Evaluate for signs and symptoms of anemia (e.g., pallor, easily fatigued, dyspnea on exertion, syncope, dizziness).
		11c. Monitor lab data, particularly red-cell count, hemoglobin, hematocrit, red-blood-cell indices, reticulocyte count, platelet count, peripheral blood smear, bone marrow aspirate/biopsy.
		Intervention:
		11a. Encourage adequate fluid and nutritional intake, emphasizing foods high in iron and protein. Consult dietician for specific caloric and hydration needs.
		11b. Review current medications with physician to determine modifications where appropriate.

Table continued on following page.

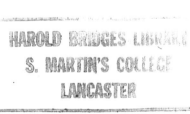

NURSING CARE PLAN FOR THE IMMUNOCOMPROMISED PATIENT (continued)

Problem	Expected Outcome	Nursing Care
		11c. Organize activities to allow adequate periods of rest. Monitor fatigue pattern so that activities may be scheduled during peak energy periods.
		11d. Monitor for evidence of active bleeding (e.g., black tarry stools, hematuria, blood in sputum, petechiae, ecchymosis, etc.).
		Patient/S.O. Teaching:
		11a. Instruct patient and S.O. regarding importance of nutrition in prevention and treatment of anemia. Obtain dietary consult as indicated.
		11b. Discuss contribution of medications in development of anemia and assist in selecting acceptable OTC alternatives when possible.
		11c. List signs and symptoms of anemia to report to physician or nurse (pallor, fatigue, dyspnea on exertion).
12. Potential for bleeding related to disease process and/or treatment.	12A. Patient exhibits no evidence of bleeding.	**Assessment:**
	12B. Patient and S.O. verbalize understanding of risk factors for bleeding, strategies to minimize risk, signs and symptoms to report to health care professionals.	12a. Obtain patient history, including factors that increase risk of bleeding (e.g., personal or family history of bleeding disorders, autoimmune disease that causes platelet destruction, aplastic anemia, OTC and prescription medications including chemotherapy, radiation therapy to bone marrow).
		12b. Inspect skin for ecchymoses, petechiae, hematomas.
		12c. Inquire about recent episodes of abnormal bleeding (e.g., gums and oral cavity, hematuria, tarry stools or bright red blood in stools, unusually heavy menses, epistaxis, altered levels of consciousness).
		Interventions:
		12a. See Intervention 7b above for oral hygiene plan.

12b. Monitor platelet count and initiate safety measures as indicated (e.g., padded side rails, ambulation with assistance only).

12c. Minimize invasive procedures (e.g., avoid IM injections, coordinate labs to reduce number of venipunctures, discourage use of tampons).

12d. Review current medications with physician to determine appropriate modifications.

12e. Implement measures to control bleeding episodes (e.g., application of pressure or ice packs).

Patient/S.O. Teaching:

12a. Discuss contribution of medications to impairment of platelet function and assist in selecting acceptable OTC alternatives when possible.

12b. List signs and symptoms of thrombocytopenia to report to physician or nurse (unusual bleeding from gums, heavy menses, blood in urine or stool, tarry stools, "coffee grounds" emesis, easy bruising, development of petechiae).

12c. Outline measures to reduce risk of bleeding, including use of electric shavers and water-soluble lubricants during intercourse.

SELECTED BIBLIOGRAPHY

Goodman, M., & Stoner C. (1991). Mucous membrane integrity, impairment of, related to stomatitis. In J.C. McNally, et al. (Eds.), *Guidelines for oncology nursing practice.* Philadelphia: W. B. Saunders, 1991.

GLOSSARY

Absolute granulocyte count (AGC)–includes only cells capable of immediate phagocytic function; the percentage of mature neutrophils plus the percentage of "band" neutrophils can be estimated as follows: total white-cell count × (segmented neutrophils + bands) = AGC; absolute neutrophil count.

Absorptive endocytosis–invagination of the phagocytic cell around the target and sealing of the target within a vesicle, forming a vacuole; primary mechanism of cellular ingestion.

Accelerated phase–first phase of the terminal stage of chronic myelogenous leukemia.

Acquired immunity–immunity that every individual's body normally makes or can receive as an adaptive response to invasion by foreign proteins; occurs naturally or artificially and is either active or passive.

Acquired immunodeficiency syndrome (AIDS)–a pathologic condition resulting from chronic infection with the human immunodeficiency virus (HIV); includes positive HIV culture, immune system changes, and physical symptoms.

Active immunity–occurs when antigens enter the body and the body responds by making specific antibodies against those antigens; natural active immunity or passive active immunity.

Acute lymphocytic leukemia (ALL)–acute leukemia; originates from the lymphoid stem-cell line.

Acute myelogenous leukemia (AML)–acute leukemia; originates from the myeloid stem-cell line; can be myelocytic, monocytic, erythrocytic, or megakaryocytic.

Acute rejection–a type of graft rejection that occurs between 1 week and 3 months after transplantation, caused by both antibody-mediated and cellular mechanisms, that leads to organ destruction.

Adherence–the third step of phagocytosis; direct contact of the phagocyte with its intended target, which is facilitated by opsonization.

Afterloading–technique in brachytherapy in which an implant, without the radioactive isotope, and position-holding devices, are placed within an organ or body cavity.

Agglutination–antibody-binding reaction; binding of multiple antigen molecules to each antibody unit; slows the movement of antigen through extracellular fluids and enhances the defensive action of other leukocytes.

Agranulocytes–term formerly used for referring to lymphocytes, monocytes, and macrophages.

AIDS-related complex (ARC)–presence of a positive HIV culture and immune system abnormalities, including diminished T helper/inducer to T suppressor ratio.

Alkylating agents–antineoplastic agents that are not cell-cycle specific; they cause cross-linking of DNA, which results in disruption of cell division.

Allogeneic transplantation–a graft that comes from a donor source who is not genetically identical to the recipient.

Alpha rays–type of gamma radiation; rays are heavy and slow, easily transfer energy to their surroundings, and quickly lose their ability to penetrate.

Alternative complement pathway–a mechanism for complement activation initiated when the presence of carbohydrate groups on microorganisms triggers the cleavage and binding of the C3 protein; this pathway permits complement fixation in response to microorganisms in the absence of antibodies.

Amyloidosis–comprehensive term for a variety of conditions associated with tissue infiltrates comprised of insoluble proteins and/or protein–polysaccharide complexes.

Anamnestic response–secondary immunologic response.

Antibiotics–a class of antineoplastic drugs, with bacteriocidal action, that inflicts damage by interrupting DNA and/or RNA synthesis of tumor cells.

Antibody–one of five types of proteins that participate in actions that neutralize, eliminate or destroy antigen; structurally, a Y-shaped molecule constructed of two light and two heavy chains of protein joined by disulfide bridges; also called *immunoglobulin* or *gamma globulin.*

Antibody–antigen binding–the fifth stage of antibody-mediated immunity; characterized by antigen recognition by the two Fab antibody fragments, and the binding of each of those fragments to an antigen molecule, usually with hydrogen bonds, to form an immune complex.

Antibody-binding reactions–the sixth stage of antibody-mediated immunity; specific reactions, initiated by the formation of an immune complex, that cause antigen neutralization, elimination and/or destruction, including agglutination, lysis, complement fixation, precipitation, and inactivation/neutralization.

Antibody-mediated immunity (AMI)–characterized by antigen-antibody actions to neutralize, eliminate, or destroy foreign proteins; formerly called *humoral immunity.*

Antibody production and release–the fourth step of antibody-mediated immunity; production by the plasma cell of antibody specific to that against which the parent B lymphocyte was sensitized.

Antigenic determinant–the "universal product code" of an antigen; the protein markers on the surface of an antigen that are uniquely specific to that antigen.

Antigen-processing cell (APC)–macrophage, other leukocyte, or nucleated body cell that engulfs and degrades nonself proteins, attaches them to the APC's major histocompatibility complex proteins, and presents the antigen to M H C-compatible T cells.

Antigen recognition–the second step of antibody-mediated immunity; the recognition of antigen as nonself by an unsensitized B lymphocyte, with the cooperation of T cells and macrophages.

Antigens–cell-surface proteins unique to each individual and can be recognized as foreign by the immune system of another person.

Antihormone drug–receptor antagonists that compete with hormones at their receptor sites; may be a monoclonal antibody.

Antimetabolites–chemotherapeutic agents that exert their greatest cytotoxic effects on cells that are in S phase; they exert their effects by competing with, replacing, or antagonizing normal metabolites.

Antitoxin–antibodies directed against a specific antigen that are derived from the serum of an animal injected with a specific toxoid followed by subsequent injection with the specific toxin; one of the agents used to confer artificial passive immunity; also called *antivenin.*

Antivenin–see *antitoxin.*

Artificial active immunity–type of active immunity that occurs when small amounts of specific antigens (toxoids or vaccines) are deliberately placed in the body to promote an active antibody response; used to confer immunity against diseases that could cause death or permanent disability; lasts many years, but may require a booster.

Artificial passive immunity–type of passive immunity that involves the injection of one person with antibodies produced in another person or animal; provides temporary protection lasting only days to a few weeks; agents used include intravenous immune globulin, antitoxins, antivenins, and human hyperimmune sera.

Attenuated vaccine–vaccine made with live virus or bacteria that have undergone laboratory manipulation to decrease their ability to grow in humans; used to confer artificial active immunity.

Attraction–the second step in phagocytosis; the process by which chemotaxins, leukotaxins, and other elements of extracellular fluid attract leukocytes to a site of tissue injury or foreign protein invasion.

Autologous bone marrow transplant (ABMT)–graft in which the donor and recipient are the same person.

Band neutrophils–less mature neutrophils not yet capable of phagocytic action.

Basophils–leukocytes that release histamine, heparin, and other vasoactive amines in response to tissue damage during inflammation; the basic pH of their cytoplasm causes blue staining with Wright's stain; they make up less than 0.5% of the total white-cell count.

Beam radiation–see *teletherapy.*

Bence Jones proteins–monoclonal immunoglobulin light chain proteins excreted in the urine of persons with multiple myeloma.

Beta rays–type of gamma radiation; heavier rays with moderate to high-speed, high-linear-energy-transfer potential that do not penetrate well.

Blast phase–second phase of the terminal stage of chronic myelogenous leukemia; leukocyte and differential counts show increases in immature or "blast" cells, which proliferate rapidly and interfere with production of other hematopoietic cells (blastic crisis).

B-lymphocyte primary immunodeficiency syndrome–primary immunodeficiency syndromes characterized by compromised antibody-mediated immunity; include Bruton's agammaglobulinemia, common variable immunodeficiency, and IgA deficiency.

B lymphocytes–leukocyte category that includes plasma cells and memory cells and participates in antibody-mediated immunity; primary function is to become sensitized to antigen and secrete antibodies specific to that antigen.

Bone marrow transplant (BMT)–procedure in which bone marrow is removed from a donor by needle aspiration and given to the recipient by intravenous infusion.

Booster–repeated small doses of antigen placed in the body in order to maintain artificial active immunity.

Brachytherapy–a type of radiation delivery in which the source of radiation is within the patient; requires the radiation source to come in direct and continuous contact with the target.

Bruton's agammaglobulinemia–primary B-lymphocyte immunodeficiency syndrome; characterized by lack of circulating B-lymphocyte plasma cells and antibodies; inflammatory response and cell-mediated immunity are intact; X-linked recessive disorder.

Bursa of Fabricius–an area of lymphoid tissue in birds where the maturation and differentiation of committed lymphocyte stem cells occurs.

Carcinogenesis–the exposure of a normal cell to a carcinogenic substance that causes DNA breaks and rearrangements.

Cell-mediated immunity (CMI)–type of immunity provided by leukocytes that recognize nonself cells and respond either by exerting direct immunologic activities or by inducing the cytotoxic activities of other cells; also regulates activities of antibody-mediated immunity and inflammation; also known as *cellular immunity;* critical components include helper, cytotoxic, and suppressor T cells.

Cellular ingestion–the fifth step of phagocytosis; the bringing of the target cell into the phagocyte by absorptive endocytosis.

Chemotaxin–a chemical substance that acts as a magnet to attract leukocytes to the site of tissue damage or foreign invasion.

Chemotherapy–the treatment of disease through the use of chemical agents; a major component in medical management of cancer.

Chronic lymphocytic leukemia (CLL)–chronic leukemia in which malignant changes occur in the lymphocytes, some of which produce immunoglobulins.

Chronic myelogenous leukemia (CML)–chronic leukemia in which malignant changes occur in the hemopoietic system at the stem-cell level; characterized by a chronic stage and a terminal stage with an accelerated phase and a blast phase.

Chronic rejection–a type of graft rejection in which functional tissue of the transplanted organ is replaced with fibrotic, scar-like tissue.

Class I antigens–human leukocyte antigens coded for by the genes HLA-A, HLA-B, and HLA-C.

Class I genes–a class of genes in the major histocompatibility complex that code for the human leukocyte antigens.

Class I MHC proteins–surface–membrane proteins expressed on cytotoxic T lymphocytes and all nucleated body cells.

Class II genes–a class of genes in the major histocompatibility complex that code for Ir proteins that control or regulate immune function.

Class II MHC proteins–surface–membrane proteins expressed on helper T lymphocytes, tissue macrophages, and dendritic cells.

Class III genes–a class of genes in the major histocompatibility complex that code for proteins that regulate complement synthesis and activity.

Classical complement pathway–a mechanism for complement activation that begins with the activation of C1q when antibody–antigen binding takes place.

Colony-stimulating factor (CSF)–a substance released by tissue macrophages to enhance inflammation; stimulates bone marrow to decrease leukocyte generation time from 14 days to just a few hours.

Commitment–irreversible selection of a maturational pathway by a pluripotent stem cell, induced by lymphopoietic factor.

Common variable immunodeficiency–primary B-lymphocyte immunodeficiency syndrome; characterized by little or no antibodies but normal numbers of circulating B lymphocytes.

Complement fixation–antibody-binding reaction; a mechanism of opsonization and enhancement of phagocytic adherence to target cells; binding of IgM or IgG to antigen provides a binding site for C1q to bind, initiating the complement cascade; major complement proteins are labeled C1 through C9; there are 20 complement components currently identified.

Complement-mediated cytolysis–see *membrane lysis.*

Complement-mediated lysis–see *membrane lysis.*

Conditioning–process of preparing a patient for bone marrow transplant in which intensive chemotherapy and sometimes radiotherapy are used to obliterate the patient's own bone marrow.

Consolidation phase–second phase of medical management of acute lymphocytic leukemia; begins immediately after person enters remission; goal of chemotherapeutic treatment is to destroy any residual leukemic cells.

Corneal transplant–see *keratoplasty.*

Cytokines–low-molecular-weight protein hormones synthesized by leukocytes; induce and/or regulate inflammatory and immune responses through pleiotrophic or specific actions on responder cells; include monokines and lymphokines.

Cytotoxic T cell–T lymphocyte that, following initial exposure to an antigen, selectively destroys nonself cells, including virally infected cells, grafts, and transplanted organs; lymphocytes that express MHC Class I proteins; also called *cytolytic T cells, Tc cells,* and *CTL cells.*

Degradation–the seventh step of phagocytosis; destruction of ingested target by granular and lysosomal enzymes.

Denaturation–the laboratory process of heating or exposure to formaldehyde; used in the conversion of toxins to toxoids.

Derepression–activation of oncogenes.

Differential count–the percentage of a particular type of white cell in the total white-cell count.

DiGeorge's syndrome–primary T-lymphocyte immunodeficiency syndrome due to incomplete embryonic development of the third and fourth pharyngeal pouches; characterized by deficiency in cell-mediated immunity due to an absent or rudimentary thymus gland, but normal inflammatory response- and antibody-mediated immunity.

Dose–amount of radiation exposure absorbed by a recipient cell or tissue.

Electromagnetic radiation–type of ionizing radiation used for cancer therapy; includes gamma radiation and roentgen radiation.

Engraftment–the process of a transplanted organ's acceptance by the host's body; also called a *take*.

Eosinophils–leukocytes whose major function is regulation of inflammatory reactions, histamine release in allergic responses, and destruction of parasitic larvae; their acidic cytoplasm stains red with Wright's stain; they make up 1 to 2% of the total white-cell count.

Erythropoietin–erythrocyte growth factor secreted by kidney cells in response to hypoxia.

Exposure–the first step of an immune response (phagocytosis, antibody-mediated immunity, or cell-mediated immunity); exposure of leukocytes to substances released by internal tissue damage and/or the presence of foreign proteins; also, the amount of radiation delivered to a recipient cell; also called *invasion*.

Extramedullary hematopoiesis–uncontrolled synthesis of cellular blood components in sites where hematopoiesis does not normally occur after fetal life, such as spleen and liver.

First response–primary immune response to antigen.

Fractionation–the delivery of several small doses of radiation to achieve optimal prescribed dosage with the least amount of effects to normal tissue.

Gamma radiation–type of electromagnetic radiation; produced intranuclearly by decay of radioisotopes that release energy in the form of gamma rays, beta rays, and alpha rays.

Gamma ray–type of energy produced by gamma radiation; very light rays with low energy transfer potential that travel rapidly, can be concentrated, and penetrate deeply.

Graft-versus-host disease (GVHD)–a series of immunologic responses, mounted by the host of a transplanted organ, with the purpose of destroying, eliminating, or neutralizing these non-self cells; also called *organ rejection*. In bone marrow transplantation, GVHD manifests as the destruction of host cells by the grafted immune system cells.

Granulocytes–leukocytes with small granules (lysosomes) and vesicles within the cytoplasm, includes eosinophils, basophils, and neutrophils.

Gray (Gy)–used to describe absorbed dose of radition; 100 rad (calculated as joules/per kilogram).

Helper cells–T lymphocytes that assist in recognition of nonself, and secrete factors, cytokines, and lymphokines that regulate leukocytes in inflammatory, antibody-mediated, and cellular defensive actions against antigens; lymphocytes that express MHC Class II proteins; also called *inducer T cells, T4 cells,* and *CD4 cells.*

High mitotic index–a term used to indicate tumors that have large numbers of cells in the active growth phase.

Histocompatibility–matching between donor and recipient to find the donor that most closely matches the HLA antigens of the recipient; HLA-A, HLA-B, and HLA-C compatibility are determined using antibodies; HLA-D compatibility is determined through donor-recipient mixed lymphocyte culture.

HIV-antibody-positive–presence of antibodies to human immunodeficiency virus determined by enzyme-linked immunosorbent assay (ELISA), Western blot, and immunofluorescence assay (IFA).

HIV-culture-positive–presence of live human immunodeficiency virus in the blood (antigenemia).

Hormone–naturally occurring chemical, secreted by endocrine glands and picked up by capillaries, that exerts its effect on specific target tissue.

Homograft–type of transplant in which donor tissue is derived from the same species as the recipient, e.g., bone marrow grafted into humans comes from human donors; may be syngeneic, allogeneic, or autologous.

Host–person receiving a donated organ.

Hot implantation–the procedure in brachytherapy of inserting radioactive sealed radiation sources into body tissues or cavities.

Human histocompatibility antigens–see *human leukocyte antigens.*

Human hyperimmune sera–agent used to confer artificial passive immunity; includes specific human hyperimmune sera and nonspecific human hyperimmune sera.

Human immunodeficiency virus (HIV)–retrovirus that is the causative agent for acquired immunodeficiency syndrome; selectively infects immune system cells expressing CD4 molecules.

Human leukocyte antigens (HLAs)–genetically determined, unique identification proteins on the surface of all nucleated cells that enable cells of the immune system to distinguish between "self" and "nonself" cells, tissues, and proteins; the four major HLA antigens are HLA-A, HLA-B, HLA-C, and HLA-D; these determine the "tissue type" of the individual.

Human transplantation antigens–see *human leukocyte antigens*.

Humoral immunity–see *antibody-mediated immunity*.

Hyperacute rejection–a type of graft rejection that begins immediately after transplantation in which antigen–antibody complexes form within the vessels of the transplanted organ and initiate a blood clotting cascade that leads to cellular destruction and organ loss.

Hyperfractionation–fractionation technique in which smaller doeses of radiation are administered several times each day, usually at least 6 hours apart, to achieve a normal total dose.

Hyperviscosity syndrome–symptoms due to increased concentration of abnormal blood proteins in persons with multiple myeloma; characterized by bleeding tendency, dilation and segmentation of retinal and conjunctival veins, neurologic symptoms, and distention of peripheral vessels, increased vascular resistance, and cardiac failure.

IgA deficiency–most common primary B-lymphocyte immunodeficiency syndrome; characterized by lack of circulating or secretory IgA; normal numbers of circulating B lymphocytes, plasma cells and B lymphocytes with surface IgA are present.

Immune complex–antigen–antibody formation that stimulates a permissive and catalytic role in initiating reactions that neutralize, eliminate, or destroy antigen.

Immunity–protection provided by the immune system's recognition of "self" and "nonself," and its ability to remove or destroy nonself cells, which include infected, debilitated, or malignant self cells, bacteria, viruses, fungi, protozoa, pollens, helminths, spores, and cells from other people or animals.

Immunocompetence–full immunity that requires adequate function and interaction of the inflammatory response, antibody-mediated immunity, and cell-mediated immunity.

Immunoglobulin A (IgA)–antibody on mucous membranes and outer-body skin surfaces that provides the first line of defense in preventing antigens from entering the body; most IgA is present in body fluids and secretions; comprises less than 15% of total serum immunoglobulins; dimeric structure, with molecular weight of 155,000; also called *secretory immunoglobulin.*

Immunoglobulin D (IgD)–antibody whose specific function is not clear, called the "mystery protein"; probably moderates IgM activity; found in plasma, but not serum, in concentrations of less than 1%; molecular weight, 180,000; has shortest life span (half-life of approximately 2 to 3 days).

Immunoglobulin E (IgE)–antibody that binds the surface of basophils and mast cells, causing degranulation and release of vasoactive amines, and the manifestations of allergic and immediate hypersensitivity reactions; comprises less than 1% of total serum immunoglobulins; monomeric structure, molecular weight, 180,000.

Immunoglobulin G (IgG)–antibody primarily responsible for acquired natural and acquired artificial sustained immunity; through antigen binding, neutralizes and opsonizes antigen and stimulates activation of complement; most abundant antibody type, comprises more than 75% of total serum immunoglobulins; monomeric structure, molecular weight of 160,000; only antibody that crosses placenta because of its monomeric structure; antibody with longest life span (half-life of approximately 30 days).

Immunoglobulin M (IgM)–antibody that responds to the presence of bacteria in the blood; efficient at precipitation and agglutination and the activation of complement; large molecule, molecular weight of 180,000 with pentameric structure; comprises 10% of total serum immunoglobulins; found on surface of red blood cells, it determines the major blood groups, A, B, and O; levels increase during antoimmune responses.

Immunosenescence–age-associated decline in immune responsiveness.

Inactivation–antibody-binding reaction; binding of antibody to antigen that interferes with the function of the active site by covering it or by inducing a change in the active site's physical configuration; does not result in immediate destruction of antigen.

Induction phase–first phase of medical management of acute leukemias; goal of chemotherapeutic treatment is to achieve a remission.

Inflammation–a nonspecific immune response to invasion or injury generated by neutrophils, macrophages, eosinophils, and basophils that provides immediate, short-term protection; occurs in three functional stages (I, II, and III).

Innate immunity–a genetically determined characteristic of an individual, group, or species that cannot be developed after birth and is not an adaptive response to injury or invasion by foreign proteins.

Intravenous immune globulin (IVIG)–antibodies obtained from the serum of a pool of at least 1000 different individuals; one of the agents used to confer artificial passive immunity.

Invasion–the first step of phagocytosis; exposure of leukocytes to substances released by internal tissue damage and/or the presence of foreign proteins; also called *exposure.*

Ionizing radiation–type of radiation that, during cellular or tissue absorption, causes "kicking out" of an orbital electron from the atom of elements, resulting in ionization and release of energy; includes particulate radiation and electromagnetic radiation; type of radiation used for treatment of malignancy.

Keratoplasty–surgical removal of an individual's diseased corneal tissue and replacement with tissue from a human donor cornea; corneal transplant.

Killed vaccine–vaccine made with actual virus or organism that is killed to prevent proliferation after it is injected into the body; used to confer artificial active immunity.

Lamellar keratoplasty–partial thickness corneal transplant in which the superficial cornea is removed and replaced with donor tissue.

Leu-3–monoclonal antibody to the T4 lymphocyte membrane protein.

Leukapheresis–the removal of white blood cells.

Leukemia–malignancy of the hematopoietic and/or lymphopoietic systems, characterized by excessive cellular growth and incomplete cellular maturation; classified as either myeloid or lymphoid and acute or chronic.

Leukocytes–white blood cells of the immune system that originate in the bone marrow, mature at other body sites, and protect the body from invasion by foreign microorganisms.

Leukotaxin–a chemical substance that acts as a magnet to attract leukocytes to the site of tissue damage or foreign invasion.

Lymphocytes–leukocytes that provide sustained immunologic protection; include B lymphocytes and T lymphocytes; they make up 25 to 30% of the total white-cell count.

Lymphocyte sensitization–the third step of antibody-mediated immunity; the process by which a B lymphocyte "learns" to respond only to the identical antigenic determinants of one specific antigen, then divides to form a plasma cell and a memory cell.

Lymphokines–cytokines synthesized by T lymphocytes.

Lymphopoietic factor–cytokine, thought to induce commitment to lymphocyte differentiation of the pluripotent stem cell.

Lysis–antibody-binding reaction; disruption of antigen's membrane surface that results from antibody binding to membrane-bound antigens of foreign proteins; permits rapid changes in the intracellular environment of the foreign protein.

Lysosomes–intracellular granules composed of enzymes that degrade proteins and cellular debris.

Macrophages–final maturational stage of monocytes present in large numbers in body tissues; main function is nonspecific ingestion and phagocytosis of foreign proteins and microorganisms during inflammation.

Maintenance phase–third phase of medical management of acute leukemias; low-dose chemotherapeutic treatment is given in a series of cycles from months to years.

Major histocompatibility complex (MHC)–the gene region, located on chromosome 6, that contains Class I, Class II, and Class III genes; codes for the production of MHC proteins.

Malignant transformation–the process of changing from a normal cell to a cancer cell; occurs through carcinogenesis.

Marker proteins–antigens present on the cell-membrane surface that can be used to identify immune system components, such as T-lymphocyte subsets.

Membrane attack mechanism–see *membrane lysis*.

Membrane lysis–direct action of complement fixation that occurs wherever the membrane is surrounded by activated complement and results in a membrane lesion that destroys or neutralizes the antigen; also called *complement-mediated cytolysis, complement-mediated lysis,* or *membrane attack mechanism*.

Memory–see *sustained immunity*–the ability of B-lymphocyte memory cells to retain specific sensitization and antibody production over time.

Memory cell–B lymphocyte that remains sensitized to a specific antigen and can secrete increased amounts of immunoglobulins to the antigen the next time it is exposed to it.

Metabolites–cofactors that play essential roles in critical cell processes, for example, vitamins.

MHC–major histocompatibility complex.

MHC proteins–surface proteins expressed on the membranes of lymphocytes, tissue macrophages, dendritic cells, and all nucleated body cells; include Class I and Class II proteins.

MHC restriction–the requirement by T lymphocytes that only antigens presented by APCs with MHC proteins identical to the T cell's will be recognized.

Minor antigens–genetically determined antigens that, with major antigens, form the individual's specific "tissue type."

Mixed lymphocyte culture (MLC)–method of determining HLA-D compatibility in which donor and recipient live lymphocytes are mixed and incubated in culture; mitosis indicates incompatibility.

Monoclonal origin of cancer–the concept that groups of cancer cells can arise from a single transformed normal cell.

Monocytes–intermediate-phase leukocytes released from bone marrow prior to maturation into macrophages; main function is complement activation and limited phagocytosis during inflammation; they make up 2 to 4% of the total white-cell count.

Monokines–cytokines synthesized by mononuclear phagocytes, including macrophages, neutrophils, eosinophils, and monocytes.

Mononuclear phagocytic system–the tissue macrophage system, formerly called the *reticuloendothelial system (RES)*.

Mucositis–the development of open sores on mucous membranes.

Multiple myeloma–malignant condition of B-lymphocyte plasma cells characterized by uncontrolled proliferation of a single clone of plasma cells, and profound depression of antibody-mediated immunity.

Myeloid metaplasia with myelofibrosis–a myeloproliferative disorder in which failing bone marrow results in decreased hematopoiesis and hypocellularity and the stimulation of extramedullary hematopoiesis.

Myeloproliferative disorders–diseases that result from abnormal proliferation of all or part of the cell types derived from the committed myeloid stem cell; includes chronic myelogenous leukemia, polycythemia vera, myeloid metaplasia with myelofibrosis, and essential thrombocytopenia.

Natural active immunity–type of active immunity that occurs when antigen enters the body, without human assistance, and the body responds by making antibodies against that antigen.

Natural killer cell–lymphocyte that nonspecifically attacks nonself cells, including grafts and transplanted organs and especially body cells that have undergone mutation and become malignant; has some T-lymphocyte characteristics, but not a true T lymphocyte; also called *NK cell.*

Natural killer cytotoxic factor (NKCF)–substance secreted by natural killer cells that is attracted to nonself cells that NK cells recognize and attack, and enhances their cytotoxic effects.

Natural passive immunity–a type of passive immunity that occurs with the transfer of antibodies from mother to fetus through the placenta or to the infant through colostrum or breast milk.

Neutralization–see *inactivation.*

Neutrophils–leukocytes whose major function is nonspecific ingestion and phagocytosis of microorganisms during inflammation; neutral pH of their cytoplasm causes light purple staining with Wright's stain; they make up 55 to 70% of the total white-cell count.

Nonspecific human hyperimmune sera–antibodies obtained from the serum of a large pool of individuals; no one antibody type is guaranteed to be present, but because of the large pool, usually all types of antibodies are present; an agent used to confer artificial passive immunity.

OKT3–monoclonal antibody to the human T-cell CD3 surface antigen.

OKT4–monoclonal antibody to the T4 lymphocyte CD4 membrane protein.

Oncogenes–early embryonic genes capable of causing cancer if turned on again (derepressed) after development is complete; normal genes that are part of every cell's normal makeup and were critically important in early development.

Opportunistic infection–infection often caused by normal flora in persons lacking natural killer cells, neutrophils, and macrophages to differentiate "self" from "nonself"; occurs in persons infected with human immunodeficiency virus.

Opsonins–substances that coat a target cell, changing its surface charge, in preparation for phagocytosis.

Opsonization–the mechanism of enhancement of phagocytic adherence to target cellular debris or foreign proteins.

Organ rejection–see *graft-versus-host disease.*

Osteoclast-activating factor (OAF)–a cytokine associated with bone resorption, local destruction, and secondary hypercalcemia; present in areas of bone adjacent to myeloma cell deposits in patients with multiple myeloma.

Passive immunity–the transfer of circulating antibodies from one person to another to provide immediate immunity of short duration.

Penetrating keratoplasty–corneal transplant in which the full thickness of the cornea is removed and replaced with donor tissue.

Phagocytosis–the process by which leukocytes engulf cellular debris and/or foreign proteins and destroy them through a series of intracellular degradative events.

Phagolysosome–organelle, formed by the fusion of lysosomes and phagosomes, that participates in the phagocyte's lytic destruction of target cells.

Phagosome formation–the sixth step of phagocytosis; formation of vacuoles or phagolysosomes containing cytoplasmic granules of the phagocyte and beginning destruction of target cells by degranulation.

Plant alkaloids–antineoplastic agents that interfere with the formation of microtubules, preventing spindle formation and chromosomal separation necessary for cell division; include vinca alkaloids.

Plasma cell–B lymphocyte that becomes sensitized to antigen and immediately secretes antibodies against the antigen to which it was sensitized.

Pleiotrophic–widespread effects within the immune system of some cytokines, which sets immunomodulation in motion.

Pluripotent stem cell–immature cell that has the potential to mature into any type of differentiated blood cell.

Poietins–chemicals that stimulate the stem cell's commitment to a specific maturational pathway and induce maturation.

Polycythemia vera–myeloproliferative disorder characterized by hypercellularity of the bone marrow and overproduction of all myeloid cells, especially erythrocytes.

Precipitation–antibody-binding reaction; formation of large, insoluble antibody–antigen complexes that can be acted on and cleared by other nonspecific leukocytes.

Primary immunodeficiency syndrome–syndrome caused by congenital problems present at birth.

Primary response–immune response to the first invasion of the body by an antigen that results in the production of antibodies and acquired immunity to that antigen; first response.

R (roentgen)–absorbed dose of radiation; unit of radiation that can ionize a certain amount of air; 1R = a dose less than 1 rad or less than 0.01 Gy.

rad–radiation absorbed dose; used to describe absorbed dose of radiation.

Radiation therapy–use of radiation to destroy malignant cells with minimal exposure of normal cells to the cell-damaging effects of radiation.

Recognition–the fourth step of phagocytosis; the differentiation of "self" from "nonself" by the phagocytic cell.

rem–roentgen equivalents in man; used to describe absorbed dose of radiation.

Remission–clinically defined as an absence of leukemic cells in the bone marrow.

Respiratory burst–destruction of a target cell by a phagocyte through the formation of oxygen metabolites that exert oxidation damage.

Responder cell–cell with specific surface receptors for cytokine binding that changes its activity in response to the presence of a cytokine.

Retrovirus–class of virus that differs from ordinary viruses in the presence of reverse transcriptase and RNA as the only genetic material.

Reverse transcriptase–complex of enzymes, present in retroviruses, that increases the efficiency of viral replication once the virus enters a host cell.

Roentgen radiation–type of electromagnetic radiation; produced extranuclearly by linear acceleration with electrical machines.

Secondary response–increased immune response on reexposure to an antigen in which memory cells rapidly produce antibodies to clear the antigen and prevent symptoms of the disease; anamnestic response.

Secretory immunoglobulin–see *immunoglobulin A.*

Segmented neutrophils–fully mature neutrophils capable of immediate, effective phagocytosis; this count is a reliable measure of a person's susceptibility to infection.

Self-tolerance–the ability of the immune system to distinguish "self" from "nonself."

Severe combined immunodeficiency syndrome (SCIDS)–primary T and B lymphocyte immunodeficiency; characterized by lack of antibodies and circulating lymphocytes with generalized impairment of immunity and inflammation; two patterns of inheritance include X-linked recessive and autosomal recessive patterns.

Shift to the left–a condition in which the majority of the neutrophil population present in the blood are less mature forms that are further to the left on the maturational pathway; this indicates that bone marrow production of mature neutrophils cannot keep pace with the presence of infectious microorganisms.

Simulation–a "dry-run" done on a simulator prior to teletherapy to define and refine positions, exposures, and intensities; the simulator mimics beam distribution, but produces only weak, superficial radiation.

Specific human hyperimmune sera–antibodies obtained from the serum of persons exposed to a specific antigen and producing the antibody directed against that antigen; an agent used to confer artificial passive immunity.

Specificity–a property of plasma cells characterized by the fact that the lymphocyte produces only antibodies specific to the antigen that originally sensitized the parent B lymphocyte.

Split course–technique of teletherapy in which half the dose of radiation is delivered daily, with a 2- to 3-week rest before the other half is administered.

Stage I–first stage of inflammatory response, also called *vascular stage;* occurs primarily at the vascular level and involves tissue macrophages; phase one is characterized by vasoconstriction at the site; phase two is characterized by hyperemia and swelling at the site.

Stage II–second stage of inflammatory response, also called *cellular exudate stage;* characterized by neutrophilia, secretion of factors into interstitial fluid, and formation of exudate.

Stage III–third stage of inflammatory response, also called *stage of tissue repair and replacement;* leukocytes induce division of healthy cells and revascularization and collagen formation of scar tissue.

Stem cell–an immature, undifferentiated, pluripotent cell produced by the bone marrow.

Suppressor cells–T lymphocytes that assist in regulation of cell-mediated immunity by preventing the formation of autoantibodies or the overreaction in response to exposure to non-self antigens; also called *Ts cells, T8 cells,* or *CD8 cells.*

Sustained immunity–see *memory.*

Syngeneic transplantation–a graft that comes from a donor source who is genetically identical to the recipient, so that all HLA antigens, major and minor, are perfectly matched.

T and B primary immunodeficiency syndromes–primary immunodeficiency syndromes characterized by compromised antibody-mediated and cell-mediated immunity; includes Wiskott–Aldrich syndrome and severe combined immunodeficiency syndrome.

T lymphocyte–leukocyte that participates in cell-mediated immunity; includes helper cells, cytotoxic cells, and natural killer cells.

T-lymphocyte primary immunodeficiency syndrome–primary immunodeficiency syndromes characterized by compromised cell-mediated immunity; includes DiGeorge's syndrome.

Teletherapy–a type of radiation delivery; the actual radiation source is external from the patient and remote from the tumor site; also called *beam radiation.*

Toxins–substances produced by an infecting organism rendered harmless by denaturation and converted into toxoids.

Toxoids–substances with the same antigenic determinants as toxins that are introduced into the body to confer artificial active immunity.

Transplantation–removing all or part of an organ from one person and placing it in the body of another.

Universal product code–the protein markers on the surface of a cell that are uniquely specific to that cell; the cell's antigenic determinants.

Vaccine–preparation made with altered virus or bacteria used to confer artificial active immunity; there are two types: killed vaccines and attenuated vaccines.

Venoocclusive disease (VOD)–complication of liver graft-versus-host disease in which liver blood vessels are occluded due to immune reactions that cause fibrin build-up in the vessels.

Virion–part of a virus that contains the genetic material of the virus.

Virus–cellular parasite that enters the host nucleus and uses the cellular machinery of the host cell to replicate by splicing viral DNA into the human cellular DNA.

Wedging–the use of wedge-shaped pieces of different types of metal that absorb radiation differently to direct radiation beams more accurately to the target site.

White-cell count–total number of white cells in a cubic microliter (μl) of blood.

Wiskott–Aldrich syndrome–T and B primary immunodeficiency syndrome characterized by thrombocytopenia, depletion of circulating lymphocytes, and progressive loss of cell-mediated immunity; X-linked recessive disorder.

INDEX

Note: Page numbers in *italics* indicate figures or illustrations; page numbers followed by a t indicates tables.